ATLAS OF THE DIFFICULT AIRWAY
A Source Book

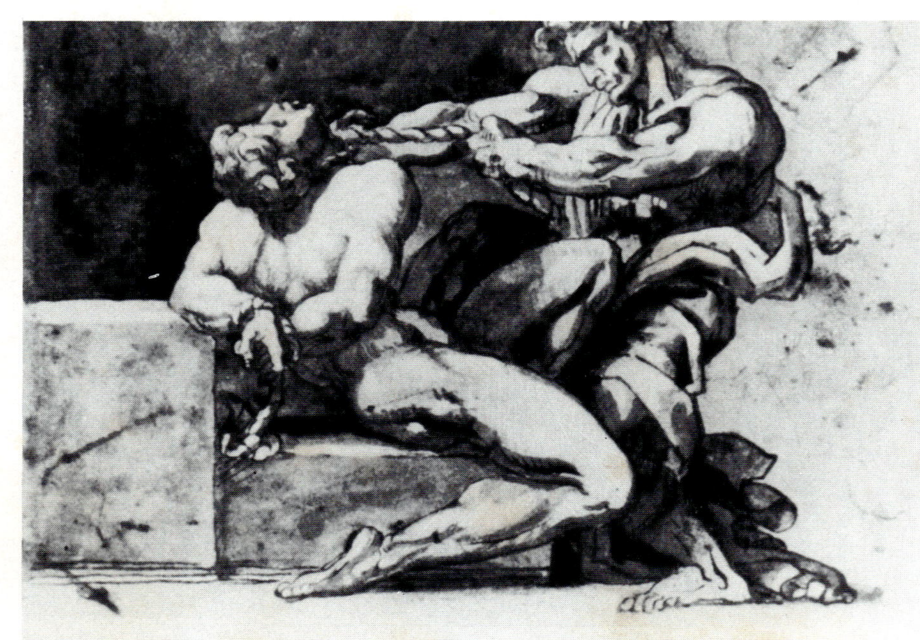

The difficult airway

Atlas of the Difficult Airway
A Source Book

**MARTIN L. NORTON, M.S.P.H.
(SAN ENG), M.D., J.D., D.AN.**
*Professor, Department of Anesthesiology
Associate Professor (Anesthesia)
Department of Otorhinolaryngology
University of Michigan Medical Center
Ann Arbor, Michigan*

**ALLAN C.D. BROWN, M.B., Ch.B.,
F.F.A.R.C.S.**
*Associate Professor, Department of Anesthesiology
University of Michigan
Ann Arbor, Michigan*

EDITORIAL ASSOCIATE:
Jeanne T. Fitzgerald, M.A., D.A.

MEDICAL ARTIST:
Jaye Schlesinger, M.F.A., M.I.

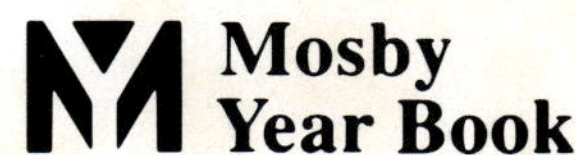

**Mosby
Year Book**

St. Louis   Baltimore   Boston   Chicago   London   Philadelphia   Sydney   Toronto

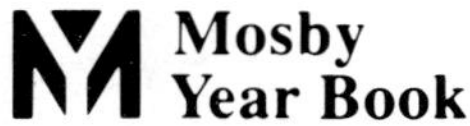

Dedicated to Publishing Excellence

Sponsoring Editors: Susan Gay/Richard Lampert
Assistant Managing Editor, Text and Reference: Jan Gardner
Production Project Coordinator: Yvette Sellers/Karen Halm
Proofroom Manager: Barbara Kelly

1   2   3   4   5   6   7   8   9   0 CL MV MV CL 95   94   93   92   91

Library of Congress Cataloging-in-Publication Data
Norton, Martin L.
    Atlas of the difficult airway : a source book / Martin L. Norton.
      p. cm.
    Includes bibliographical references and index.
    ISBN 0-8151-6425-4
    1. Respiratory organs—Obstructions—Atlases. I. Title.
    [DNLM: 1. Intubation, Intratracheal—atlases. 2. Laryngoscopy—atlases. 3. Lung Diseases, Obstructive—atlases. 4. Lung Diseases, Obstructive—diagnosis—atlases. 5. Respiration, Artificial—atlases. WF 17 N886a]
RC776.03N67 1991
616.2—dc20   91-10559
DNLM/DLC   CIP
for Library of Congress

To my wife, Shirley H. Norton, without whose encouragement, _______________
*unbelievable patience, and understanding nothing could have
been accomplished; and to my mother, Julia Kaufer Norton,
who believed in me and started me on the pathway to the
study of medicine.*

If there be no knowledge, how can there be discernment?
(Talmud Yerushalmi, Berakhot)

CONTRIBUTORS

ALLAN C. D. BROWN, M.B., CH.B.,
F.F.A.R.C.S.
Associate Professor of Anesthesiology
Department of Anesthesiology
University of Michigan
Ann Arbor, Michigan

ALPHONSE BURDI, PH.D.
Professor, Department of Anatomy
 and Cell Biology
Research Scientist
Center for Human Growth
 and Development
University of Michigan
Ann Arbor, Michigan

WILLIAM L. ESCHENBACHER, M.D.
Medical Director
Pulmonary Laboratory
Methodist Hospital
Houston, Texas

JOHN FLEETHAM, M.D., F.R.C.P.(C)
Associate Professor of Medicine
Head, Respiratory Division
The University of British Columbia
Vancouver, Canada

JEFFREY KYFF, D.O., D.AN.
Staff Anesthesiologist
Department of Anesthesiology
Henry Ford Hospital
Detroit, Michigan

FRANK LONDY, R.R.T.
Department of Radiology
University of Michigan
Ann Arbor, Michigan

ALAN A. LOWE, D.M.D., DIPORTHO,
PH.D., F.R.C.D.(C)
Professor and Head
Department of Clinical Dental Sciences
The University of British Columbia
Vancouver, Canada

MARTIN L. NORTON, M.S.P.H. (SAN
ENG), M.D., J.D., D.AN.
Professor, Department of Anesthesiology
Associate Professor (Anesthesia)
Department of Otorhinolaryngology
University of Michigan
Ann Arbor, Michigan

GEORGE UPTON, D.D.S., M.S.
Professor, School of Dentistry
University of Michigan
Ann Arbor, Michigan

NIALL WILTON, M.B., B.S.,
M.R.C.P., F.F.A.R.C.S.
Assistant Professor
Department of Anesthesiology
University of Michigan
Ann Arbor, Michigan

FOREWORD

From the earliest period in their training, the importance of the airway is emphasized to anesthesiologists, otolaryngologists, and others involved in its management. As young physicians move from those frightening first attempts at endoscopic examination, mask ventilation, and endotracheal intubation, they come to realize that the majority of patients they are asked to care for have "easy" airways, and they come to trust themselves and their skills.

Increasing experience and clinical maturation allow them to develop the clinical judgment needed to recognize patients who will present problems with airway management. Many of these patients are easily recognized. The patient with a severe postsurgical or congenital deformity, for example, is readily identified. With more experience, the nascent endoscopist can anticipate difficulty with more subtle anatomic variations. Most of these patients may be managed with a bit of advance planning and perhaps the assistance of a colleague.

There is a lingering problem of significant consequence, however. Every respiratory endoscopist, no matter how experienced, realizes that in certain patients airway management and endotracheal intubation not only are difficult but are essentially impossible. Every anesthesiologist has felt the cold panic when he or she first realizes that the usual anatomic structures cannot be visualized and control of the airway established. It also becomes clear that a fraction of these are not detectable by customary examination procedures. In such situations a more scientific approach to airway evaluation and management becomes necessary.

Drs. Norton and Brown and their contributors have spent the last few years intensively studying patients with abnormal airways referred to the Difficult Airway Clinic at the University of Michigan Medical Center Department of Anesthesiology. This clinic, the first of its type, is in the process of establishing a registry of patients who represent the broad spectrum of anatomic and functional abnormalities of the upper airway.

Evaluation of these patients is carried out utilizing an extended range of techniques. In addition to the history of previous airway difficulty or suggested potential problems and conventional physical examination of the upper airway, the Clinic also has available to it various means of direct examination, including fiberoptic studies utilizing high-resolution video recording (for later review and teaching), conventional as well as dynamic fluoroscopic analysis, and multiplane still photography. Many patients are also evaluated by selected pulmonary function testing, particularly flow-volume loop recordings.

To decrease the amount of clinical empiricism involved in airway evaluation, each patient referred to the Clinic has a series of specific anatomic measurements recorded. These measurements are validated and correlated with the studies noted above, to permit development of a database containing both normal and abnormal anatomic and functional profiles of the upper airway.

An important goal of this work is the formation of evaluative criteria for patients suspected of being at risk for airway catastrophe. Based on these criteria, a management plan has been developed to provide the safest approach to securing the airway for induction of anesthesia and for nonoperative airway management.

This atlas is a compilation of information and visuals obtained from patients studied, together with the experience, thoughts, and suggestions of the several co-contributors. Its intent is to provide the prudent endoscopist with an understanding of the upper airway in its many variations, especially those that make airway control difficult. It also presents examples of the more unusual anatomic and functional syndromes that may be seen in a busy anesthesiologic and endoscopic referral practice.

Finally, it suggests a protocol for the clinical evaluation of such patients and for the development of a care plan that maximizes patient safety. This is an important undertaking and introduces objective observation and recording into an issue that has been too long a subject of "clinical" impressions.

JAY S. FINCH, M.D.
Former Chairman and Professor
Department of Anesthesiology
University of Michigan
Ann Arbor, Michigan

ACKNOWLEDGMENTS

The material contained herein is the result of many years of interest and experience with the problem of the difficult airway. To this has been added the collective presentations of the annual seminars on The Difficult Airway presented at the Towsley Center for Continuing Medical Education, University of Michigan Medical Center, Ann Arbor, from 1988 to the present, and the results of an ongoing study of patients at the Difficult Airway Clinic of the Department of Anesthesiology, University of Michigan Hospitals. We have, at all times, had a continued participatory interaction with the Departments of Radiology, the Pulmonary Function Testing Service, the Sleep Apnea Clinic, and the Department of Otorhinolaryngology.

The visual presentations include a collection of teaching materials from past years and from the archives of our Clinic. The subjects of this presentation have, after extensive discussion and explanation, graciously granted permission for their pictures and cases to be reproduced herein for the education of health professionals and the resultant benefit of future patients we are so honored and privileged to serve.

MARTIN L. NORTON
ALLAN C. BROWN

CONTENTS

PART I

> Errors are not in the art but in the artificiers.
> *Philosophiae Naturalis Principia Mathematica*
> Sir Isaac Newton, 1687

Since the beginning of anesthesiology its practitioners have recognized the occasional patient with an airway that is difficult or impossible to maintain patent under the depressant effects of anesthetic agents. With the introduction of muscle relaxant drugs into anesthetic practice, intubation of the trachea for ventilatory support became an integral part of anesthetic technique. However, this change also demonstrated the existence of another group of occasional patients whose airway anatomy makes intubation difficult or impossible with standard anesthetic techniques. These two groups are not mutually exclusive. Some airways may be difficult to maintain under mask anesthesia but are easily intubated. Other airways are difficult to intubate, but may be maintained with mask anesthesia for the duration of an operation. Some are difficult to manage in both respects.

The problem in characterizing the difficult airway is to first define what is meant by "difficult." Most anesthesiologists, usually during their early years of practice, will remember the patient whose airway they were unable to intubate after multiple attempts. After requesting assistance from a senior colleague, they were mortified to see the endotracheal tube passed with the first attempt! This leads to the conclusion that experience with the standard techniques for securing an airway must play some part in defining what is difficult.

The first section of this atlas examines the problem of the difficult airway: the results of failure to manage the airway as a justification for all that follows and the published incidences of difficulty with the limitations of the definitions used. Chapters 2 and 3 review basic techniques and equipment used in maintaining an airway that have to fail in competent hands before the label "difficult" airway may be applied. Chapter 4 is a partisan plea to treat those patients with a demonstrated or suspected difficult airway as a group, with a medical condition of serious import justifying a separate and exhaustive preoperative evaluation.

Chapter 1

Problem of the Difficult Airway in Perspective

Martin L. Norton

The results of a failed airway intubation are dramatically demonstrated in a study by the American Society of Anesthesiologists (ASA) Committee on Professional Liability.[1, 2] An analysis of approximately 1,541 closed malpractice insurance claims for all types of surgical procedures revealed that respiratory mishaps accounted for 34% of the claims. Three mechanisms of injury accounted for three fourths of the adverse respiratory events: (1) inadequate ventilation, 38%; (2) unintentional esophageal intubation, 18%; and (3) "difficult" intubation, 17%. Of all of the respiratory mishaps studied, 66% of the patients died and 9% had permanent brain damage. The balance of injuries were grouped as "other" (e.g., airway obstruction, bronchospasm, aspiration, premature or unintentional extubation, inadequate inspired oxygen delivery, and endobronchial intubation).

Still other studies have concluded that failure to secure a patent airway was the predominant cause of anesthesia-related maternal death in recent years.[3–5] When obstetric cases alone were analyzed, and despite the fact that regional anesthesia was the predominant technique used in cesarean section (with epidural anesthesia frequently administered in routine deliveries), respiratory-related problems were the most common critical incident reported (14% involved difficult or esophageal intubation). Other authors have found similarly related problems.[6, 7]

The ASA report clearly demonstrates that respiratory problems are the most common cause of brain damage and death during anesthesia, with unintentional intubation of the esophagus a major cause. This excellent study involved only closed insurance claims that actually led to a lawsuit, and thus its research findings are somewhat skewed. The data did not include other cases of morbidity that never reached the point of legal action or manifest insurance claim. Imagine the number of cases that never came to litigation and the magnitude of the problem truly begins to take shape, leading to the conclusion that respiratory-related mishaps of the airway are a major source of patient risk.

Contrary to the categorization of the ASA committee, we are convinced that esophageal intubation rightfully belongs in the category of difficult intubation; otherwise, what rationale can we give for the rate of improper placement? (If not in the difficult airway grouping, then the level of teaching and practice of endotracheal intubation is deplorable!) Figure 1–1 shows correct and incorrect loci for endotracheal intubation.

This position is supported by the International Committee for Prevention of Anesthesia Mortality and Morbidity 1988 summary report by Dr. Gaisford Harrison (personal communication, 1988). Harrison came to the conclusion that over the years there has been improvement in response to problems associated with monitoring of vital signs and using the intellect, but problems associated with manual skills have not substantially improved.

We must ask ourselves why we do not continue to build on the legacy that has come down to us from the early days of anesthesiology. Examine the contributions by the giants of the past. Sir William MacEwen,[8] a Scottish surgeon, is often erroneously reported to have been the first to perform endotracheal intubation, in 1880. In fact, endotracheal intubation, more or less as we know it, was first accomplished by Kirstein[9] with the aid of a laryngoscope in 1895. However, this was preceded by blind nasal intubation (originally described by Desault, Surgeon in Chief of the Great Hospital of Humanity in Paris in 1814,[10] and popularized by Magill and Rowbotham in the 1920s[11] and by tactile intubation, practiced by Kite in the 18th century and described by Herholdt and Rafn[12] in 1796. They mention passing a catheter blindly over their fingers, which were placed behind the epiglottis into the windpipe.

Above all, we are indebted to the father of clinical endoscopy, Chevalier

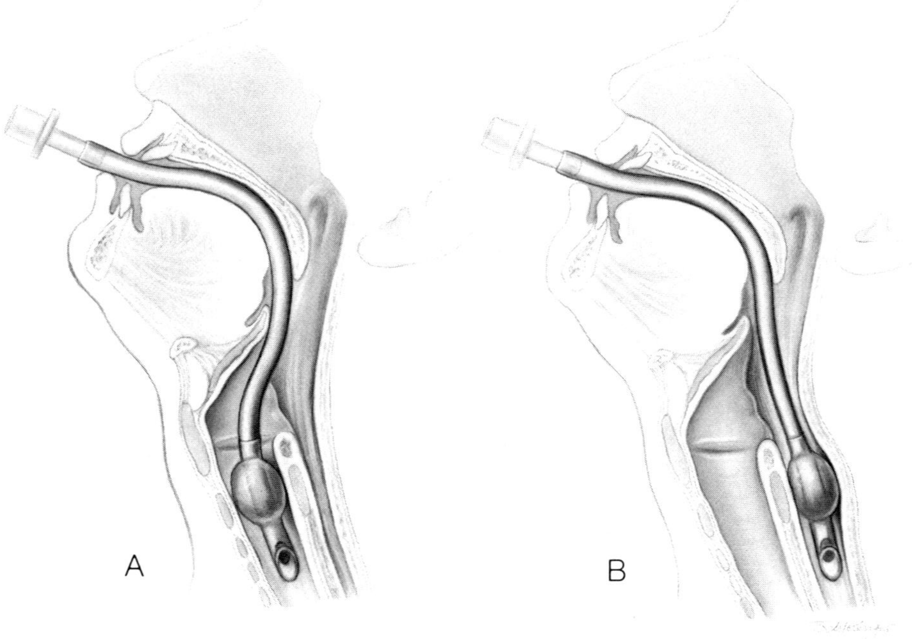

FIG 1–1.
Loci of endotracheal intubation. Correct **(A)** and incorrect **(B)** placement of tube.

Jackson, for his teaching, instrumentation, and clinical textual material. Although the modern endoscopist who is not familiar with flexible fiberoptic techniques cannot be considered as practicing state-of-the-art intubation, it is no less important that facility with both straight and curved rigid laryngoscopes and rigid bronchoscopic instrumentation be part of the armamentarium.

Moving into the 21st century does not mean discarding the knowledge and skills of those who came before us. Stylet, light reflective (Flexilume), and retrograde techniques should also be learned and applied where suitable as well. Table 1–1 gives a listing of older intubation techniques and contemporary techniques that are their heirs.

No reliable study of the clinical practitioner's experience with difficult intubations has been done in recent times, nor has the true incidence of unintentional esophageal intubation been determined. What is more, we do not have information on delayed recognition of unintentional esophageal intubation that did not result in catastrophe. The few studies of note[13, 14] suffer from the problems of varying definitions of the difficult airway, the most glaring omission being a lack of clear, prospective, reproducible criteria for identification of a difficult airway.

The question of who is responsible for what arises among surgeons, anesthesiologists, and other specialists requiring access to the airway. Our experience has shown that the problem does not reside in the hands of one specialty. Yes, we want to hear about problem cases in advance—and at our convenience; then we fail to give the problem the medical consideration it deserves. We act as technicians, not physicians. This is where a professional attitude, manifesting itself through thorough examination and evaluation based on an understanding of anatomy and biomechanics, can contribute most.

The profession, and above all the patient, cannot accept such ego-driven statements as, "I can handle airway problems. I don't need someone else to tell me," or, "I know a difficult airway when I see it." We must recognize that airway problems are primary and usually precede other considerations of surgery. Let us remember the A of the ABCs (Airway, Breathing, Circulation) of cardiorespiratory management.

We have come to recognize that a wide disparity in airway management

TABLE 1–1.

Historical and Contemporary Intubation Techniques

Older Techniques	Newer Techniques
Bougie	Laryngeal mask/airway
Oral hook	Guide wire
Retrograde	Fiberoptic stylet laryngoscope
Whistle catheter	Flexible laryngoscope
Light wand	Bullard laryngoscope
Digital	Flexible bronchoscope
Endotrol tube	Flexible stylet
Mirror/prism	Jet catheter/stylet
Cricothyroidotomy	
Rigid bronchoscope	

skills and abilities exists among modern anesthesiologists, otolaryngologists, and other endoscopists. The notion that they can insert a tube in any airway demonstrates that many of our colleagues have shifted focus from the ABCs of resuscitation to the esoteric world of calculated doses (which are often given whether or not patient response shows a need), microspheric cardiac studies, and end-tidal carbon dioxide pressure (Pco_2) values seen on a screen, without consideration of the meaning of the pattern visualized, among other examples.

Endotracheal intubation is a matter of particular sensitivity for the anesthesiologist and otolaryngologist, compounded by the fact that we do not have any real criteria for defining endoscopic and intubation skills. Of equal import is the failure of surgeons to recognize the problem except in the most obvious situations. The surgeon often assumes that access to the airway is a simple mechanical problem solved by a simple, mechanically minded "gas passer" of lesser stature sitting at the head of the table. Of course, if things do not work out, "We can always do a tracheostomy," potential complications of tracheostomy notwithstanding (Table 1–2).[15]

In certain cases the anesthesiologist may find it impossible to introduce an endotracheal tube after anesthesia has been induced. There may be no immediate life, limb, or organ-saving emergency making it necessary to proceed with the surgery, but the surgeon may insist on doing a tracheostomy (which is the surgeon's prerogative) so as not to lose his or her place on the booking schedule. Often the reason for the problem appears to carry no weight in surgical considerations. Worse still, that the same patient may *in the future* present the same airway access dilemma does not give the surgeon pause to consider a proper evaluation of the reasons for the intubation difficulty. This mentality emphasizes convenience rather than concern for the patient's welfare.

It is time for the medical profession to reassess goals, with patient care considerations uppermost. It is time our specialties matured, so that we can come to terms and recognize that management of the difficult airway presents very special problems and solutions. That time is not the night before surgery or the moment the patient is put on the operating table. It must be done in advance through a consultancy service, such as the Difficult Airway Clinic (University of Michigan Medical Center, Ann Arbor). Assessment of the difficult airway is

TABLE 1–2.

Some Tracheostomy Complications*

1. Infection
2. Opening of fascial planes (infection, aerodissection around larynx, trachea, mediastinum)
3. Tracheal stenosis
4. Pneumothorax (especially on right)
5. Hemorrhage, hematoma, innominate (brachiocephalic) artery fistula
6. Difficulties of access (tumors, obesity)
7. Cosmesis (keloid and other scar formation)
8. Injury to structures adjacent to trachea (damage to recurrent laryngeal nerves, entrance into major vessels, laceration of esophagus or tracheoesophageal fistula)
9. Failure to cannulate the airway
10. Long-term complications from the use of endotracheal or tracheostomy tubes (pressure necrosis, tracheomalacia, ball valve obstruction, granulation tissue)

*Adapted from Stauffer JL, Olson DE, Petty TL: *Am J Med* 1981; 70:65–76.

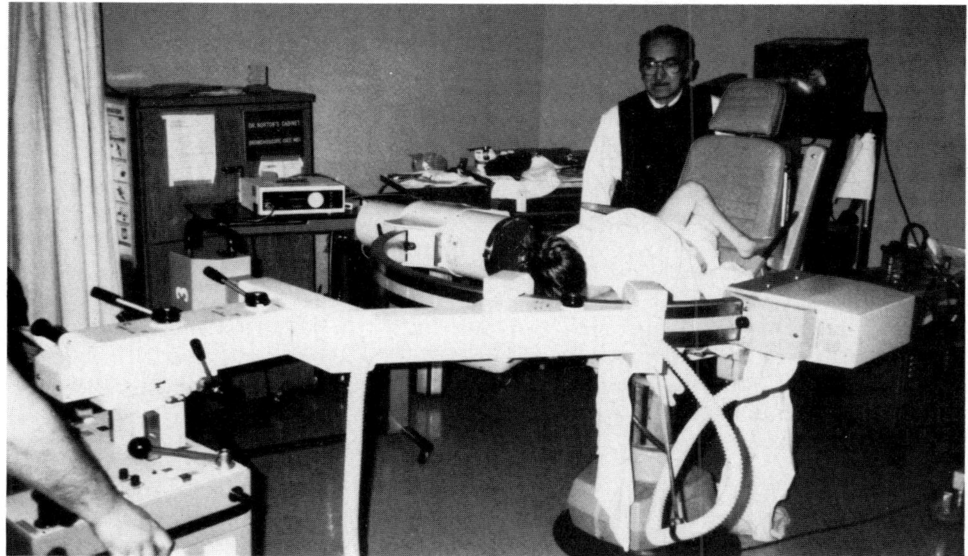

FIG 1–2.
Difficult Airway Clinic setting.

as important as a preoperative electrocardiogram. This assessment can be achieved only by providing sufficient time for proper and considered evaluation and planning for the final objective.

With this information, the growing availability of flexible fiberoptic instruments, and attention to the problem as exemplified by our development of a difficult airway evaluation clinic (Fig 1–2),[16, 17] this catastrophic incidence can be reduced. The difficult airway is of concern to every physician, and especially to anesthesiologists, otolaryngologists, oral surgeons, plastic surgeons, orthopedists, and our colleagues in medical specialties such as rheumatology, neurology, and pulmonary medicine.

REFERENCES

1. American Society of Anesthesiologists, Committee on Professional Liability: Preliminary study of closed claims. *ASA Newslett* 1988; 4(52):8–10.
2. Caplan RA, Posner K, Ward RJ, et al: Adverse respiratory events in anesthesia: A closed claims analysis. *Anesthesiology* 1990; 72:828–833.
3. Endler GC, Mariona FG, Sokol RJ, et al: Maternal death as a result of anesthesia — the Michigan experience. *Am J Obstet Gynecol* 1988; 159:187–193.
4. Chadwick HS, Posner K, Ward RJ, et al: A review of anesthesia malpractice claims [abstract]. *Anesthesiology* 1989; 71:A942.
5. Caplan RA, Ward RJ, Posner K, et al: Unexpected cardiac arrest during spinal anesthesia: Closed claims analysis of predisposing factors. *Anesthesiology* 1988; 68:5–11.
6. Holland R: Anesthesia related mortality in Australia, in Pierce EC, Cooper JB (eds): *International Anesthesiology Clinics.* Boston, Little, Brown & Co, 1984, pp 61–71.

7. Caplan RA, Todd DP: Respiratory mishaps: Principal anesthetic of risk and implications for anesthesia. *Anesthesiology* 1987; 67:A469.

8. MacEwen W: Clinical observations on the introduction of tracheal tubes by the mouth instead of performing tracheotomy or laryngotomy. *BMJ* 1880; 2:163.

9. Kirstein A: Autoskopie des larynx und der trachea. *Berl Klin Wochenschr* 1895; 32:475.

10. Bichat X: *The Surgical Works, or Statement of Doctrine and Practice of P. J. Desault.* Philadelphia; T Dobson, 1814, pp 229–234.

11. Magill JW: Technique in endotracheal anesthesia. *BMJ* 1930; 1:817–819.

12. Herholdt JD, Rafn CG: *An Attempt at an Historical Survey of Life-Saving Measures for Drowning Persons and Information of the Best Means by Which They Can Again Be Brought Back to Life.* Copenhagen, H Tikiobs, 1796. (Reprinted by the Scandinavian Society of Anesthesiology, Aarhus, Denmark, Stiftsbogtrykkerie, 1960.)

13. Sia RL, Edens ET: How to avoid problems when using the fiberoptic bronchoscope for difficult intubations. *Anesthesia* 1981; 36:74.

14. Aro L, Takki S, Aromaa U: Technique for difficult intubation. *Br J Anesthesiol* 1974; 43:1081.

15. Stauffer JL, Olson DE, Petty TL: Complications and consequences of endotracheal intubation and tracheostomy. A prospective study of 150 critically ill adult patients. *Am J Med* 1981; 70:65–76.

16. Norton ML, Wilton N, Brown AC: The Difficult Airway Clinic. *Anesth Rev* 1988; 15:25–28.

17. Norton ML, Brown ACD: Evaluating the patient with a difficult airway for anesthesia. *Otolaryngol Clin North Am* 1990; 23:771–785.

Chapter 2

Normal Practice of Endoscopy and Intubation

Martin L. Norton

EXAMINATION

Of crucial importance is the need to do a thorough examination of areas that have not been completely studied by the referring physician. Indeed, it is necessary to repeat parts of the history and physical examination. There is truth to the often made comment, "I cannot visualize what is written on the chart unless I see it for myself."

This is particularly true when evaluating the airway, because other medical specialists do not always give attention to some of the factors that anesthesiologists must. For example, a patent nasal passage for intubation includes consideration of the outside diameter of the tube to be inserted, particularly in children. Some anesthesiologists are reluctant to examine children in the awake state. They may have forgotten (or never learned) the ear, nose, and throat examination skills practiced by the family physician or otolaryngologist!

Examination must include a history specifically related to the area of concern as well as other systems affected. It requires the art of visualization. It is interesting that indirect laryngoscopy originated with Manuel Garcia, a professor of singing at the Paris Conservatoire. In 1855 he read a paper before the Royal Society of Laryngology in England entitled "Observations on the Human Voice,"[1] based on patient self-examination of his vocal cords with a dental mirror. Auscultation, palpation, and other exercises of the art of visualization add up to the physical diagnosis.

Problems such as tonsillar enlargement, glossoptosis (posterior and downward apposition of the base of the tongue, with resultant airway obstruction), or nasal passage obstruction are readily visualized with the simple and painless use of the otoscope and nasal or other speculae. Such tools are used routinely in the pediatrician's office. In the infrequent case where it is necessary, appropriately small doses of midazolam, ketamine, or other medication can be given, but always with the precautions of postexamination observation and the availability of airway support equipment. It is fallacious to call the latter "awake intubation." This is medicated intubation, and in some cases borders on light general anesthesia.

The anesthesiologist must never wait until the moment of surgery to do an appropriate examination. Such strategy speaks ill of our profession by endangering the patient! One of the reasons for establishing the Difficult Airway Clinic (University of Michigan Medical Center, Ann Arbor) is to avoid the problems that ensue from last-minute examinations.

POSITIONING THE PATIENT

Dripps et al.,[2] in their classic text followed Jackson and Jackson[3] in describing the axes of intubation as oral, pharyngeal, and tracheal. By opening the mouth properly and extending the cervical vertebrae at the atlantoaxial joint and flexing the lower cervical vertebral joints, these axes (especially tracheal and pharyngeal) can be brought together. This is the basis for placing the head in the "sniffing," or "pecking," position by means of a pad under the head for adults.

You will note in Chapter 10, however, that the area described (atlantoaxial joint) is not the site of most movement (flexion-extension) of the neck. In fact, this site lies between C-4 and C-7. Adding to the problem, endoscopists often put too large a pad under the head, thus limiting the available opening of the mouth. Similarly, what has become almost a reflex motion, that of snapping the head to extreme extension by pulling up the chin and pressing down and backward on the cranium, must be decried. As a consequence, the airway narrows despite the greater room available to open the mouth. In addition, there is great risk of physician-induced trauma (euphoniously called iatrogenic) in older patients and those with osteoporosis, Paget's disease, rheumatoid arthritis (with atlantoaxial instability), or other potential odontoid-peg problems.

Of particular importance is the relationship of the hyoid cartilage and its attached musculature. This "bone" is related specifically to the attachment of the middle constrictor and hyoglossus muscles at the greater cornua of the hyoid along with the suspensory effect of the body of the hyoid with attached geniohyoid and with the genioglossus muscles shifting the base of the tongue anteriorly, thus opening the airway.

Anesthesia, sedatives, ethanol, and vagally mediated volume feedback from the lungs all suppress motor output to the genioglossus in animals. Sleep deprivation has been shown to depress the phasic respiratory activity of this muscle in normal humans. In unanesthetized cats and sleeping human infants, neck position influences genioglossal activity and pharyngeal configuration. Neck flexion reflexly activates genioglossal discharge, which tends to maintain airway patency.

MONITORING CORRECT PLACEMENT OF ENDOTRACHEAL TUBE

The end point of endotracheal tube placement must be closely monitored. The risk of esophageal insertion is real, and there are severe consequences to lack of recognition of this misplacement. Much of this monitoring is based on suspicion. The following should be observed during tube placement:

1. Top of the endotracheal tube cuff at or just below the level of the vocal folds.
2. With the use of translucent tubes, fogging with expiration and clearing on inspiration. However, this may also appear from the gases within the upper gastrointestinal tract and thus is not a reliable sign.
3. Movements of the chest during assisted inspiration, especially the left side of the thorax, should follow.
4. Comparative breath sounds determined by auscultation at the level of the fourth and fifth intercostal spaces at the middle to anterior axillary line. (Note: The practice of listening over the second or third intercostal space in the midclavicular line is fraught with the danger of deception from transmitted sounds from the trachea or even the esophagus.)
5. Gurgling sounds in the stomach during assisted ventilation. (This step should be performed by auscultation of the epigastrium in conjunction with no. 2 as well.)
6. End-tidal CO_2 monitor for pattern of ventilation and level of CO_2 return. This is the penultimate guide, but although it does clearly indicate esophageal intubation, it does not clearly verify endobronchial intubation.
7. Level of red blood cell hemoglobin saturation using the pulse oximeter or other techniques of transcutaneous oxygen saturation monitoring. This may be a late sign, but it is certainly quicker and more accurate than the item 8.
8. Skin or mucosae for cyanosis (a very late sign).
9. Confirmation by visual identification (flexible fiberoptic endoscopy) of the carina or bronchopulmonary segments (most useful when using double-lumen tubes).
10. Confirmation of tube positioning by radiologic means (x-ray), although this may take more time than is safe.

Above all, constant vigilance and suspicion are the keystones when monitoring tube placement. We must also keep in mind that any change in patient position on the table mandates rechecking all parameters of endotracheal tube position.

NASAL PASSAGE

Direct examination using a nasal speculum is rarely done. The common practice appears to be to determine nasal airway patency by asking the patient about ease of respiration while occluding one or the other of the nares or while passing a long cotton-tipped swab probe saturated with cocaine or a lidocaine-epinephrine solution. Passage of the long swab demonstrates only that there is enough room for a 2 or 3 mm instrument; it does not yield information as to obstructions using (in adults) a nasotracheal tube with 6 mm inside diameter or

6.3 mm outside diameter. It does give some guidance about the direction of the inferior ethmoid passage, but does not produce accurate measurements and certainly does not indicate the diameter of the passageway or its adequacy for passage of varying size endotracheal tubes. Even rhinomanometric values have not been reliable as a means of distinguishing between normal and abnormal passages based on rhinoscopic evaluation.[4]

Nasal resistance values also are unreliable. Traditional medical practice has long taught the necessity of knowing the anatomy (Fig 2–1), physiology (especially the functional suspension of the hyoid, Fig 2–2), and pharmacology of the area of concern. Similarly, a proper diagnostic examination includes visualization, wherever possible, and the use of ancillary diagnostic methods to further illuminate understanding of the passageway in the specific patient. I have found the use of the otoscope with its long speculum especially advantageous in visualizing the nasal passageways, especially the regions of the nasal vestibule, turbinates, and the choanae. Nasal septal deviations, turbinate and conchael malformations, and simple polyps may be clearly visualized using this method.

Of particular note is the palatal arch (hard palate). If the palate is significantly highly arched (Fig 2–3) the floor of the nose bulges to the nasal lumen as a result. Possibly as a secondary phenomenon, the nasal septum is often buckled and deflected to one side or the other. The septal spurs impinge on the shelflike turbinates and complete the picture of nasal obstruction.

In children, and some adults, hypertrophied adenoid tissues and tonsils present complications. The current deemphasis on tonsillectomy and adenoidectomy during childhood appears to have resulted in more obstructive tonsillar masses in adults, and these occasionally complicate nasotracheal intu-

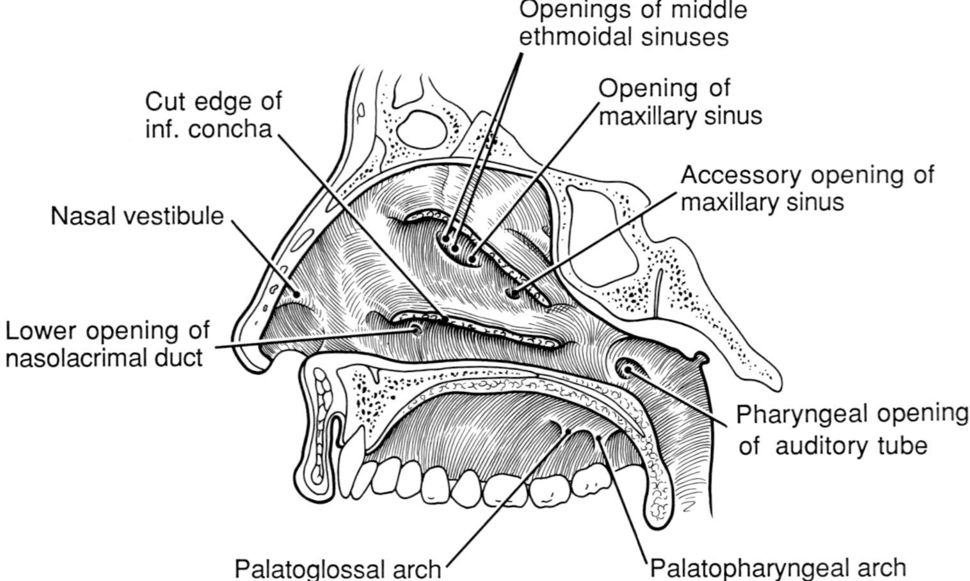

FIG 2–1.
Anatomy of the nasal passage.

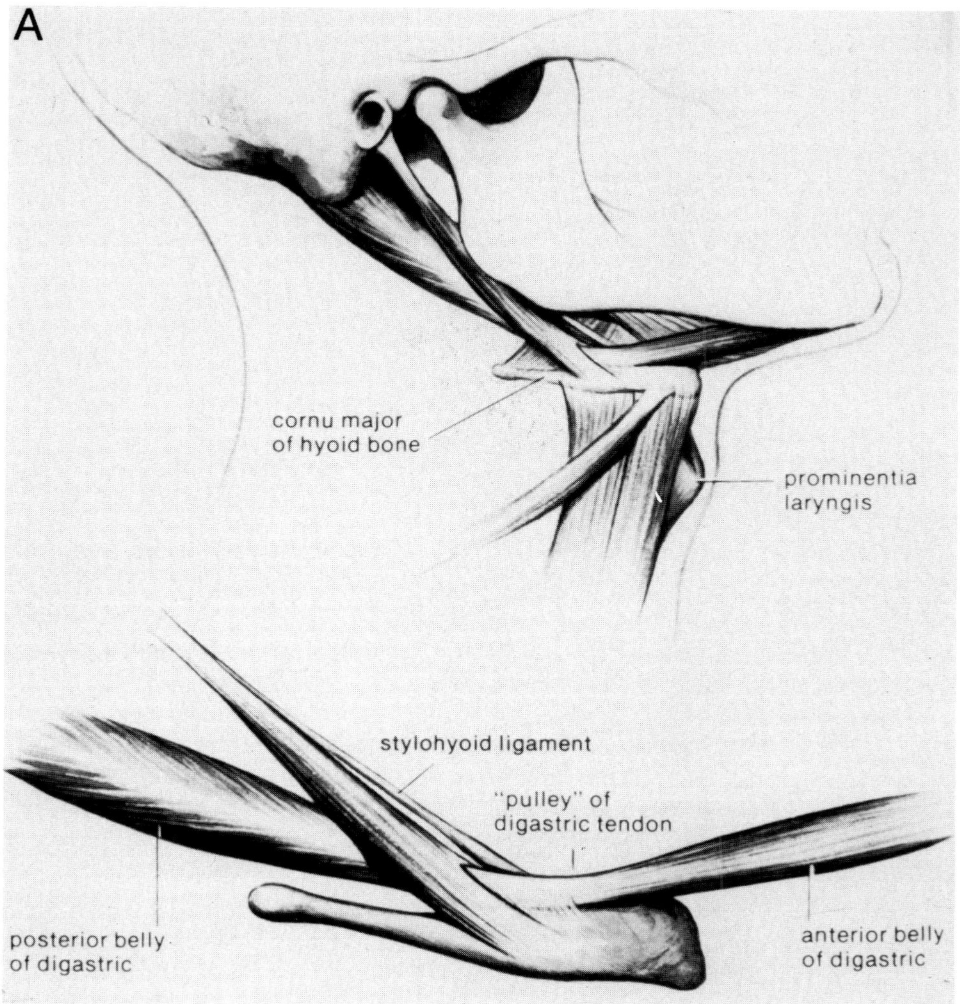

FIG 2–2.
Functional suspension of the hyoid. **A,** suspension; **B,** function.

bations. The contribution of these masses to sleep apnea is yet to be fully elucidated.

An upper respiratory tract infection or allergy, often manifested by nasal polyps, also compromises the patency of the nasal airways.

After visualization, we use graded sizes of soft, very well lubricated nasopharyngeal tubes to reinforce visual observations and to stretch up the diameter of the nasal passages. We start with a small nasopharyngeal tube (about 6.0 mm for adults) and progress to one size larger than the nasotracheal tube that I wish to insert.

This is particularly important in view of another consideration: the nasal passage is highly vascular. We therefore must be concerned about potential severe hemorrhage from trauma and the fact that the definitive endotracheal tube will soften in the nasal passage over a period of time, leading to the risk

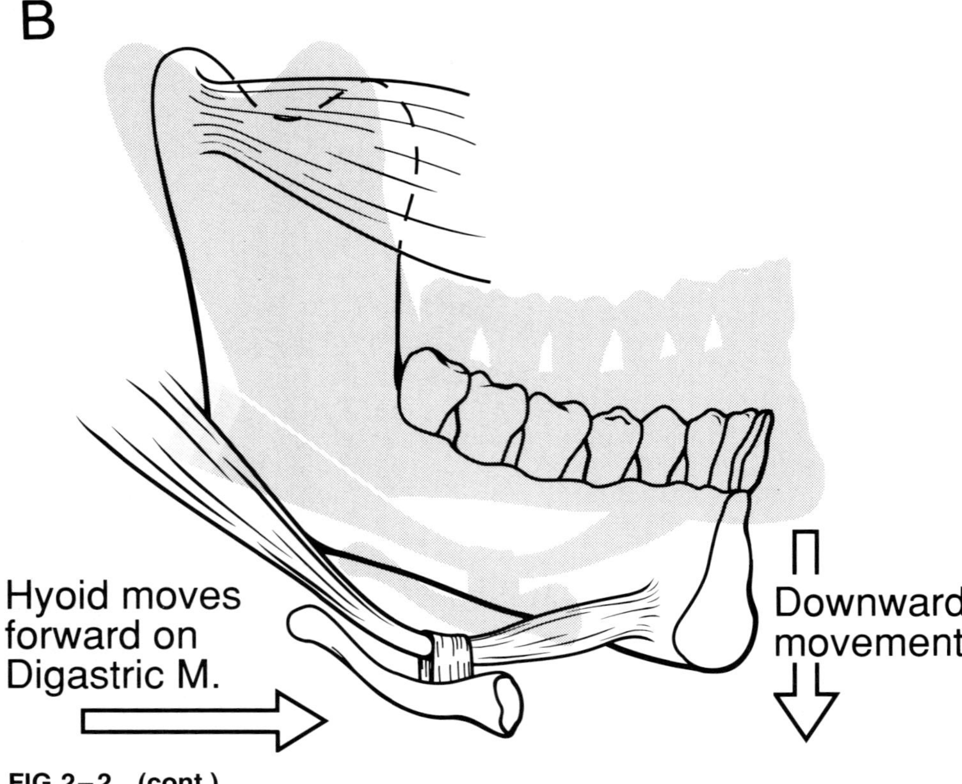

FIG 2–2   (cont.).

of kinking or at least decreasing the internal diameter of the available imposed airway.

Today there is less concern about tube size and its relationship to rheologic patterns than in previous years. The response we hear is that any problem in this regard would be picked up by the end-tidal CO_2 monitor.[5] This could be true, in part, if the end-tidal pattern were closely monitored. With major kinking the plateau portion of the end-tidal capnograph will show the usual obstructive signs (i.e., the sudden drop to a low level). However, this is best seen in spontaneously breathing patients, whom we are rarely dealing with at this point.

In addition, the patient should be properly prepared. In most situations the patient is most comfortable in the sitting or semi-Fowler position. For fiberoptic laryngoscopy and bronchoscopy the upright sitting position is best, because of the suspension of the larynx. (We have been using a dental chair to great advantage, because of its familiarity to patients and ideal adjustability.)

A small dose of fentanyl or midazolam is of value to calm the patient. We then spray a mixture of 4% lidocaine mixed with 4% cocaine into the nasal passages.

As a precaution, intravenous barbiturates and a source and system for providing controlled oxygen are available. We also have a pulse oximeter attached to each patient being examined, and in appropriate patients an electrocardio-

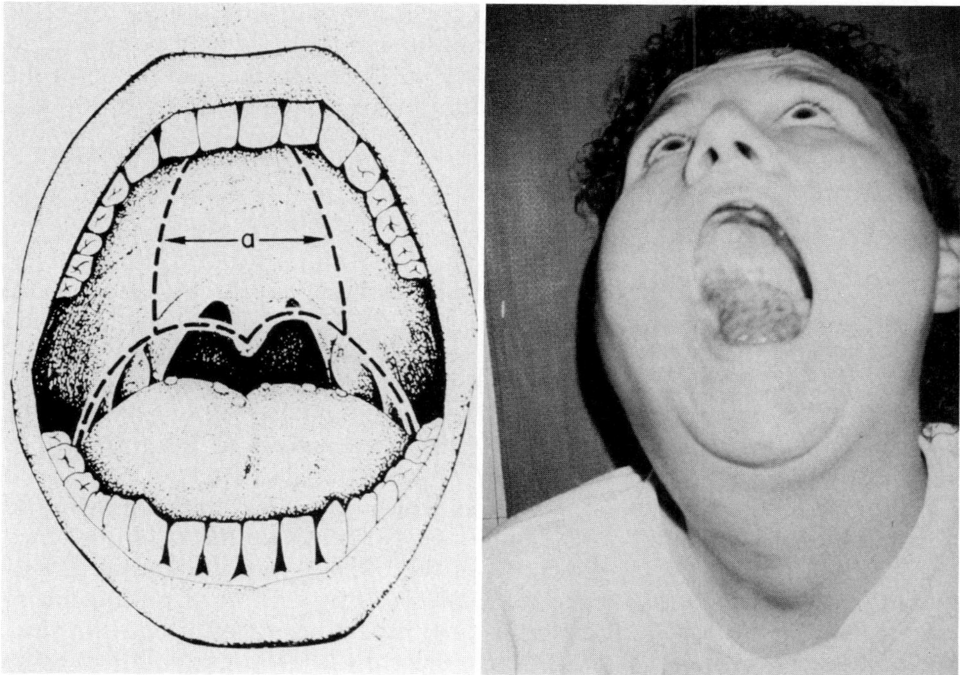

FIG 2–3.
Depiction of a significantly high arched palate.

graph and blood pressure cuff (Dynamap) are used as constant recording monitors.

Nasotracheal intubation airway management has become the procedure of choice in intensive care units (long-term intubation) and for plastic surgical and orosurgical procedures. Many of our colleagues in these specialties are particularly adamant about the need for nasoendotracheal intubation.

However, there are also negative aspects other than the risk of hemorrhage and the need for a smaller than optimum sized airway. Among these are the risk of reflex otic pain or internal ear infection (usually serous otitis) related to the proximity of the pharyngeal orifice to the auditory canal, trauma to the posterior nasopharynx, and impingement of the endotracheal tube or endoscope on hypertrophied tonsillar or adenoidal tissue while the breathing tube is being advanced down past the soft palate and uvula. In addition, the tube is often further kinked by pressure of the inferior conchae of the turbinates. It is important to note that although dental surgery is easier (for the surgeon) on the patient whose airway is intubated through the nose, there are few dental operations that cannot be performed with an orotracheal tube positioned behind the third molar and running along the buccal pouch and out of the mouth. We must remember that the convenience and comfort of the surgeon cannot take precedence over medical considerations of risk to the patient.

There is an important difference between the adult and the infant in that the large infant tongue is apposed to the palate during quiet respiration. Also, the glottis is much higher, resting between the third and fourth cervical vertebrae in the neonate and next to the sixth cervical vertebra in the adult. Furthermore, in the child the glottis is funnel shaped, and the narrowest portion internally lies at the cricoid cartilage, not the vocal folds. Further indication of the differences between the adult and pediatric larynx can be found in the Appendix.

FIBEROPTIC INTUBATION

Flexible fiberoptic laryngoscopy is the most recent approach to the difficult airway. It must not be pursued as an afterthought or after endoscopy has failed with other techniques. This approach requires careful evaluation of the patient's anatomy, proper preparation of the passages, adequate anesthesia (topical or general), correct positioning of the patient, and an endoscopist with the requisite skill and experience. Table 2–1 lists those situations where fiberoptic endoscopy is recommended.

Further intubations of the airway in which prior intubations have failed should be postponed until the patient's tissues have had time to recover from the incident trauma and to allow time for thorough reevaluation of the airway per the procedures described for the Difficult Airway Clinic. Failure to do so risks complications that include but are not limited to the extreme risk of unrecognized entrance into the superior mediastinum by laceration of the thin membrane at the level of the cricopharyngeus decussation.

We believe the endoscopist must perform at least 100 flexible fiberoptic intubations before he or she can be considered an expert in this field. Every residency program in anesthesiology should provide the opportunity for the house officer to attempt at least 25 fiberoptic intubations. We suggest at least 25 practice intubations in teaching models, followed by at least 25 intubations in the airways of patients scheduled electively for nasotracheal intubation. This

TABLE 2–1.

Intubations Where Fiberoptic Endoscopy is Recommended

Unstable bridge work	Arthritis in airway or
Mandibular hypoplasia	neck
Temporomandibular	Laryngeal tumors
joint disease	Radical neck
Congenital	dissection
abnormalities	Neck masses
Swallowing dysfunction	Radiation therapy to
Vocal fold paralysis	upper airway
Mallampati class III or	Cicatricial
IV	burns/phemphigoid
Collagen vascular	Old tracheostomy
disease of neck or	Foreign body
pharynx	History of difficult
Myopathy/myositis	intubation
Morbid obesity	
Unstable neck	
fractures	
Fixed neck	

should then be followed by at least 10 orotracheal intubations. The patients included in this mix should include both awake (topical anesthesia) and lightly anesthetized (vocal folds functioning) subjects. Indications for awake fiberoptic evaluation are somewhat controversial; Table 2–2 lists these indications.

These requirements further imply the considered understanding of the anatomy and pathophysiology of the nasopharynx as well as the oropharynx. Once again we are reminded of the basics of medicine, anatomy, physiology, and pharmacology.

A classic case wherein the fiberoptic instrument is of specific use is in the patient with glossoptosis. Glossoptosis is defined as tongue pressure on the cervical portion of the spinal column. Posterior positioning of the tongue causes pressure on the glottis. This closes the glottis if the mouth is shut, and limits it even with mouth open. The airways to the nasopharyngeal space are also closed. Consequently, patients with glossoptosis are forced by anatomic mechanics to breathe and eat with an open mouth.

Severe glossoptosis can often be recognized by the habitus of the patient: the head bends forward, the shoulders hang, the body seems bent and collapsed, the thighs appear excessively relaxed, and the facial expression is adenoidal. The teeth of the maxillary jaw are forward with reference to those of the retrograde mandibular jaw. The mouth responds to the condition of the weak receding chin by hanging open during breathing. The dull appearance of the patient combined with sloppy posture may suggest deficient mental development. However, we must caution that this conclusion is not necessarily true. Children seem physically and psychologically stunted in growth because they constantly feel indisposed and are ventilating poorly, although not seriously ill.

The differential diagnosis must also include macroglossia and its causes. Often these patients have a clear history of sleep apnea. However, this history must be sought, because this is one syndrome that is often missed. The fact that these patients are often subjected to veloplasty or mandibular advancement procedures, or both, makes this syndrome of particular interest to otolaryngologists, plastic surgeons, oral surgeons, and anesthesiologists.

The insertion of a fiberoptic instrument through the oral route is reputedly more difficult than through the nasal route. We have found this not necessarily so. The key to success is the use of an appropriate oropharyngeal airway combined with proper topical anesthesia. We have found the Berman intubating airway (Fig 2–4) most useful, although the smaller sizes are not currently available. (Others have found the use of the Ovassapian airway, also pictured in

TABLE 2–2.

Controversial Indications for Awake Fiberoptic Intubation

Facial trauma	Status asthmaticus
Dental disease	Evolving respiratory failure
Epiglottitis	Severe coronary disease
Unstable neck	Full stomach
Pharyngeal mass	Obstetric anesthesia
Mediastinal mass	Sepsis/shock
Bronchopleural fistula	

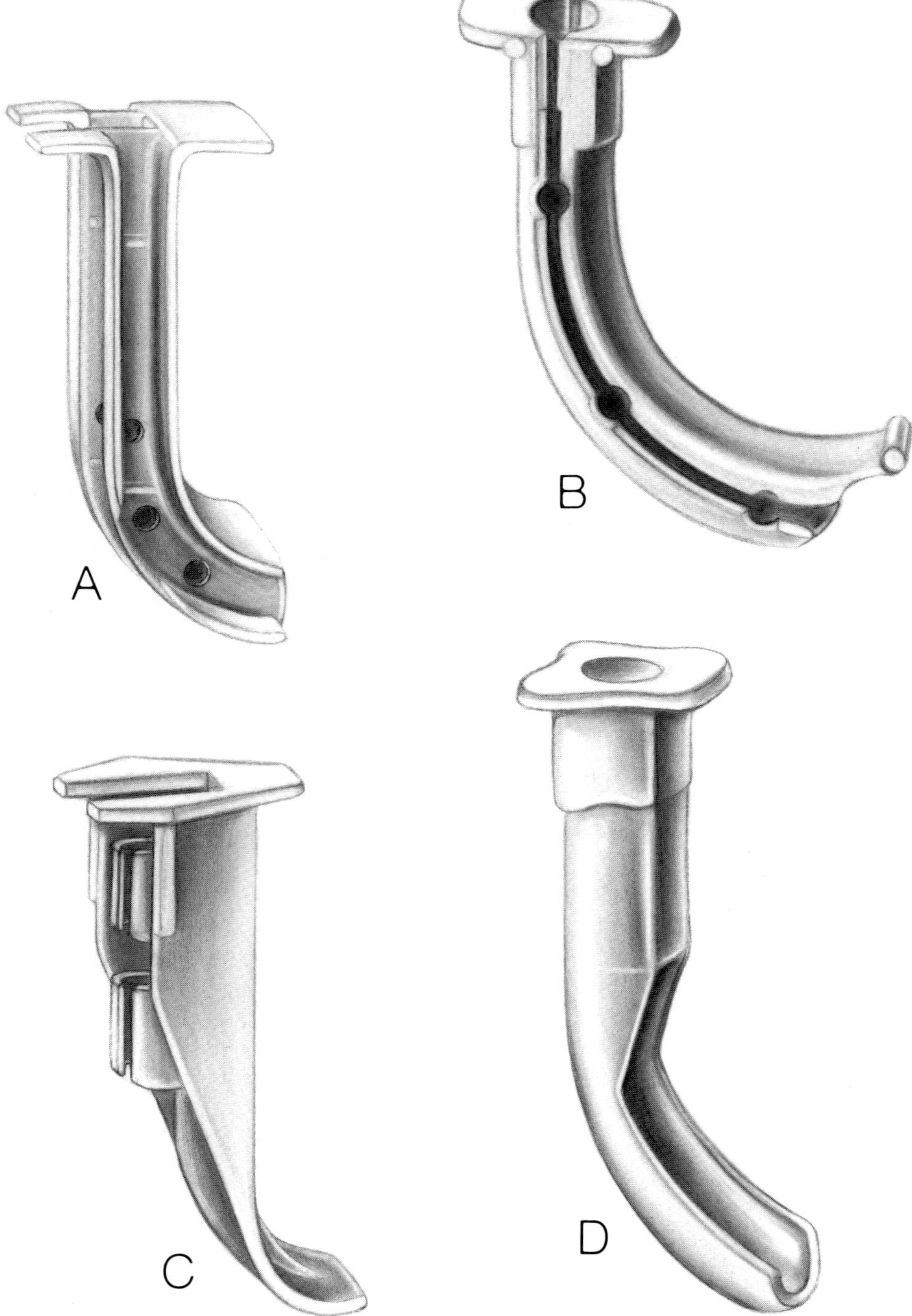

FIG 2–4.
A, Luomanen intubating airway; **B,** Berman intubating airway; **C,** Ovassapian airway; **D,** Williams airway.

TABLE 2–3.

Lower Airway Problems Where Fiberoptic
Evaluation is Strongly Recommended

Laryngoesophageal cleft	Bronchiectasis
Tracheoesophageal fistula	Lung/airway resection
Tracheostomy/ cricothyrotomy	Severe lung scarring, tracheal distortion
Substernal thyroid-tracheal compression	Foreign body in airway
	Intratracheal lesions
	Bronchial bleeding
Anterior mediastinal masses	Recurrent atelectasis/plugging
Superior vena cava syndrome	Suspected perioperative aspiration

Figure 2–4, of equal value.) This instrument has an added lip on its undersurface that protrudes into the vallecula epiglottis but can also be inserted over the epiglottis. It has a slit along the entire side that allows for somewhat larger sizes of endotracheal tubes, or it can be used to open up the device for removal. Finally, fiberoptic endoscopy is useful in a number of lower airway situations, detailed in Table 2–3.

TECHNIQUES FOR ESTABLISHING THE AIRWAY

Several approaches can be taken in the particularly difficult intubation. One is to pass a long arterial wire (used often in the cardiac catheterization laboratory) through the suction channel of the intubating fiberoptic bronchoscope. Then the tip of the scope may be positioned for full visualization of the larynx, and the arterial wire passed under direct vision into the trachea. This is followed by passage of the fiberscope over the wire, then the endotracheal tube over the fiberscope, when indicated.

Another approach is to pass the fiberscope down to the additus laryngis transnasally, then bring the endotracheal tube down the opposite nasal passage until it can be visualized at the rima glottidis through the optics of the fiberscope. Thus the tube would be further advanced under direct fiberoptic vision.

Perhaps the most important concept to be learned is that the best patient preparation includes a careful and sympathetic explanation of what endoscopy entails, followed by a second, equally careful, step-by-step explanation during the procedure. Success probably depends more on rapport and resultant cooperation, and therefore on the temperament of patient and endoscopist, than any other factor. This takes time and cannot be done in an environment of noise, confusion, and psychological pressure!

Of great importance too is positioning of the patient. We recommend the superb reference works by Fink[6] and Fink and Demarest.[7] They certainly are the basis of consideration for efficient endoscopy and intubation. The reader will find the schematic to suggest the biomechanics of the unfolding of the lar-

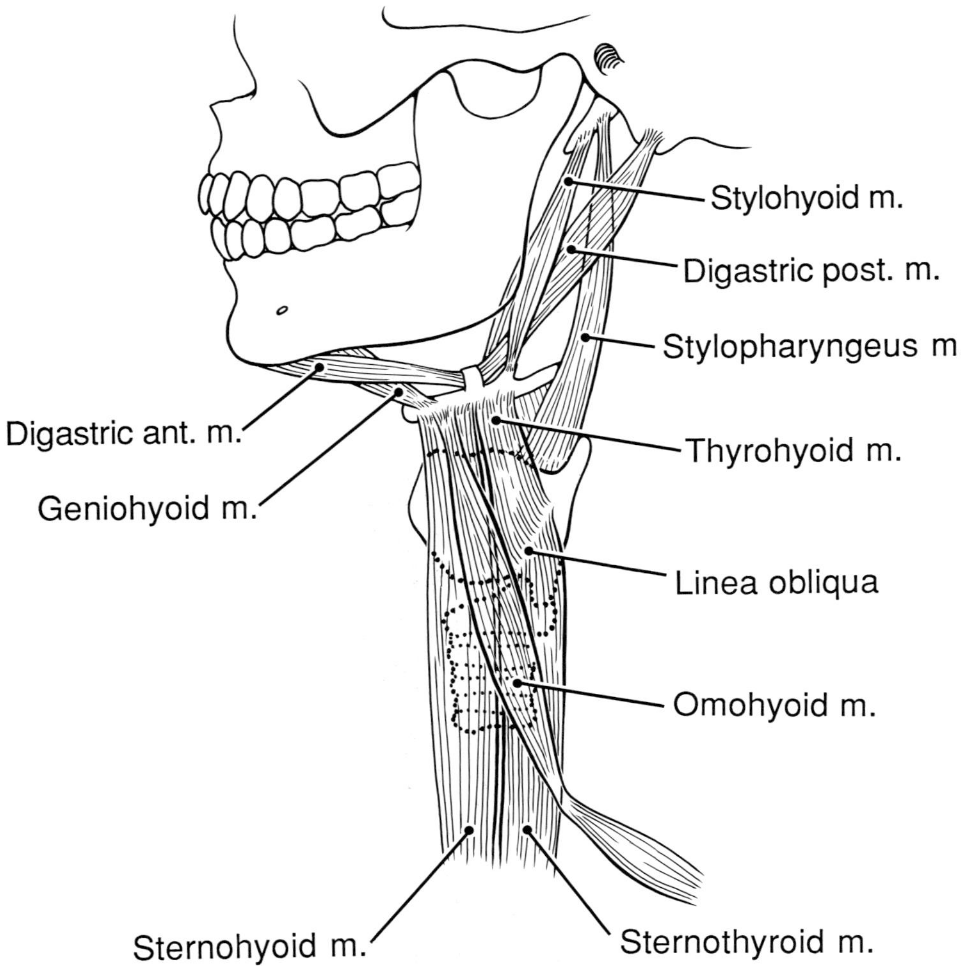

FIG 2–5.
Muscle and ligamentous supports of larynx.

ynx through utilization of its active and passive supports (Fig 2–5).* These studies present the rationale for considering the sitting position optimal for flexible fiberoptic endoscopy.

Decisions on positioning must consider the effect of the weight of the lungs and their fluid content (vasculature and cell fluid volume) when opening up the thoracic inlet as well as on the unfolding of the larynx itself. In addition, the proper manipulation of the mandible and patient cooperation in extending the tongue contribute to the efficiency of the procedure.

The sitting posture is usually comfortable for the patient and convenient for the operator. The patient's shoulders should be fully relaxed and the chin jutted forward. The tongue is protruded and held forward while the topical anesthetic is applied and during the endoscopic procedure. If the patient is fully

---

*Refer also to Figures 3 to 7 in *The Human Larynx.*[6]

conscious, constant urging to breathe deeply and slowly through the mouth can be of additional aid.

Endoscopy in the supine position is more familiar to the anesthesiologist and otolaryngologist when rigid instrumentation is used. However, changes in support of the soft tissues of the upper respiratory tract lead to collapse of the

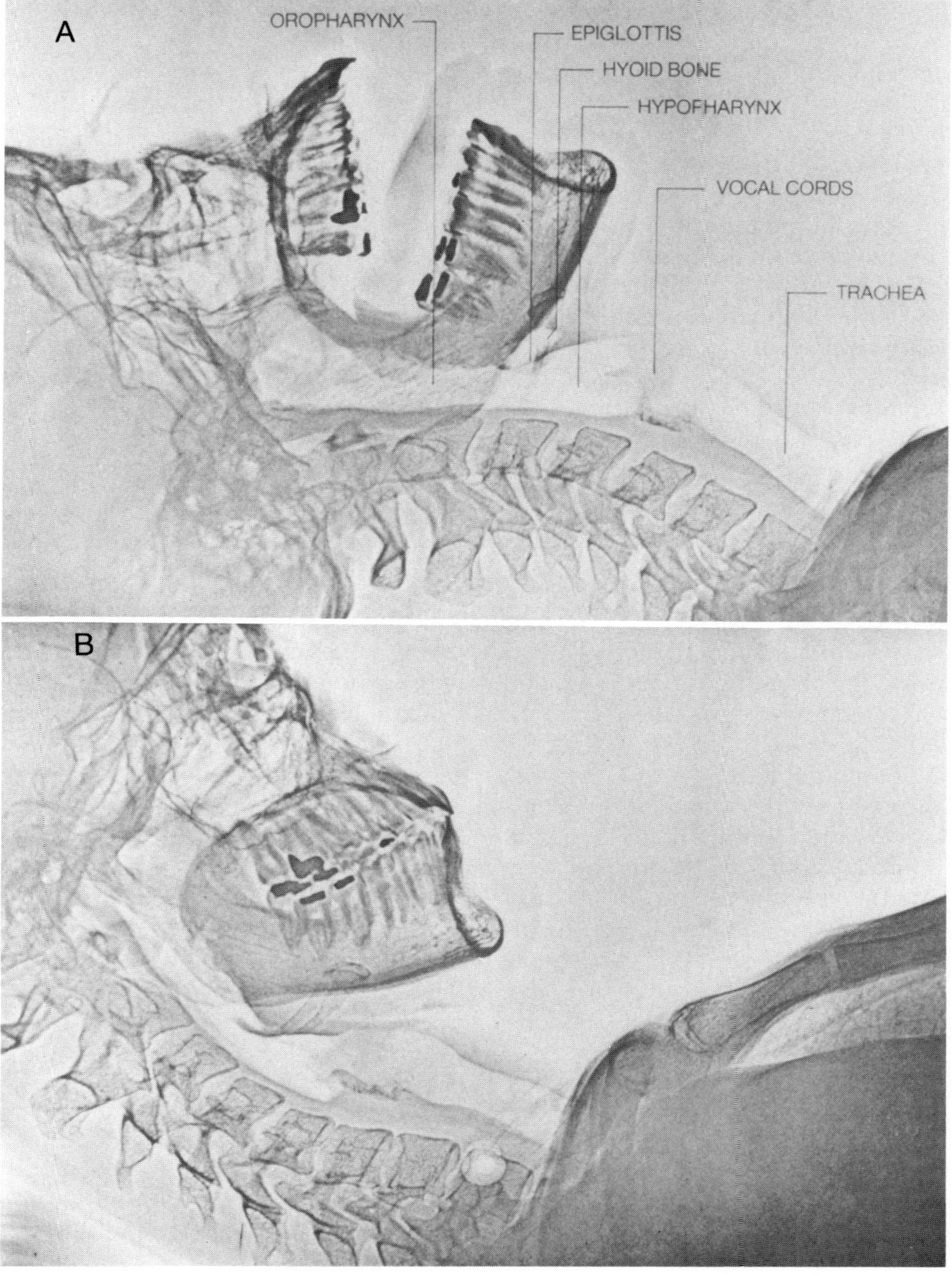

FIG 2–6.
Xeroradiographs of head and neck. **A,** extension; **B,** flexion.

pharyngeal funnel. Head position becomes crucial with ventral movement of the C6 and C7 vertebrae, presenting a further obstacle. Use of ancillary aides such as the Berman, Luomannen, or Ovassapian intubating airway or pre-placement of a nasotracheal tube to the point of maximal breath sounds can be of value in overcoming these obstacles.

Cricoid pressure is an often used maneuver, originally described by Sellick in 1961.[8] Developed to prevent regurgitant flow from the stomach into the airway, the maneuver involves applying backward pressure on the front of the cricoid cartilage, obstructing the upper esophagus, and theoretically preventing regurgitation and aspiration before intubation. Some even believe that it prevents gastric distention during positive pressure ventilation by mask. However, the patient is often positioned with the head extended in the "pecking position" (Fig 2–6).

Cricoid pressure technique was presented as an alternative to induction in the sitting position. However, anatomic distortion can occasionally result from pressure on the neck, rendering intubation more difficult, particularly in the obese or pregnant patient or in the patient with a short neck. Posterior displacement of the larynx by pressure on the thyroid or cricoid cartilage is frequently used during difficult intubations when the larynx is not readily brought into adequate viewing. This also can distort the anatomy and may require contracricoid pressure[9] to the back of the neck.

EXTUBATION

Of equal importance to endotracheal intubation are the considerations and techniques of extubation. The general rule holds that a difficult intubation means a potentially difficult extubation. Every time an endotracheal tube is removed (or a tracheostomy is decannulated), we must be prepared for a possible emergency reintubation. Examples of situations requiring emergency recannulation include, but are not limited to, tracheal collapse following total thyroidectomy of Riedel's struma, recurarization syndrome, and sedative overdose in the postanesthesia patient.

One technique we routinely use is to insert the long intubation guide (Norton Teflon or Eschmann woven) down to the level of the carina, decannulate the endotracheal tube, and leave the stylet in situ for at least 1 hour. Patients tolerate the retention of the stylet very well compared with the endotracheal tube and can even vocalize with it in place. Clinical observation of many patients over many years has demonstrated that airway obstruction (e.g., edema) following decannulation usually occurs within the first hour. If this does occur, it is simple to railroad the endotracheal tube over the long intubation guide into the trachea and thus bypass the obstruction until further treatment is provided. This approach has been and is being used routinely in both nasal and orotracheal intubations.

REFERENCES

1. Garcia M: Observations on the human voice. Paper presented to the Royal Society of Laryngology, 1855.

2. Dripps RD, Eckenhoff J, Van Dam L: *Textbook of Anesthesia*. Philadelphia, WB Saunders Co, 1969.
3. Jackson C, Jackson CL: *Diseases of the Nose, Throat, and Ear*. Philadelphia, WB Saunders Co, 1945.
4. McCaffrey TV, Kern EB: Clinical evaluation of nasal obstruction: A study of 1000 patients. *Arch Otolaryngol* 1979; 105:542.
5. Smallhout BA: *Quick Guide to Capnography and its Use in Differential Diagnosis*. Böblingen, Germany, Hewlett Packard Medical Products Group, 1983.
6. Fink BR: *The Human Larynx*. New York, Raven Press, 1975.
7. Fink BR, Demarest RJ: *Laryngeal Biomechanics*. Cambridge, Mass, Harvard University Press, 1978.
8. Sellick BA: Cricoid pressure to control regurgitation of stomach contents during induction of anesthesia. *Lancet* 1961; 2:404.
9. Crawford JS: The "contra cricoid" cuboid aid to tracheal intubation. *Anaesthesia* 1982; 37:345.

Chapter 3

Instrumentation and Equipment for Management of the Difficult Airway

Allan Brown

Martin L. Norton

An old saying suggests that the shoemaker must not blame the equipment for faulty work. An analogy for the physician could be extended to his or her care of equipment. We seem to have forgotten that equipment has a design and that we need to understand its construction and handling in relation to anatomic configuration. The problem airway occasionally becomes much more difficult as a consequence of improper instrumentation techniques.

RIGID LARYNGOSCOPE BLADES

Often anesthesiologists pass the endotracheal tube through the channel of the laryngoscope. Although this method sometimes may be useful in difficult situations, the channel was originally designed to serve as a visual pathway, and using this incorrect technique will usually obstruct vision, leading to inadvertent esophageal intubation or trauma from insertion of the tube.

Similarly, the straight blade (and the curved blade as well) was intended to be inserted along the right side of the pharynx, with the flange of the blade used to displace the bulk of the tongue to the left. This gets the tongue out of the way and provides a larger pharyngeal area through which to pass the endotracheal tube.

One part of the use of the straight blade seems to have been lost since the days of Chevalier Jackson. He taught insertion of the straight blade along the right pharyngeal area, directing it into the pharynx over the pathway delineated by the molar dentition and tonsillar area, bypassing the right root of the tongue and lifting up the epiglottis from the lateral side by making a small C-shaped motion with the tip of the blade. This simple maneuver allows one not only to bypass the bulk of the tongue but also to elevate the epiglottis, even if the epiglottis is floppy, long, or bulky (e.g., from epiglottic cyst, hemangioma, or other lesion).

In patients with dentition, the jaw should not be depressed when it is opened and the laryngoscope blade should not be inserted into the mouth. The optimum opening of the mouth should be with a motion that approximates the gliding motion of the temporomandibular joint (TMJ). Thus we advise a thumb-over-index finger approach, with the index finger on the maxillary dentition as far to the right as possible and the thumb placed on the lower dentition. The resultant motion is C shaped, with the mandible opening in a semicircular fashion following the configuration of the TMJ.

In essence, the resultant motion should be the same as for the elevation of the mandible and tongue: down, out, and finally elevated on to the laryngoscope blade. The mandible is lifted onto the blade rather than the blade being placed under the tongue. Thus, in allowing this motion the TMJ is "dislocated" anteriorly. (Because the usual intubation is done with muscle relaxants, this dislocation is readily achieved.) The larynx and its component parts are then brought superiorly and in close approximation to the lighted tip of the laryngoscope blade.

This approach is particularly applicable to the use of the straight blade, but it also is of significant use when the curved blade is inserted. We often hear about the "anterior larynx" when difficult intubation problems are discussed with clinicians. This term is incongruous in light of the fact that the most prominent cartilage of the larynx is directly under the skin. What is meant is that the tracheal cartilage is positioned higher than usual and may be enfolded within the arch of the hyoid cartilage, thus narrowing the additus laryngis.

STRAIGHT VS. CURVED BLADE LARYNGOSCOPES

We hear constantly of advocates of straight vs. curved blade rigid laryngoscopes; thus an analysis of their origin, application, advantages, and disadvantages appears warranted. Certainly there is a place and a need for both types. The choice of instrumentation (Fig 3–1) in the airway is as important as any other facet of the diagnostic-therapeutic plan.

In the early era of anesthetic and laryngologic endoscopy the most common type of blade was exemplified by the Wisconsin (Foregger) blade. Subsequently the Macintosh blade came into vogue.[1]

The technique for insertion of the straight blade is as follows: The laryngoscope should be held in the left hand with the thumb and first finger of the right hand separating the lips and teeth and preventing the lips from being caught between blade and teeth. The blade is then inserted on the right side of the mouth, advancing it alongside the molars until the root of the tongue is reached (near the tonsillar pillars). The straight blade must *never* be inserted in the midline. After insertion on the right side of the mouth, the tip of the blade is deflected toward the midline under the right root of the tongue, serving to visualize the epiglottis. The tip of the blade is inserted under the epiglottis (dorsal surface) and advanced a few millimeters. The proximal end of the blade is moved toward the midline only far enough to allow passage of the endotracheal tube or bronchoscope.

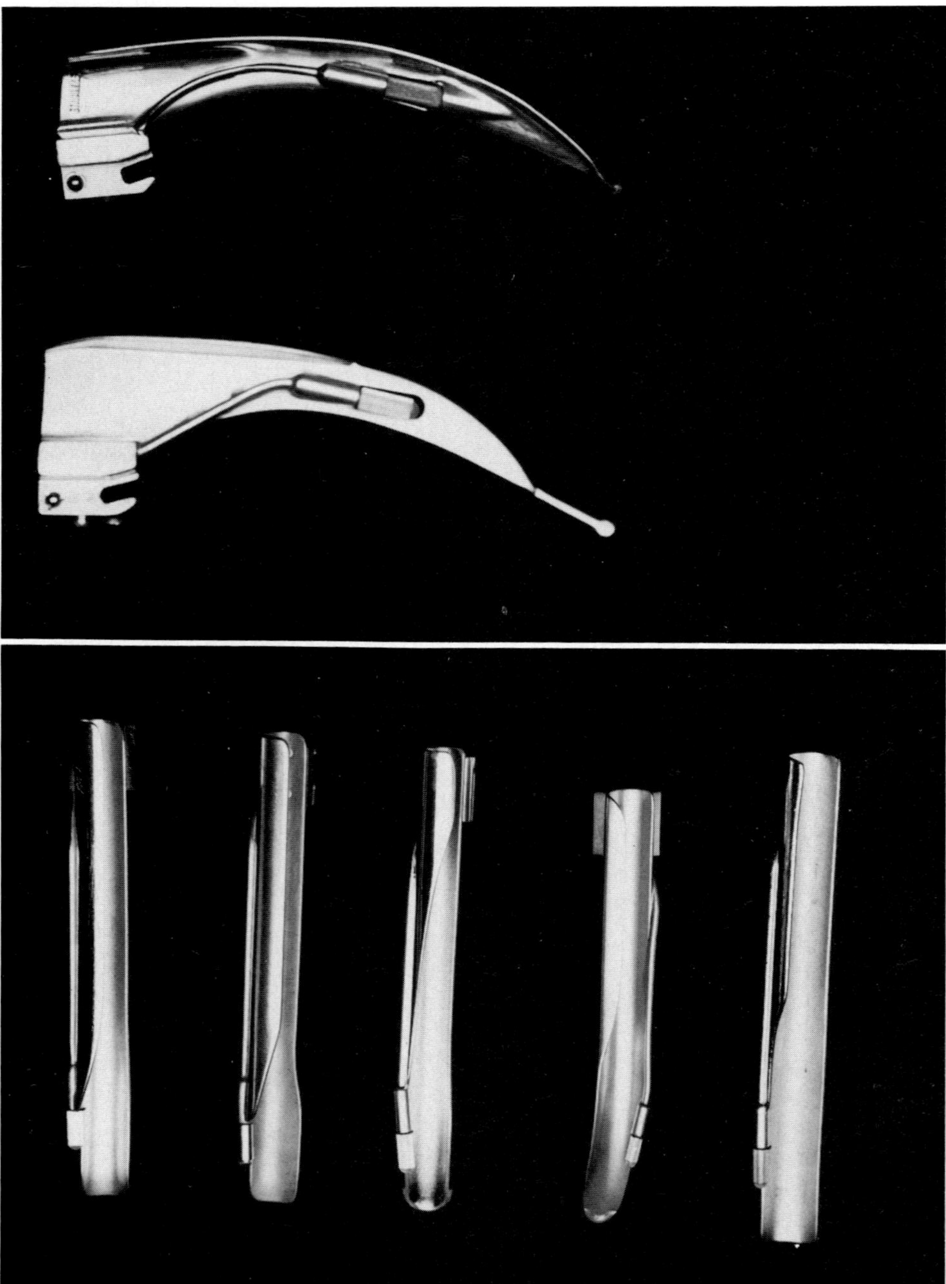

FIG 3–1.
Choice of instrumentation in airway.

Rarely it may be necessary to reverse this to a left-handed approach. This would be applicable for bulky tumors of the right side of the tongue and right tonsillar fauces, particularly if friable. An upward and outward lift of the instrument in a 45-degree angle from the face should provide exposure of the rima glottidis. Overinsertion of the blade results in elevation of the larynx as a whole rather than exposure of the glottic opening. Occasionally the blade will expose the esophagus, which is recognizable by its oval opening and lack of arytenoid cartilages.

The tip should never be advanced without visualization and identification of the orifice and tissues being approached. The three rules of endoscopy are identify, identify, and identify. The risk relates to the cricopharyngeus decussation at the level of the C-6 and C-7 vertebrae (posterior wall of the esophagopharynx), where there is only a thin layer of fibrofascial tissue that can readily be perforated and lead to a potentially life-threatening mediastinitis, particularly if the trauma is unrecognized.

The technique with the curved blade approach is the same, through the right pharyngeal pouch, except that exposure of the glottic opening should not be obtained through elevation of the laryngoscope blade placed under the laryngeal surface of the epiglottis. Rather, the tip of the blade remains in contact with the tongue and rests in the area between the epiglottis and base of the tongue (vallecula). Elevation causes retraction of the epiglottis toward the blade and exposure by the pull on the glossoepiglottic ligament. If the tip of the blade is inserted too deeply, retraction cannot occur and exposure becomes difficult.

The theoretical advantages of a curved blade are derived from the fact that the sensory innervation of the laryngeal surface of the epiglottis arises from the superior laryngeal branch of the vagus nerve (X). Stimulation of this surface by the blade may lead to reflex vocal fold spasm and coughing. Conversely, innervation of the pharyngeal surface is derived from the glossopharyngeal nerve (IX). Stimulation of this surface is less likely to cause laryngeal spasm. However, this does not account for the minor branch interdigitations of the ninth and tenth nerves in the dorsal ganglion of the vagus, the nucleus salivatarius, and the glossopharyngeal ganglion. Further, any stretching of the mucosae of the dorsal surface of the epiglottis is similarly reflected in the mucosal tissue of the ventral surface, thereby still producing activation of both nerve endings to some degree. In fact, when healthy subjects were fully anesthetized before their airways were intubated, no variation in cardiovascular response could be demonstrated.[2] However, the curved blade does allow more room for the passage of the tube than the average straight blade in patients with large bulky tongues (macroglossia), prominent mandibular dentition, and some mandibular jaw malformations.

Sometimes exposure of the glottis is not so good as that obtained with the straight blade, as in cases of floppy epiglottis, and it is evident that an intubating stylet or guide must be used in a high proportion of patients. Despite this, in short, thick-necked individuals and those with a more superiorly situated larynx the curved blade may prove to be the instrument of choice.

STYLETS AND GUIDES

Long intubation guides are used occasionally when direct rigid laryngoscopy does not permit visualization of more than the arytenoids or perhaps demonstrates only an air bubble. Sometimes they are even inserted blindly (by tactile sensation) along the laryngeal surface of the epiglottis.

A plethora of stylets is available for insertion of endotracheal tubes. Most of these will keep the tube in a predetermined, flexed position. However, the most useful ones are the long, semiflexible, intubation stylets, better described as guides: the British (Eschmann woven brown), the Norton (Teflon), and the JEM77400 (Instrumentation Industries, Inc., Bethel Park, Pa.) white or clear hollow tubes (Fig 3–2).

The hollow guide provides a lumen, purportedly for the patient to breathe through during the manipulative phase of intubation. However, the length and cross-sectional diameter of the lumen often create a great deal of resistance, resulting in excessive ventilatory efforts for the patient. Thus its value is questionable. In addition, the tube tends to kink.

These guides may be used for changing tubes as well as providing guidance for blind or direct vision in situations where the immediate insertion of the endotracheal tube is limited by size of the evident airway or visual obstructions. Our experience also has indicated that quality control of the guides may not be sufficient to guarantee that the distal end is smooth. We have had sev-

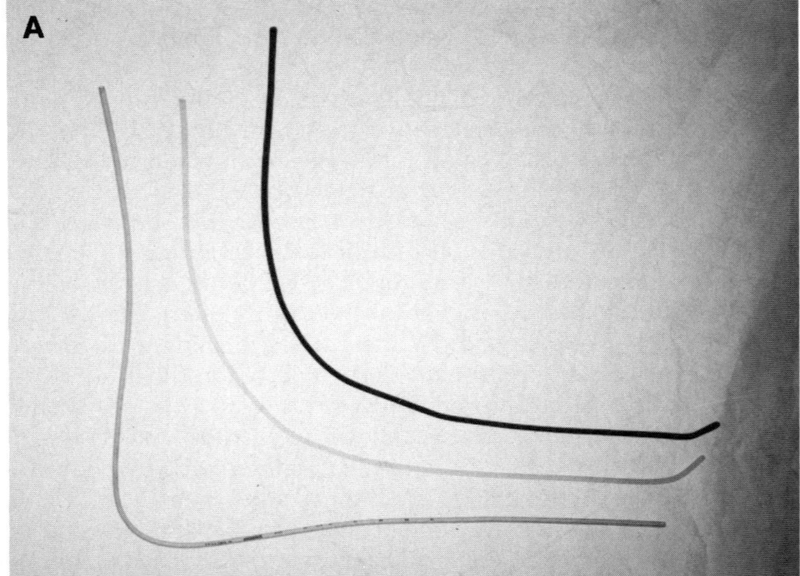

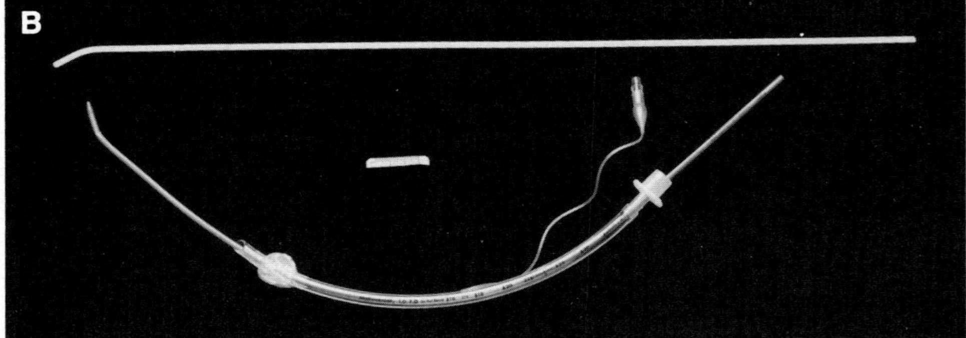

FIG 3–2.
A, array of guides. **B,** Norton intubation guide.

eral indications of mucosal tears, probably secondary to rough distal ends. We also note that unless the guides are relatively stiff, they may whip out of the airway during the threading of the endotracheal tube. In this sense the long guides act more as a stylet by molding the threaded endotracheal tube in the direction of the airway. Note that the tubes should be threaded over the introducer with a rotary motion.

We have used these guides in extubations of adult airways where there are demonstrated or potential difficulties for reintubation, such as found in intensive care units. Here, after the usual suction and other precautions the intubation guide is inserted through the extant endotracheal tube. The tube is then extubated over the guide. The guide is left in situ for a time after the endotracheal tube is removed. If the patient's airway needs to be reintubated during this time, it is simple to thread the replacement tube over the long guide. Patients tolerate the guide very readily and can even talk around it. Note that the diameter of the guide is only a few millimeters and therefore, in relation to the average adult endotracheal tube, presents a negligible obstruction to closure of the vocal folds.

These long guides should be used with caution. There is a remote risk of forcing the long guide into a bronchopulmonary orifice and segment, causing disruption of the wall of the peripheral bronchus and resultant pneumothorax. This could occur if the proximal end of the guide catches on the edge of the endotracheal tube Rovenstine adapter or if too small an endotracheal tube is threaded over the guide. This instrument should never be inserted against resistance. The endotracheal tube should be significantly larger than the guide, and it is imperative to remove the endotracheal tube adapter to allow unimpeded threading and passage without force. Consideration of the possibility of complications must always be a part of stylet- and guide-assisted maneuvers.

Many types of rigid laryngoscope blades are described in the literature; most are rarely used today. With the advent of fiberoptic laryngoscopes, rigid blades are less commonly used for the difficult airway. We describe herein some of the examples for the sake of completeness. However, we specifically recommend the Snow and Eversole blades for limited uses. We have not fully described all aspects of these blades. Further study will reveal differences even in our standard Macintosh blades, such as the height of the flange, which is crucial in situations where the patient has prominent maxillary dentition.

THE FIBEROPTIC ENDOSCOPE*

The development of the fiberoptic endoscopes has initiated a new era in airway management (Fig 3–3).

Diagnostic indications for the use of the fiberoptic endoscope (see Table 2–1) include sampling of airway secretions, assessment of airway patency, pre-

*We have used the Olympus BF3C10 pediatric and the BF20 adult bronchoscope attached to an Olympus OTV-F2 camera, projecting onto a Sony TV screen and attached to a VCR for tape recording. These instruments have added markings to indicate depth of insertion. (Courtesy of Olympus Corporation, Tokyo; Hiroyuki Furihata, Manager, Endoscope Section of Product Development, and Akio Nakada, Design Engineer, Research and Development.)

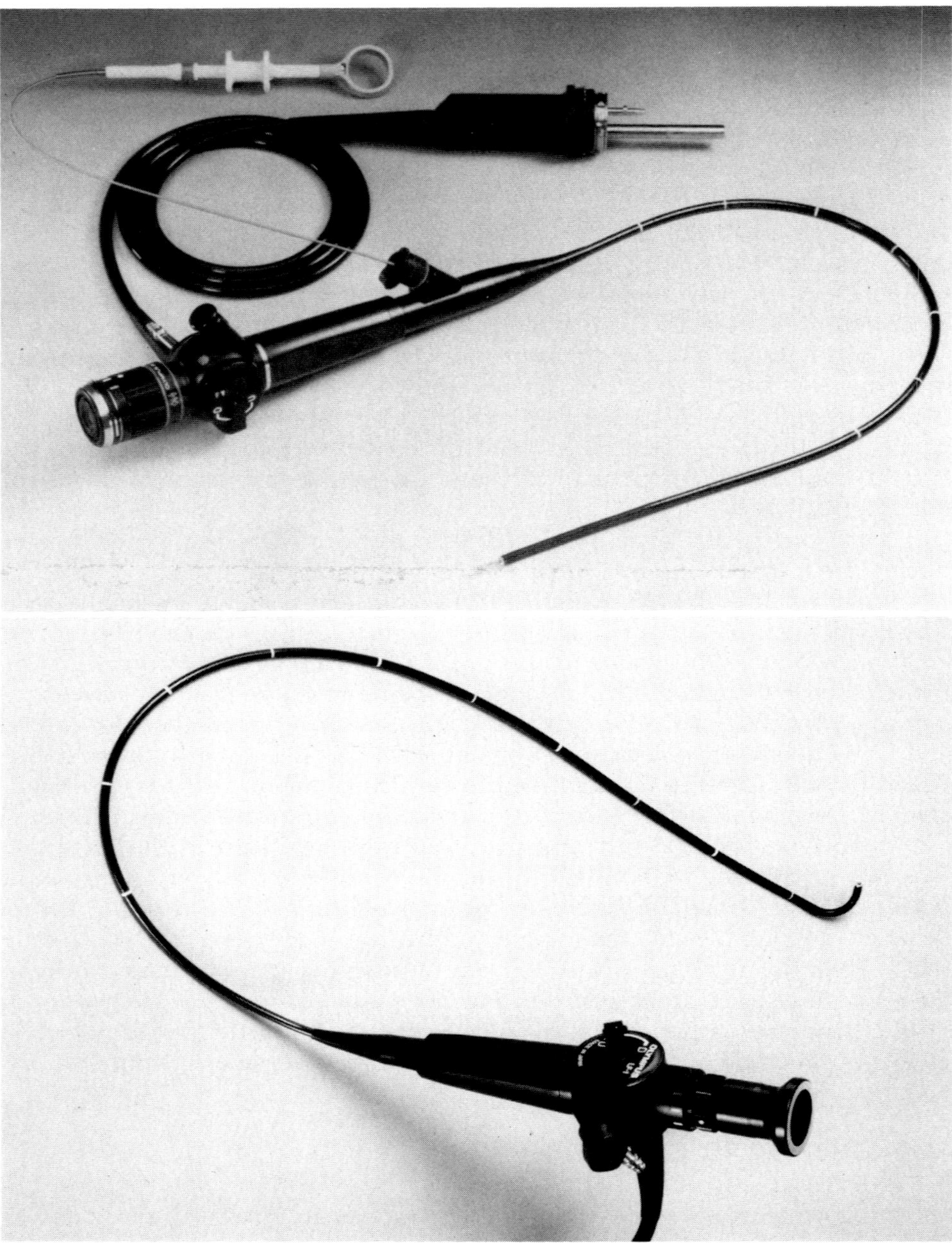

FIG 3–3.
Fiberoptic endoscope. (Courtesy of Olympus Corporation, Tokyo.)

operative and postoperative laryngeal evaluation, assessment of airway damage after smoke or steam inhalation, endotracheal intubation, determination of the locus of double-lumen endotracheal tubes, evaluation of the nasopharynx, and other pulmonary applications.

The instrument has a particular application following smoke inhalation.

(See Chapter 14 for a further discussion of the fiberoptic in management of burns.)

The care of the fiberoptic instrument deserves special emphasis. In addition to the usual admonition never to bend the fiberoptic bundles to an extreme or to bang them against anything, it is imperative never to apply torsion force to the instrument.

Not enough emphasis is given to immediately flushing the suction channel and washing the outside of the fiberoptic scope (see Appendix 3–A). We also suggest passing a wire as soon as possible to mechanically clear mucus and blood and prevent blood clots and debris from plugging the channel. Keep in mind that this channel must be kept clear for suction or insufflation of oxygen.

The outside of the fiberscope also requires some attention. It should never be forced through a small endotracheal tube; this will wrinkle the outer protective coating of the bronchoscope and may permanently damage the exterior. Similarly, as soon as the fiberscope is removed from the patient, it should be washed in cold water, then in a soapy solution, followed by a second rinse in cold water.

Maintenance cannot be overemphasized, because the cost of most fiberscopes is in the range of $9,000 to $15,000. Repairs are costly and a significant factor in the consideration of health care costs.

REFERENCES

1. Macintosh RR: *Lancet*, February 1943.
2. Cozantis DA, Nuuttila K, Merrett JD, et al: Influence of laryngoscope design on heart rate rhythm changes during intubation. *Can Anaesth Soc J* 1984; 31:155.
3. Sackner MA: Bronchofiberscopy. *Am Rev Respir Dis* 1975; 111:62.
4. Townsend TR, Wee S, Koblin B: An efficacy evaluation of a synergized glutaraldehyde-phenate solution in disinfecting respiratory therapy equipment contaminated during patient use. *Infect Control* 1982; 3:240–244.
5. Bageant RA, Marsik FJ, Kellogg VA, et al: In-use testing of four glutaradehyde disinfectants in the cidematic washer. *Respir Care* 1981; 26:1255–1261.
6. Centers for Disease Control: Guidelines on environmental control: Part I. Bethesda, Md, Department of Health and Human Services, 1982.

APPENDIX 3–A

Care of the Fiberoptic Bronchoscope [3-6]

Step 1

Prepare a 1 L mixture of glutaraldehyde (Sporicidin) as follows:

1. Measure 5 mL of 25% glutaraldehyde solution and pour into a 1 L Sporicidin mixing bottle.
2. Measure 60 mL of Sporicidin buffer solution and pour into the 1 L Sporicidin mixing bottle.
3. Top off Sporicidin mixing bottle to the 1 L line with tap water. Mix.
4. The Sporicidin mixture is now ready for use.
5. Rinse out graduated cylinder after use.

Step 2

Clean the fiberoptic bronchoscope as follows:

1. Clean immediately after use. Wash suction valve and suction valve cover with soap and water. Soak these pieces in Sporicidin for at least 10 minutes.
2. Insert the channel cleaning brush into the biopsy port and brush several times with soap and water. Brush the port until all debris is removed.
3. Wash the entire scope with soap and water, *avoiding the eyepiece.* The eyepiece should be capped to protect lens, as should the light source probe.
4. Soak the bronchoscope in Sporicidin for at least 10 minutes. The port areas can be soaked during this time by placing the tip of the syringe in each port, drawing the Sporicidin up into the syringe.
5. After soaking the bronchoscope for 10 minutes, rinse the bronchoscope, including the suction valve, suction valve cover, suction channel, and the ports.
6. Wipe dry all parts and reassemble. It is preferable to hang up the bronchoscope (1) to drip dry the channels and (2) to prevent shaping or kinking. Bronchoscopes should not be soaked for more than 45 minutes. Soaking the scope beyond this time causes the sheath to become brittle.

Chapter 4

Difficult Airway Clinic

Martin L. Norton

Allan C.D. Brown

The Difficult Airway Clinic was established at the University of Michigan in May 1987[1]; we believe it to be the first formally established unit for evaluation of upper airway problems related specifically to endoscopy and airway management. This unit was originally developed to identify factors that lead to failed intubations, traumatic intubations, case cancellations, and catastrophic consequences alluded to in the anesthesia risk management closed malpractice case report.[2] The objectives laid out and accomplished were:

1. To provide presurgical evaluation of potential or known intubation problems.
2. To identify and evaluate patients at risk.
3. To present recommendations for airway management.
4. To expedite, through development of a comprehensive plan, operating room management of the difficult airway.
5. To provide experience-based reassurance to the patient and the physician of available methods for airway problem identification and management.
6. To accumulate research data on prospective, reproducible criteria for the difficult airway syndrome.
7. To encourage teaching of endoscopic skills, with particular emphasis on flexible fiberoptic techniques.

The parameters studied are indicated in Figure 4–1; Table 4–1 indicates the categories of patients; Figure 4–2 depicts the patient referral process.

The key to success in this clinic is the fact that we insist on seeing patients at the time they are first considered for elective surgery. This strategy avoids the pitfall of having to wait until the night before or morning of surgery to

UNIVERSITY OF MICHIGAN MEDICAL CENTER

Department of Anesthesiology

AIRWAY CLINIC RECORD SHEET

Patient Identification Stamp

| DATE | Video # |
| Referred by: | |

CONSENT TO: Procedures ☐ Photography ☐

PHOTOGRAPHY   ⇨ Apply markers ⇦

	AP	LAT
Head in comfort position:	☐	☐
Head fully extended:	☐	☐
Head fully flexed:		☐

Full–face mouth open: ☐

Lateral head–neck–shoulder: ☐

MEASUREMENTS

	L	cms	R
TMJ to angle of ramus:			
Angle of ramus to mentum:			

degrees

HEAD GONIOMETER

DENTITION: Dentures ☐   Protrusion ☐
comments: ________________________

PULMONARY FUNCTION TESTS ☐

Mullers test ☐

	cms
Maximum interdental opening at central incisors:	
Alveolar ridge separation between first molars:	U
	L
Mentum to hyoid:	
Mentum to sternal notch:	
TMJ to opposite TMJ:	
Angle of ramus to opposite angle:	
Ramus to thyroid prominence: (vertical plane)	

Malampatti ☐

PATIENT GROUP

SEX: M F   WEIGHT   HEIGHT

AGE: ☐

Pounds   Feet/ins.

BODY TYPE: ☐

RACIAL GROUP

1: Caucasian ☐
2: Black ☐
3: Amer.Indian ☐
4: Asian ☐
5: Oriental ☐

KNOWN ABNORMALITY RELATED TO:

Unknown: ☐

Syndrome: ☐

Disease: ☐

Traumatic: ☐

FIG 4–1.
Difficult Airway Clinic record sheet.

evaluate the airway. Our examination procedure is detailed in Table 4–2, and a decision tree for guiding clinical evaluation is depicted in Figure 4–3.

Ancillary but critical studies may include magnetic resonance imaging and digitized computed tomography tongue volume, among others.

Consultation with our Sleep Apnea Clinic and Division of Otorhinolaryngology is in order in a number of cases. When we do screening pulmonary function testing (PFT), the emphasis is on reviewing air flow loops for signs of upper airway obstruction in the sitting and supine positions.

ENDOSCOPY

Indirect ☐   **Topical Drugs:**(& technique)   **I.V. Drugs:**

Direct ☐   ________________   ________________

Fiberoptic ☐   ________________   ________________

________________   ________________

FINDINGS: (nasopharynx, oropharynx & larynx)

____

____

____

____

____

____

STUDIES   **CONSULTATIONS**

________________   ________________

________________   ________________

________________   ________________

________________   ________________

SUMMARY & RECOMMENDATIONS   **AIRWAY ALERT GIVEN TO PATIENT:** ☐   W   N

____

____

____

____

____

____

____

____

____

____

____

____

Report sent to: Signature: ________________ M.D.

assisted by: ________________ Date: ________

FIG 4–1 (cont.).

Ordinary photography has value only in the obvious craniofacial abnormality situation, and more often than not is deceptive when the patient appears "normal." Of significant value is the practice of camera VCR reproduction of the endoscopy and fluoroscopy, with presentation of the picture on a television screen viewer. We use this for both teaching the endoscopic technique and for viewing with consulting colleagues to review unusual findings or confirm endoscopic impressions. One of the considered conclusions that must be

PATIENT REFERRAL

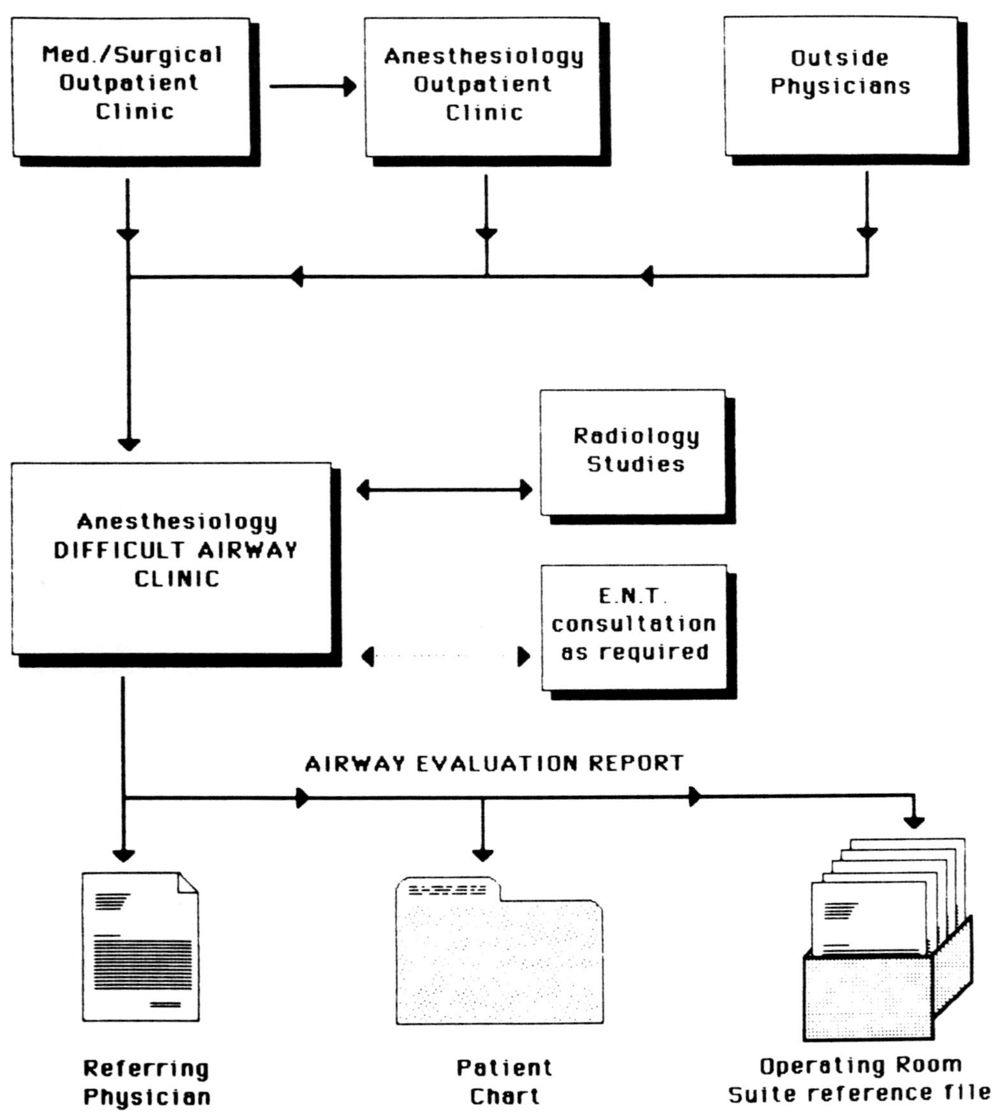

FIG 4–2.
Patient referral process.

drawn each time is whether the fiberoptic intubation route is preferable to a preoperative tracheostomy.

Considerations such as mental state of the patient during manipulation, likely postoperative status including nursing care requirements, and probability of the need for repeated tracheotomies (with consequent risk of tracheal stenosis) for future surgery must be given due weight. On the other side of the ledger, we must consider hazards of arytenoid dislocation and trauma to the

TABLE 4–1.

Categories of Patients With Difficult Airway Problems*

I. Primarily soft tissue
  A. Glossoptosis or macroglossia: acromegaly, achondroplasia, obesity, amyloidosis, Bechwith-Wiedemann syndrome, lymphangioma, hemangioma, Hurler's syndrome (gargoylism; also Hunter's syndrome, including all mucopolysaccharidoses), some cases of Pierre-Robin and Treacher Collins syndrome
  B. Superior larynx: normal pediatric patients, achondroplasia, micrognathia
  C. Pharyngeal anatomic distortions: post–radical neck dissection, glossectomy, laryngectomy surgery, and most inflammatory pharyngeal diseases, including tumor formations (e.g., Sturge-Weber syndrome)
  D. Inflammatory diseases: quinsy, retropharyngeal abscess, epiglottitis, leprosy, diphtheria, Epstein-Barr mononucleosis, croup, pharyngouveitis
  E. Miscellaneous: sleep apnea, burns, trauma
II. Primarily hard tissue
  A. Chondrocalcinosis (larynx), acromegaly
  B. Cervical vertebral limitation: Engelmann's disease (osteopathia hyperostotica scleroticus multiplex), osteoarthritis, fibrofascial myositis ossificans progressiva, Marie-Strümpell rheumatoid arthritis, Klippel-Feil syndrome, post–cervical spinal fusion, Hurler's and Hunter's syndrome, ankylosing spondylitis of either osteoarthritic or other etiology
  C. Micrognathia: Pierre-Robin mandibulofacial dysostosis, Crouzon's craniofacial dysostosis, Treacher Collins syndrome, Hallermann-Streiff syndrome, hypoplastic bony development secondary to rheumatoid arthritis
  D. Temporomandibular joint limitation: osteoarthritis, Treacher Collins syndrome, some rheumatoid syndromes
  E. Odontoid-peg disease: atlantoaxial instability, osteoporosis, Paget's disease, Morquio's syndrome

*This listing is only partial and representative of the most frequent conditions. Almost all conditions mentioned are mixed in nature. Therefore, regardless of category, the patient should be examined and managed with the understanding that it is rare to find one purely causative factor for a given difficult airway problem.

vocal folds during endotracheal tube advancement as well as trauma to the nasal passage.

Although there is much that can be done to relieve discomfort with fiberoptic endoscopy and tracheostomy, we would be remiss not to recognize the psychological aspect and that there is significant discomfort during either procedure. As a result of the data obtained from our clinic, we have established a scaled set of criteria for evaluation of the difficult airway (Table 4–3). We have not yet been able to set criteria for the parameters of ego, individual skill levels, planning for endoscopy, and response to the stress of extraneous pressures (e.g., surgical impatience) imposed on the endoscopist. Furthermore, only years of experience with this scale can validate the system. However, we do believe that this scale is a necessary first step in developing a more rational system of criteria. The concept is based on the fact that no single factor can be uniformly designated as the absolute criterion of the difficult airway syndrome. Indeed, we have never seen a patient with only one of the scaled criteria.

The application of grading schemes is discussed in the work of Wilson et al.[3] The concept yet to be explored is at what confidence level these criteria can

TABLE 4–2.

Examination Procedure at Difficult Airway Clinic

1. Stamp consultation request
   a. Photographic consent
   b. Procedure consent with patient's identification card
2. Review referral chart
3. Take photographs
   a. Lateral open- and closed-mouth views
   b. Anteroposterior open- and closed-mouth views
4. Take measurements, including:
   a. Temporomandibular joint to angle of ramus
   b. Angle of ramus to mentum
   c. Interdental opening at central incisors
   d. Mentum to hyoid
   e. Mentum to thyroid notch
5. Flex and extend neck: Measure angulation with head goniometer or protractor.
6. Dynamic fluoroscopy sequence
7. Examine nose: Patency of nasopharyngeal pathway, right and left.
8. Check oral patency.
   a. Mirror laryngoscopy: Results, possible limits.
   b. Direct laryngoscopy: Results.
9. Perform fiberoptic examination: Nasopharyngolaryngoscopy, possible limits.
10. Order lateral and anteroposterior x-ray studies.
    a. Results as needed
    b. Other tests
    c. Dynamic fluoroscopy
11. Complete consult sheets: Make recommendations.
12. Put originals of consult on chart: Copies of all forms filed alphabetically in anesthesia holding room open file.

TABLE 4–3.

Projected Difficult Endoscopy Prognostic Signs*

Sign	Score
Micrognathia with acute mandibular angles	5
Glossoptosis or basal macroglossia	4
Difficulty with prior laryngoscopy	3
Adverse sign (3+ or 4+)	2
Long, high-arched palate associated with long, narrow dental arch	2
Temporomandibular joint limitation	4
Short muscular neck with full dentition	2
Protruding maxillary dentition with premaxillary overgrowth	2
Increased alveolomental depth	1
Limited extension of the upper cervical vertebrae	2
Limited motion of lower cervical vertebrae	3
Pathologic signs of airway obstruction	3
Decreased distance between hyoid and thyroid cartilages	2
Decreased distance of epiglottis from posterior wall of pharynx	3
Skill of the intubationist	±5
Intubationist ego	±5
Planning for endoscopy	±5
Müller's sign (3–4)	

*Scale ranges from 1 to 5, with 1 being best and 5 being worst.

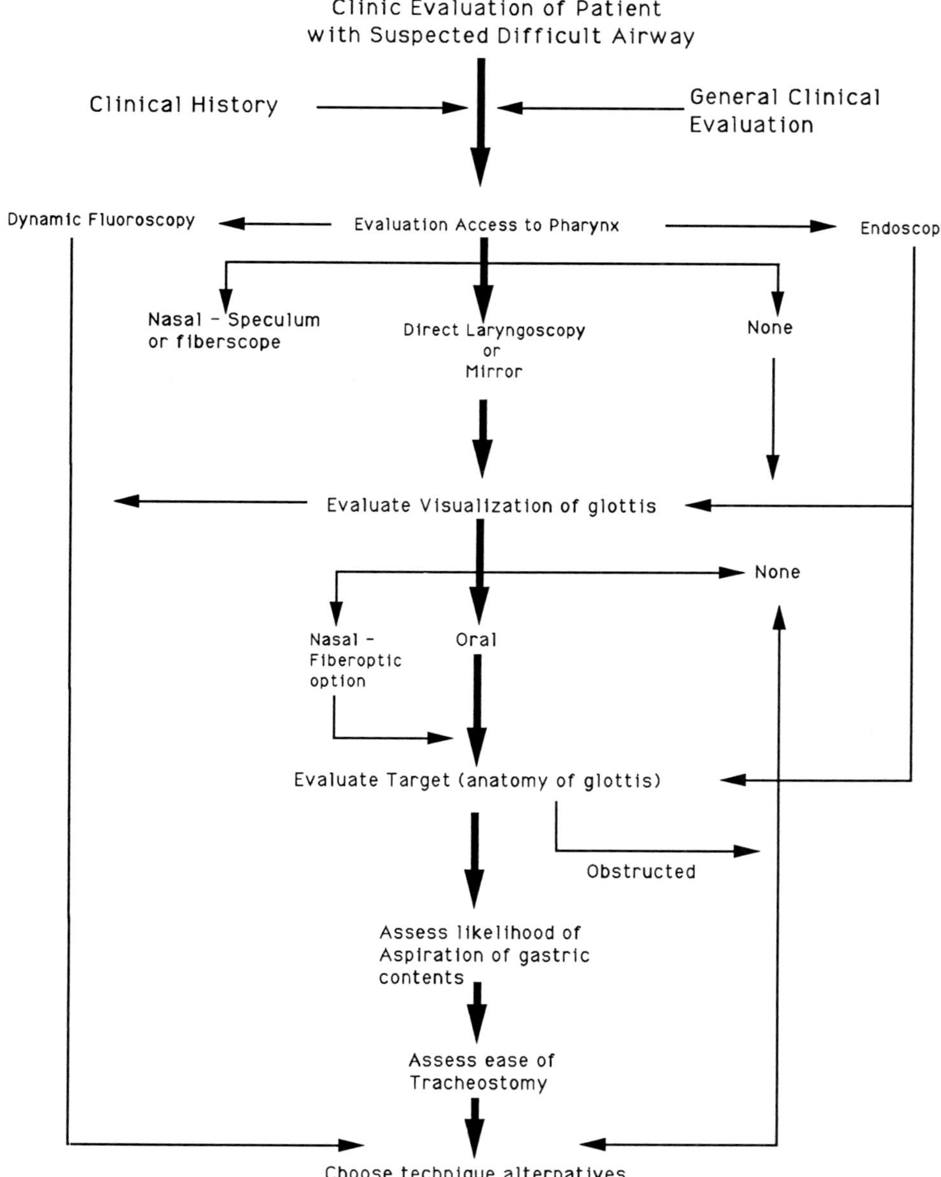

FIG 4–3.
Decision tree for clinical evaluation of suspected difficult airway.

be applied; that is, at what level will the risk to normal population become unacceptable? Wilson and associates give an example of a test that picks up 75% of high-risk patients. They state that if 10,000 patients are anesthetized per year and the incidence of difficult laryngoscopy is 1.5%, one might expect 150 difficult laryngoscopies, and 9,850 nondifficult laryngoscopies.

With a false positive rate of 12.1%, 1,191 patients per year would be falsely classified as at risk. Although we think this is an unacceptable confidence level, this very type of reasoning is the logical concomitant of the development of any form of scaling or risk value system. The ideal system would be 90% specific and 99% sensitive, but this is in practice not possible.

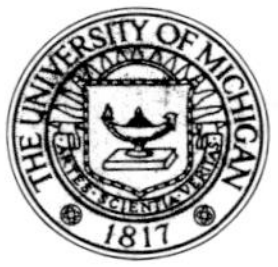

The University of Michigan

DEPARTMENT OF ANESTHESIOLOGY
1500 MEDICAL CENTER DRIVE   BOX 0048   ANN ARBOR, MICHIGAN 48109

DIFFICULT AIRWAY CLINIC
Martin L. Norton, M.D., J.D., Director
Allan C. D. Brown, Ch.B., F.F.A.R.C.S.
Niall Wilton, M.R.C.P., F.F.A.R.C.S.
Barry Powell, C.R.N.A., M.N.

Off. (313) 936-4280

**PROTOCOL
FOR SUBMISSION OF CASES FOR
REGISTRY OF THE DIFFICULT AIRWAY**

Primary Case Diagnosis: ____

Complicating Diagnoses: ____

Material Submitted: ____

a).   35 mm Slide [ ]   b). Photograph [ ]   c). Other _______________________
                                                                  specify

Brief Case History: ____

____

____

____

Suggested Pathophysiologic, anatomic, biomechanical or other basis for problem of airway

____

____

____

Outcome: Failed intubation - operation abandoned [ ]   Morbidity [ ]   Mortality [ ]

 Intubation - successful technique used: _______________________________

 Airway managed by: _______________________________

Submitting physician: _______________________________

Submitting Organization or Affiliation: _______________________________

Send to: **Martin L. Norton, M.D.
Director, Difficult Airway Clinic Registry
University of Michigan Medical Center
1500 E. Medical Center Drive
UH-1G323   Box 0048
Ann Arbor, Michigan   48109   USA**

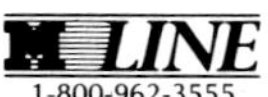

FIG 4–4.
Protocol for submission of cases to Difficult Airway Registry.

An international registry of difficult airway cases has been established at our clinic so that we can begin to accumulate the necessary data to draw better conclusions about patients with difficult airways. A copy of the protocol for registering cases is depicted in Figure 4–4.

REFERENCES

1. Norton ML, Wilton N, Brown ACD: The Difficult Airway Clinic. *Anesthesiol Rev* 1988; 15:25–28.
2. Caplan RA, Posner K, Ward RJ, et al: Adverse respiratory events in anesthesia: A closed claims analysis. *Anesthesiology* 1990; 72:828–833.
3. Wilson ME, Spiegelhalter D, Robertson JA, et al: Predicting difficult intubation. *Br J Anaesthesiol* 1988; 61:211–216.

PART II

In our description of nature the purpose is not to disclose the real essence of the phenomena but only to track down, so far as it is possible, relations between the manifold aspects of our experience.

Atomic Theory and the Description of Nature
Niels Bohr, 1934

Once the patient with a difficult airway has been identified, the specific airway problems presented have to be defined and, where possible, quantified. The airway is a space surrounded by tissues and structures. Most medical disciplines are concerned primarily with the function of the space and those pathologic processes that impinge on it. The intubationist is more concerned with the contour and consistency of the walls of the airway and the feasibility of deliberately deforming them to facilitate endoscopy. However, direct examination of a living airway is unpleasant for the patient; therefore, indirect methods must be used first before invasive techniques can be justified. An understanding of airway anatomy, what is normal and what is not, together with the many possible variations, arises from a knowledge of human embryologic origins. The anatomic sketches in Appendix A–1 show the mature anatomic relations of importance to the intubationist.

Chapters 6, 7, and 8, respectively, examine the utility of two established methods in noninvasive airway evaluation (radiographic and pulmonary function techniques) and a technique for three-dimensional analysis that shows future promise for quantitative descriptions of a difficult airway. Chapter 9 presents a brief review of upper airway function.

Chapter 5

Developmental Anatomy and Growth of the Craniofacial Area

Alphonse Burdi

The craniofacial area appears to be of more interest to a broad spectrum of medical specialties than any other single body region. For example, the anesthesiologist who must access the passages of the respiratory system not only must appreciate the morphology of the many parts and systems represented in the craniofacial complex but also needs to be mindful of temporal changes in the spatial relationships embodied in the structures of the region.

Human craniofacial development is a complex and fascinating set of events that requires sequential integration of numerous biologic steps to give rise to its final size and shape. The craniofacial complex offers a splendid example also of how fundamental morphogenic processes must take place in an integrative manner in shaping the human appearance, from conception through the aging patterns of postnatal life. Embryonic cells must proliferate, migrate, and differentiate as patternable events give rise eventually to the myriad of craniofacial structures and units, including the craniofacial skeleton, the tongue and related structures, the pharynx, and the laryngeal apparatus.

CRANIOFACIAL SKELETON

The human craniofacial skeleton can be divided into two morphologic entities: the *neurocranium,* which forms much of the skeletal case surrounding the brain; and the *viscerocranium,* which forms the skeleton of the face. The neurocranium is often divided into two regions: a membranous part, or desmocranium, consisting of flat bones that form the calvaria surrounding the brain and a cartilaginous part, or chondrocranium, from which bones of the cranial base will develop.

The sides and roof of the skull develop within the continuous sheath of mesenchyme cells surrounding the embryonic brain. Through the process of intramembranous ossification, embryonic mesenchymal cells differentiate into bone-forming osteoblast cells. As a result, a number of flat membranous bones, including the frontal, parietal, temporal, and occipital plates, are formed, which are characterized by the presence of needlelike bone spicules that radiate progressively from primary ossification centers toward their periphery.

During the period from embryo to neonate the size of the skull vault is strikingly large compared with the smaller facial region.

With further growth during prenatal and postnatal life the membranous bones enlarge by means of the combined events of (1) apposition of new bony layers on their outer surfaces, (2) coordinated resorption of bone along their inner surfaces, and (3) progressive outward displacement of all of the bones by the rapidly enlarging brain. Most of the bones that develop from the membranous neurocranium are ossified by the time of birth and are loosely connected to their neighboring bones.

At birth the flat bones of the skull are separated from each other by narrow joints of fibrous tissue called *sutures*. At points where more than two developing bones meet, the sutures are widened and are known as *fontanelles*. From a clinical perspective, the anterior and posterior fontanelles are the largest and most easily examinable. Sutures and fontanelles allow the flat bones of the skull to overlap each other during the process of childbirth.

Soon after birth the membranous bones move back to their original position to give the skull a large rounded appearance. Several sutures and fontanelles remain membranous for a considerable time after birth. Growth of these flat bones of the young skull is particularly rapid and associated with the rapid growth of the brain. Although a child at 5 to 7 years of age has nearly all of his or her brain size, some of the calvarial sutures remain patent even throughout adult life.

The overall length of the entire brain case at birth is about 65% of its total growth. By the end of the first year 82% of growth is complete, by 3 years of age 89% is complete, and by 5 years 92% of the expected postnatal size of the brain case is attained. At about 15 years approximately 98% of the definitive adult size is reached. The anterior segment of the cranial base from the anterior rim of the foramen magnum to the nasal bones is about 55% of its expected adult size at birth, and 70% by 2 years of age.

In the newborn, the width of the cranial base has grown to about 100 mm. By the sixth postnatal month the length is 150 mm, and by the first postnatal year the width of the base is approximately 125 mm. Thereafter the rate of increases in base width generally decline to less than 1 mm/year during postnatal years 3 to 14.

The midline zone of dense mesenchymal cells beneath the developing brain in the embryo progressively gives rise to skeletal elements of the cranial or skull base, or the cartilaginous neurocranium. Initially these mesenchymal cells proliferate and differentiate into cartilage-forming chondrocytes. In a short time the cartilaginous elements of the skull base are progressively ossified by later developing osteoblast cells. This skeletogenic sequence involving mesenchyme, cartilage, and bone cells is called *endochondral ossification*.

The skull base consists initially of a number of separate cartilages. When these cartilages fuse and ossify, the skull base is formed. The skull base of the young embryo consists of parachordal, hypophyseal, and otic capsular cartilages. The parachordal cartilage, or basal plate, develops from a dense group of mesenchymal cells at the cranial end of the notochord and fuses with later developing cartilage derived from the sclerotome regions of the occipital somites. This parachordal cartilage mass gives rise to the base of the occipital bone surrounding the spinal cord. The hypophyseal cartilage develops around the emerging pituitary gland and gives rise to the body of the sphenoid bone.

Otic capsules appear surrounding the developing internal ear apparatus and form the petrous and mastoid portions of the temporal bone. The most forward extension of the cartilaginous neurocranium, the nasal capsule, develops around the nasal pits and contributes to the formation of the ethmoid bone and its midline nasal septum. The cartilage of the nasal septum may play a role in the anterior growth of the face.

During the embryonic and fetal periods the skull base flexes in the region of the pituitary fossa so that the developing face is positioned between the skull base and its relatively large chest region. It doubles its length from prenatal week 10 to 14, triples its length by week 17, and is six times its original length by term. By the middle of the third prenatal month, the cartilaginous neurocranium, or skull base, appears as a unified mass of cartilage called the *chondrocranium.* As each of the definitive skull base bones emerges from the embryonic chondrocranium, cartilage zones remain between them, forming a number of cranial base synchondroses, including the sphenoocipital and sphenoethmoid *synchondroses.* These synchondroses behave as cartilaginous growth plates to increase the length of the skull base over time.

The *viscerocranium* consists of the bones of the face and is formed chiefly by a combination of mesenchymal cell proliferation in the first and second branchial arches of the embryo. Before the intramembranous development of bones in the embryonic upper facial region, the midline extension downward of the cranial base, called the *nasal capsule,* is the only skeletal support of the upper part of the face. Bones of the upper facial skeleton will undergo intramembranous ossification in the mesenchyme surrounding the cartilaginous nasal capsule.

In a sense, the nasal capsule provides a developmental template around which facial bones develop in the embryo. The first branchial arch in the embryo gives rise to a dorsal portion, the maxillary process, which extends forward beneath the region of the eyes and gives rise to the maxillary complex, the zygomatic bone, and the squamous part of the temporal bone. Bones of the palate arise from several ossification centers within the newly formed embryonic palate. In the eighth week of life, bilaterally located ossification centers in the anterior regions of the palate give rise to the premaxilla and the bony palate. The premaxillary ossification centers surround the incisor tooth germs, and the bony palate itself extends between the premaxillary centers to the depth of the soft palate. By the fourteenth prenatal week, the bony palate is well established, with a midline palatine suture extending the entire length between the maxillary and palatine bones. The squamous temporal bone eventually becomes part of the neurocranium.

The ventral portion of the first arch, known as the *mandibular arch,* gives rise to a horseshoe-shaped cartilage called *Meckel's cartilage.* This structure gives rise to most of the elements of the mandible. Mesenchymal cells surrounding Meckel's cartilage undergoes intramembranous ossification and forms the bony mandible. Over time, Meckel's cartilage atrophies except for a small portion that remains in the neonate as the sphenomandibular ligament.

The uppermost extent of the right and left limbs of Meckel's cartilage differentiate into the ear ossicles, the malleus, and the incus.

The malleus and the incus derivatives of Meckel's cartilage form a primitive, or primary, articulation between the early embryonic lower skeleton (i.e., Meckel's cartilage) and the cranial base. At about 18 weeks, with the regression of Meckel's cartilage and the progressive development of the mandibular ramus and condyle, the definitive, or secondary, temporomandibular joint later seen in both prenatal and postnatal life becomes the sole articulation between the mandible and the cranial base. The condyle arises independently at first as a carrot-shaped cartilage, extending upward and posteriorly from the newly formed mandibular body. This condylar cartilage is rapidly transformed into bone except at its upper end, where it remains as a fibrous-coated articular cartilage. The head of this cartilage soon becomes separated from the articular fossa of the temporal bone above by the temporomandibular articular disk. At birth the ramus of the mandible and its condyle form an angle of 130 degrees with the mandibular body. Later, with subsequent mandibular growth and eruption of teeth, this angle is reduced to about 100 degrees.

PATTERNS OF GROSS ANATOMY

In general the bones of the face include frontal and nasal bones and the facial bones proper, including the maxilla, mandible, zygoma, and vomeronasal complex. The larger, perpendicular portion of the frontal bone forms the forehead and front of the calvarium. Its horizontal orbital portions form the roof of each orbit and are continuous with the supraorbital rim, or brow. In the adult, the cortical plates of the supraorbital rim are often enlarged and separated to house the frontal paranasal sinus.

Bones of the upper and lower facial skeletons derive chiefly from embryonic mesenchyme. From their earliest beginnings in the embryo, they lend support to the orbital, nasal, oral, and pharyngeal cavities. The two nasal bones are small, oblong bones that meet in the midline, lending support to the root of the nose. The paired maxillary bones unite in the midline at the intermaxillary suture and anterior nasal spine to form the major skeletal framework for the maxillary jaw. They contribute parts to the orbital floors, hard palate, and lateral walls of the nasal cavities.

The body of each adult maxillary bone contains a maxillary sinus that empties into the lateral wall of the nasal cavity. The *alveolar process* of the maxillary bone is the tooth-containing region. This posteriorly incomplete ellipsoid region is smaller in the child than in the adult. This size difference is due chiefly to the fact that the child has only 8 teeth to be accommodated in this alveolar process of the maxilla, whereas the adult has 16 teeth to be accommodated. The palatine process is a horizontal projection of each maxillary bone extending toward the midline. The right and left palatine processes form the anterior three fourths of the hard palate. The two *zygomatic bones,* commonly referred to as malar, or cheek, bones, form the prominences of the cheeks and parts of the lateral wall and floor of each orbit. The temporal process of the zygomatic bone projects posteriorly and articulates with the temporal bone.

Although they are not facial bones, this is an appropriate point to discuss the paired cavities called the *paranasal sinuses*. The paranasal sinuses (with the exception of the sphenoid sinus) develop as outgrowths of the nasal cavity during the third and fourth intrauterine months. Although all of the sinuses experience their major expansions after birth, the maxillary and ethmoid sinuses are of appreciable size at birth. The frontal sinus in particular undergoes almost all of its expansion after birth. Each of the sinuses typically shows variation in size and geometric form from one individual to another. Related to these differences is the observation that the ostia connecting the sinuses with the nasal cavities have varying locations. The paranasal sinuses are located in certain cranial and facial bones surrounding the nasal cavities and are lined with mucous membranes that are continuous with the mucous linings of the nasal cavities. Paranasal sinuses are located in the frontal, sphenoid, ethmoid, and maxillary bones.

The *mandible* is the largest of the facial bones and one of the very first bones to develop in the human embryo. In the lateral view, the mandible consists of a curved, horizontal portion called the *body* and two perpendicular portions called *rami*. The angle formed at the junction of the body and the rami is larger in the young child (approximately 120 degrees) and is more acute in the adult (approximately 100 degrees). This angle is about 120 degrees in aged individuals with edentulous mandibles. Each ramus has a condylar portion that articulates with the temporal bone mandibular fossa by combined diarthrotic gliding and hinge joints, called the *temporomandibular joint.* Each half of the mandible also has an elongated, pointed process called the *coronoid process* to which the temporal muscles attach. Like the maxillary bone, the mandible has an alveolar region housing 8 teeth in children and 16 teeth in adults.

The two *palatine bones* are L shaped. The perpendicular portion of each bone forms part of the lateral wall and floor of the nasal cavity and small portions of the orbital floors. The posterior portion of the hard palate, which separates the nasal and oral cavities, is formed by the horizontal plates of the palatine bones.

In contrast to the much simpler anatomy of the nasal cavity medial wall (i.e., the nasal septum), the lateral wall of each nasal cavity is quite complex (Fig 5–1). It bounds most of the paranasal sinuses and receives their openings. The lateral walls also feature the locations of four major scrolls of bone covered by mucous membranes: the inferior, middle, superior, and supreme conchae. The spaces beneath each concha are *nasal meati* and are named according to the overlying concha, such as inferior meatus below the inferior nasal concha. The inferior and middle conchae are the largest, longest, and generally most prominent of the conchae. The superior nasal conchae are about one half their lengths. The three major nasal conchae on each side appear to converge posteriorly, and the remaining portion of the nasal cavity behind their posterior ends provides the opening into the nasopharynx. The two inferior nasal conchae are large, scroll-like bones that form part of the lateral wall of each nasal cavity and project inward toward the midline, inferior to the middle and superior nasal conchae of the ethmoid bone. The inferior nasal conchae serve the same function as the superior and middle conchae in increasing the surface area (lined with respiratory mucosa) over which air can pass to and from the lungs.

The *vomeroseptal skeleton* consists of the separate midline vomerine bone

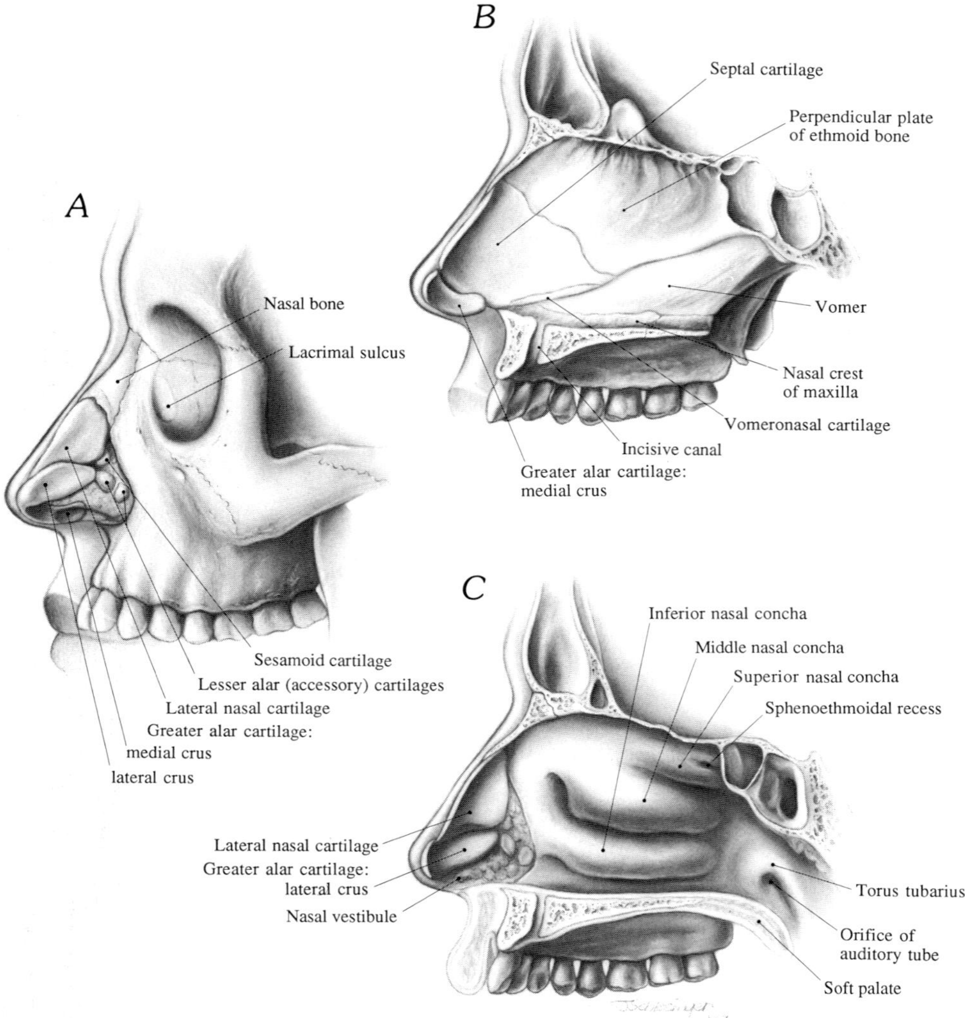

FIG 5–1.
Three views of the nasal region intended to depict the important anatomic regions. **A,** external view of nasal cartilage; **B,** midsagittal view of nasal septum; **C,** midsagittal view with septum removed to expose lateral wall of nasal cavity.

and nasal septum. The vomerine bone is a roughly V-shaped bone, and its superior troughlike portion houses the inferior and posterior portions of the nasal septum. Posteriorly the vomerine bone and the posterior portion of the nasal septum become continuous with the midline perpendicular plate of the ethmoid bone. The nasal septum itself is chiefly cartilaginous in the young child, but over time its posterior two thirds will ossify into a rigid partition between the two nasal cavities. In some cases the nasal septum can be deflected off its tongue-and-groove housing in the vomerine bone. Such a lateral deflection is referred to as a *deviated septum*. The extent of the deviation plus the size of the nasal conchae on that side can significantly reduce the size of the nasal cavity on the affected side.

TONGUE AND RELATED STRUCTURES

In general the tongue arises in the ventral wall of the embryonic oropharynx from the inner lining of the first four branchial arches. It appears in embryos at approximately 4 weeks in the form of two lateral swellings and one triangular median swelling, the *tuberculum impar*. These swellings arise from the first pharyngeal arch. A second median swelling, the *copula,* is formed by mesodermally derived mesenchyme of the second, third, and part of the fourth arches. Finally, a third median swelling, formed by the posterior part of the fourth arch, marks the development of the *epiglottis*.

Immediately behind this latter swelling is the laryngeal orifice flanked on either side by the *arytenoid swellings*. With further growth during the sixth and seventh weeks, the lateral swellings overgrow the tuberculum impar and merge with each other, thus forming the anterior two thirds of the body of the tongue. The plane of fusion between the lateral tongue swellings is marked on the tongue surface as the median sulcus of the tongue and within the tongue mass as the median septum. The posterior part of the root of the tongue originates from the second, third, and part of the fourth pharyngeal arches. The line of fusion between the anterior two thirds and the posterior one third of the tongue is demarcated by the V-shaped groove called the *terminal sulcus*. This line is marked by the large circumvallate papillae first seen at 2 to 5 months in the prenate.

The mucosa of the tongue dorsum develops filiform and fungiform papillae much earlier, at about 11 intrauterine weeks. Taste buds themselves develop from epithelial cells at about the seventh gestational week and take on their postnatal morphology during weeks 13 through 15. Some of the tongue muscles differentiate in situ, but most develop from stem cells, or myoblasts, arising in the occipital somites. The proliferating cells migrate underneath the mucous covering of the tongue, carrying along with them fibers of the hypoglossal cranial nerve.

Between birth and adulthood, the length, breadth, and thickness of the tongue normally double. As the enlarging prenatal tongue extends upward toward the nasal cavity, the less differentiated palatal shelves are forced obliquely downward toward the floor of the common oronasal cavity at about 5 weeks. With increased development of the palatal shelves at about 7 weeks, combined with tongue contraction and a downward displacement of the mandible, the earlier vertically oriented shelves are repositioned and begin to fuse in the horizontal plane above the level of the tongue. The epiglottis is formed when the posterior third of the embryonic copula is split off from the tongue body by a transverse groove. This groove is eventually divided into the valleculae by differential growth of the median glossoepiglottic fold.

PHARYNX

The pharynx is a somewhat funnel-shaped tube that is approximately 13 cm long in the adult. It begins at the posterior nasal choanae and extends inferiorly to the level of the cricoid cartilage. It lies posterior to the nasal cavity, oral cavity, and larynx, immediately anterior to the cervical vertebrae. The upper portion of the pharynx is the nasopharynx, which lies posterior to the nasal cavity and extends downward to the level of the soft palate. The roof of the nasopharynx is in contact with the sphenoid and occipital bones of the skull base. Accordingly, the shape of the upper extent of the nasopharynx reflects the shape, or form, of the skull base. Opening into it are the two posterior choanae and the two auditory, or eustachian, tubes. The posterior wall of the nasopharynx contains the pharyngeal tonsils (i.e., the adenoids). This lymphoid tissue mass extends to a variable extent into the posterior wall and downward toward the opening of the auditory tube.

Stenosis of the nasopharynx (not to be confused with congenital choanal atresia) can be produced by scarring and contracture of the posterior pharyngeal wall in the region of the adenoids or below and may extend across the soft palate, leading to possible occlusion of the lower nasopharynx. At the level of the palate, the nasopharynx narrows and then continues as the oropharynx. This narrowing is often called the *pharyngeal isthmus,* which is bounded anteriorly by the soft palate, laterally by the palatopharyngeal arches, and posteriorly by the pharyngeal wall. Above the isthmus the posterior part of the nasopharynx is particularly wide, and the lateral extension on each side consitutes the pharyngeal recess (sometimes called either the *fossa of Rosenmüller,* or the *sinus of Morgagni*). The middle portion of the pharynx, the oropharynx, extends from the soft palate above to the level of the hyoid bone. It is contiguous anteriorly, through the fauces or oropharyngeal isthmus, with the oral cavity. This portion of the pharynx has both respiratory and digestive functions.

Two pairs of tonsils, the palatine and lingual tonsils, are found in the oropharynx. On the posterior part of the dorsum of the tongue lie irregular nodules of lymphoid tissue that collectively form the lingual tonsils. If enlarged, they may cause obstruction in the zone of transition between the oral cavity and oropharynx. The lateral wall of the oropharynx, the fauces, is occupied on each side largely by the palatine tonsils. Together the lingual tonsils anteriorly, the palatine tonsils laterally, and the pharyngeal tonsils posterosuperiorly form a ring of lymphoid or adenoid tissue about the upper end of the pharynx, known as *Waldeyer's tonsillar ring.* Generalized inflammation or enlargement of tonsillar tissue in this ring can occlude the opening between the oral cavity and oropharynx.

The fauces are bounded by the palatine arches, or faucial pillars. In the adult the posterior wall of the nasal and oral parts of the pharynx is closely related above and posteriorly to the undersurface of the occipital bone and posteriorly to approximately the first three cervical vertebrae. If the neck is hyperextended, the potential retropharyngeal space can be obliterated and the wall of the pharynx forced against the vertebral bodies. The lowest portion of the pharynx, the *laryngopharynx,* is located posterior to the laryngeal apparatus and extends downward from the hyoid bone level to the level of the cricoid cartilage where it rapidly narrows to become continuous with the esophagus.

The musculature of the pharynx consists of three overlapping constrictor muscles, superior, middle and inferior, and three pairs of more longitudinally oriented muscles extending from the skull base into the pharynx. Each constrictor muscle inserts with the corresponding muscle of the opposite side in the midline pharyngeal raphe, whereas the longitudinally oriented muscles, the palatopharyngeus, salpingopharyngeus, and stylopharyngeus, spread out on the inner surface.

Coordinated movements of the palate and pharynx normally occur during both speech and swallowing. Apposition of the soft palate and uvula to the posterior wall of the nasopharynx (i.e., the velopharyngeal valve) are necessary for proper speech. Closure of the nasopharynx during speech is rapid and involves contraction of the palatopharyngeus muscle and the contraction of muscles elevating the soft palate. Muscle activity during swallowing shows a pattern wherein the bolus is moved from the oral cavity into the relaxed oropharynx, chiefly by a sequence involving backward pressure and movement of the tongue, the elevation of the tense soft palate, and the elevation of the upper pharyngeal regions.

LARYNGEAL APPARATUS

The larynx is that short passageway that connects the pharynx with the trachea. Figure 5–2 depicts the developmental progression of the larynx. It lies in the midline of the neck anterior to the fourth through sixth cervical vertebrae in the adult. In the child its wall is composed of nine skeletal or cartilaginous structures that ossify progressively with increasing age. The three single skeletal elements are the thyroid, epiglottic, and cricoid cartilages. Of the paired cartilages, the arytenoid cartilages are the most important in humans. The paired corniculate and cuneiform cartilages are of lesser significance. The thyroid cartilage consists of two broad plates that come together anteriorly to form the anterior skeletal wall of the larynx and give it its triangular shape. It is larger in men than in women.

It is important to note that the skeletal apparatus of the larynx, most notably the thyroid cartilages, is connected to and suspended from the horseshoe-shaped *hyoid bone* by the thyrohyoid membrane. Although relatively small, this hyoid bone is an important attachment site for large tongue muscles, fibers of the middle pharyngeal constrictor muscle, and the infrahyoid strap muscles. Thus the position of the hyoid bone itself can be affected by contraction of any combination of muscles attaching to it. And because the laryngeal appparatus is suspended from the hyoid bone, the dynamic positioning and movements of the hyoid bone during such actions as chewing and swallowing can affect the location and maneuverability of the laryngeal apparatus.

The *epiglottis* is a large, leaf-shaped piece of cartilage located at the superior level of the larynx. The stem of this skeletal element is attached to the thyroid cartilage in the midline, whereas its upper leaf-shaped portion is unattached

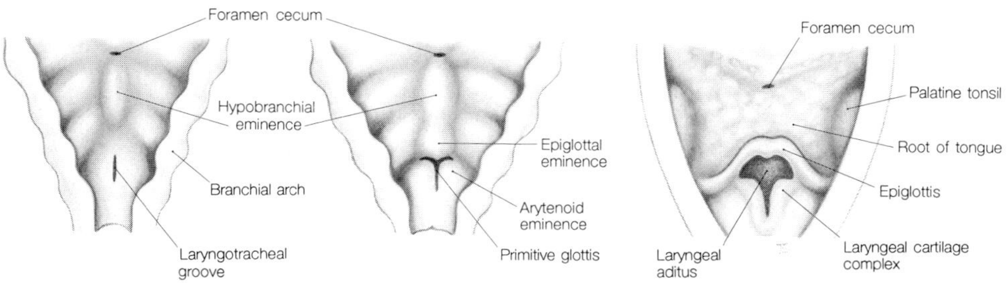

FIG 5–2.
Developmental progression of the larynx.

and can move upward and downward. During swallowing there is upward movement of the entire laryngeal apparatus plus a posterior movement of the tongue, and these combined actions serve to cause the free edge of the epiglottis to form a lid over the opening into the larynx called the glottis. The *rima glottidus* is the space between the true vocal folds in the larynx. The single cricoid cartilage is a complete ring of cartilage forming the inferior wall of the larynx. It is attached to the first cartilaginous ring of the trachea. The paired arytenoid cartilages are pyramidal and articulate with the superior border of the cricoid cartilage by a synovial joint. They attach anteriorly to the vocal folds and intrinsic laryngeal musculature and by their combined actions can move and tense the vocal folds.

The *trachea* is a tubular passageway contiguous with and extending downward from the larynx. In the adult this is about 12 cm long and 2.5 cm in diameter. Located anterior to the esophagus, it can be found at the level extending from the larynx to the fifth thoracic vertebra, at which point it divides into the right and left primary bronchi. The wall of the trachea consists of an inner mucosa, submucosa, cartilaginous layer, and outer layer of loose connective tissue. The cartilaginous layer consists of 16 to 20 horizontally oriented and incomplete C-shaped rings of cartilage stacked one on the other. The open parts of the C-shaped rings face the esophagus and permit the esophagus to expand as needed during swallowing.

Transverse smooth muscle fibers and elastic connective tissue span the ends of each C-shaped ring. The solid parts of the rings provide support so the tracheal wall can remain patent during respiration. In some situations, however, such as crushing or blunt injuries to the neck and chest, the cartilage rings can be crushed, leading to a collapse of the tracheal airway. At the point where the trachea bifurcates into the right and left primary bronchi, there is an internal ridge of cartilage called the *carina trachea.* It is formed by the posterior and somewhat inferior projection downward of the last tracheal ring. Widening and mechanical distortion of the carina, which can be seen in bronchoscopy, are serious prognostic signs because it usually indicates a carcinoma of the lymph nodes around the bifurcation of the trachea.

Chapter 6

Radiologic Techniques for Evaluation and Management of the Difficult Airway

Frank Londy

Martin L. Norton

A number of evaluative approaches can be implemented with the use of radiologic techniques, but only recently have anesthesiologists seen the need for explicit upper airway imaging.

We all are familiar with the classic lateral flat plate, using both soft tissue and standard (bone survey) densities, still a very useful means of imaging the upper airway. The use of computed tomography (CT) scanning in recent years has provided us with a valuable new tool for upper airway imaging. Of late magnetic resonance imaging (MRI) has contributed greatly to our diagnostic armamentarium. Very recently, superb work by Lowe et al.[1] using digitized CT scans has made it possible to study tongue volume. This technique offers great potential for evaluation of other soft tissues of the upper respiratory tract.

Cephalometric analysis of the airway may give further insight into what is considered normal and abnormal.

Another new technique, somnofluoroscopy, combines cineradiographic observation of the upper airway with simultaneous polysomnography,[2] a useful tool in the diagnosis of sleep apnea.

C-arm fluoroscopy, although not new, has proved to be the most useful tool for planning endotracheal intubation in patients with upper airway problems.

CT AND MRI

The wide acclaim of CT (Fig 6–1,A)[3] and MRI (Fig 6–1,B)[4] for head and neck imaging is well deserved and well documented in the literature. With regard to preendotracheal intubation studies, however, few institutions have developed specific protocols.

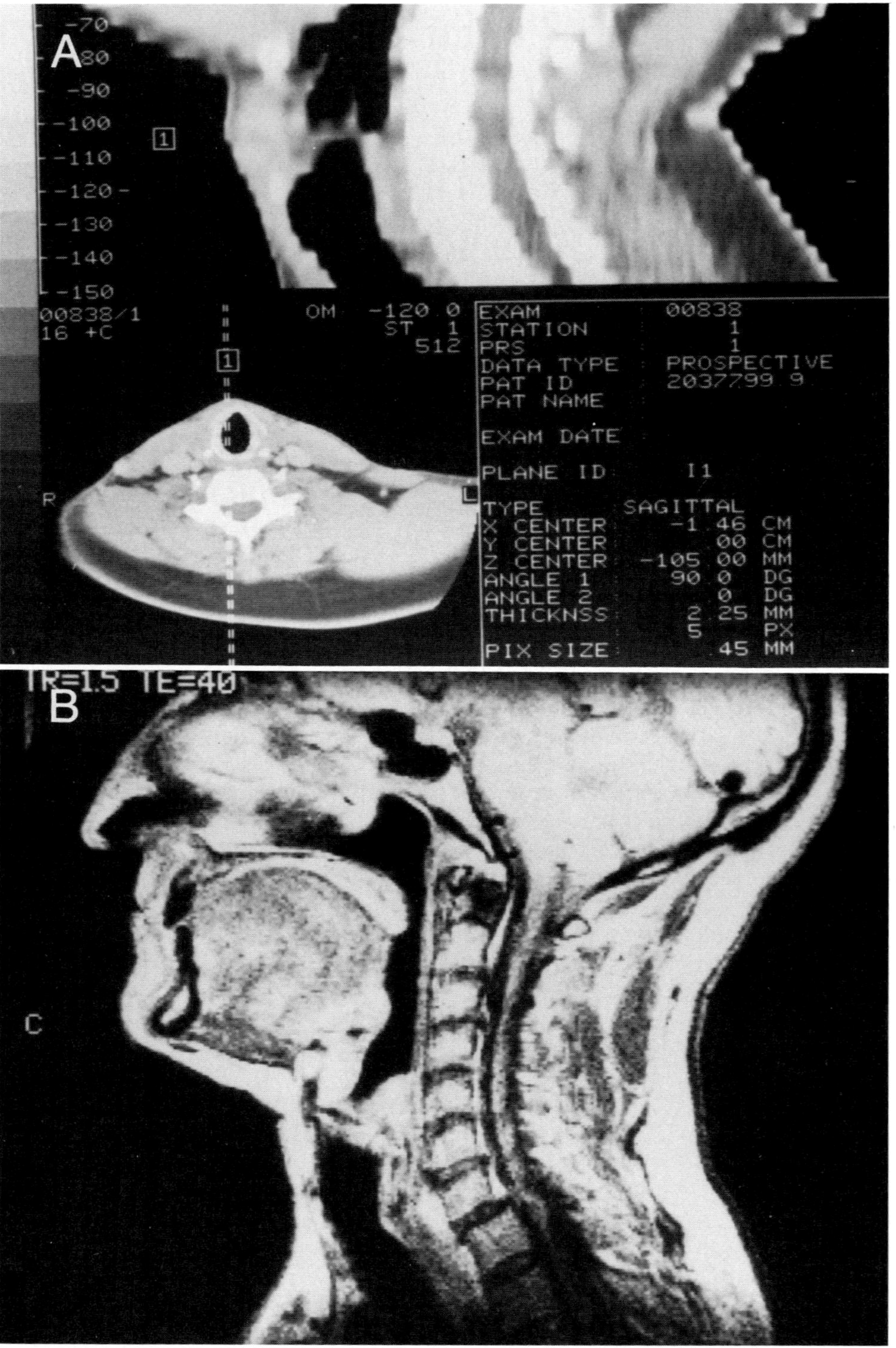

FIG 6–1.
A, CT scan. **B,** multiplanar imaging using MRI techniques.

TABLE 6–1.

Costs of Various Imaging Procedures at the University of Michigan Medical Center: 1989

Procedure	Overall Cost
Airway or neck CT	$ 837.00
Airway or neck CT in three dimensions	1,019.00
Airway or neck MRI	1,086.00
Airway or neck MRI	767.00
C-arm fluorography of airway	38.00/15min*
Plain film imaging series of TMJ	126.00
Plain film imaging series of airway	86.00
Plain film imaging of cervical spine	93.00

*Evaluation can usually be completed within 1–2 min of fluoroscopic time and 15 min of C-arm time.

Using CT we have found that 1.5 to 5 mm contiguous axial images with the gantry parallel to the vocal folds should produce optimal axial images. Viewing windows can be adjusted to further enhance the airway contrast as needed.

The greatest limitation of CT is that the scans will be in the axial plane when the patient is in a prone or supine position. For nonradiologists these images can be cumbersome to interpret. To present an easier to read, more traditional sagittal view, the computer must reconstruct the axial images. This will produce a lateral view of the airway, but is generally a choppy, poorly defined image of limited value. As CT software improves, this reconstruction shortfall will improve.

MRI offers the advantage of multiplanar views of the cartilage and soft tissues. However, it is expensive (Table 6–1), requires a relatively long time to produce the final image, and is not available everywhere. For dynamic airway evaluation MRI is usually not the method of choice. Other imaging options give as much or more information per patient dollar spent and are faster and easier to do, while allowing greater flexibility in scheduling examinations.

A new CT option coming to the market is the three-dimensional reconstruction. This method will reconstruct the CT data to produce an image that seems much like an image of a three-dimensional object photographed and projected onto a two-dimensional screen. The viewer will be able to turn the object to see it from any angle.

CEPHALOMETRY

Although we have not yet begun to use cephalometry in the Difficult Airway Clinic (University of Michigan Medical Center, Ann Arbor), we are interested in the technique and believe that it shows some promise in the imaging of these patients.

XERORADIOGRAPHY

Xeroradiography is a system that uses a dry, etchophotographic technique[5] (see Fig 2–6, A and B for an example of a xeroradiogram). It is seldom used now. Xerox Corporation is no longer producing xeroradiography equipment.

LARYNGOGRAPHY

Laryngograms (Fig 6–2) are plain film studies enhanced with contrast medium. They are of similarly historic interest as xeroradiograms because other methods, such as CT and MRI, have replaced them.

PLAIN FILM TOMOGRAPHY

Plain film tomography is a long-established modality that uses the principle of focal plane isolation through the reciprocal motion of the x-ray source and the image receptor (i.e., the film).[6] The resultant radiograph demonstrates an image that has only a narrow "layer" of the subject clearly focused. The lev-

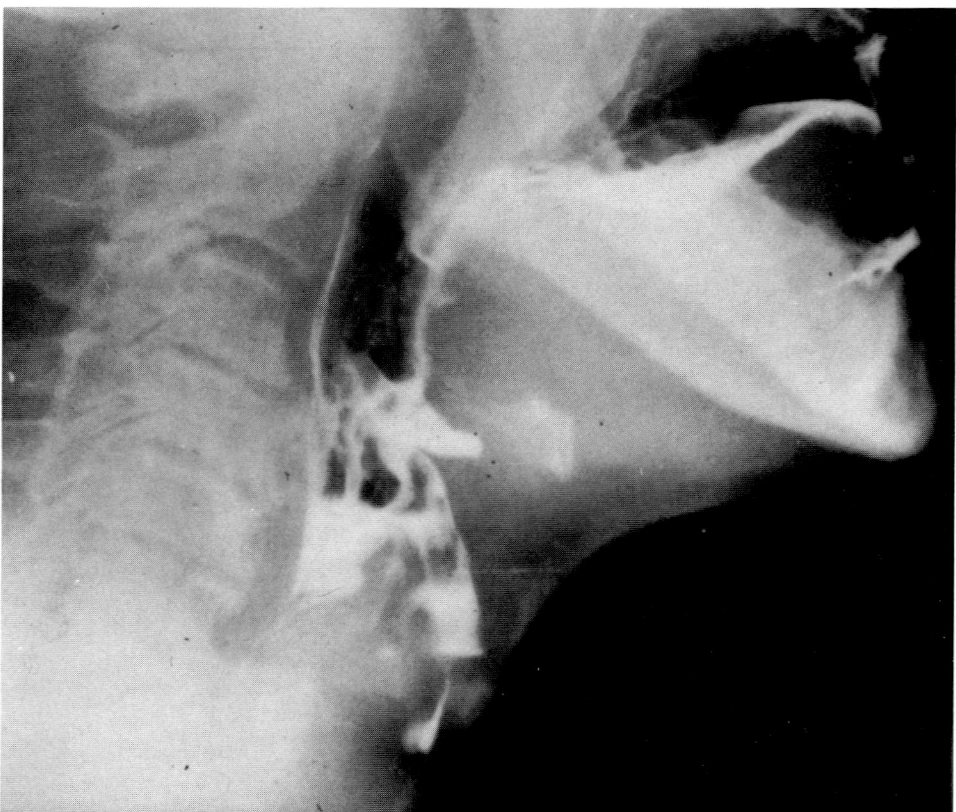

FIG 6–2.
Laryngogram.

els nearer the x-ray tube and the film are blurred, out of focus. Plain film tomography is quick and easy and does not emit a high radiation dose to the patient. Compare 135 mR/cut for plain film tomography vs. 2,232 mR/cut for CT. Plain film tomography is progressively being replaced by the greater detail and definition provided by CT and MRI for imaging of tissues in the neck.

PLAIN FILM RADIOGRAPHY (Table 6–2)

At the Difficult Airway Clinic we have made use of several methods, but have obtained the greatest amount of information from the plain film radiograph and C-arm fluorography. The lateral soft tissue neck view is the plain film technique we use most often (Fig 6–3). All plain films are taken with

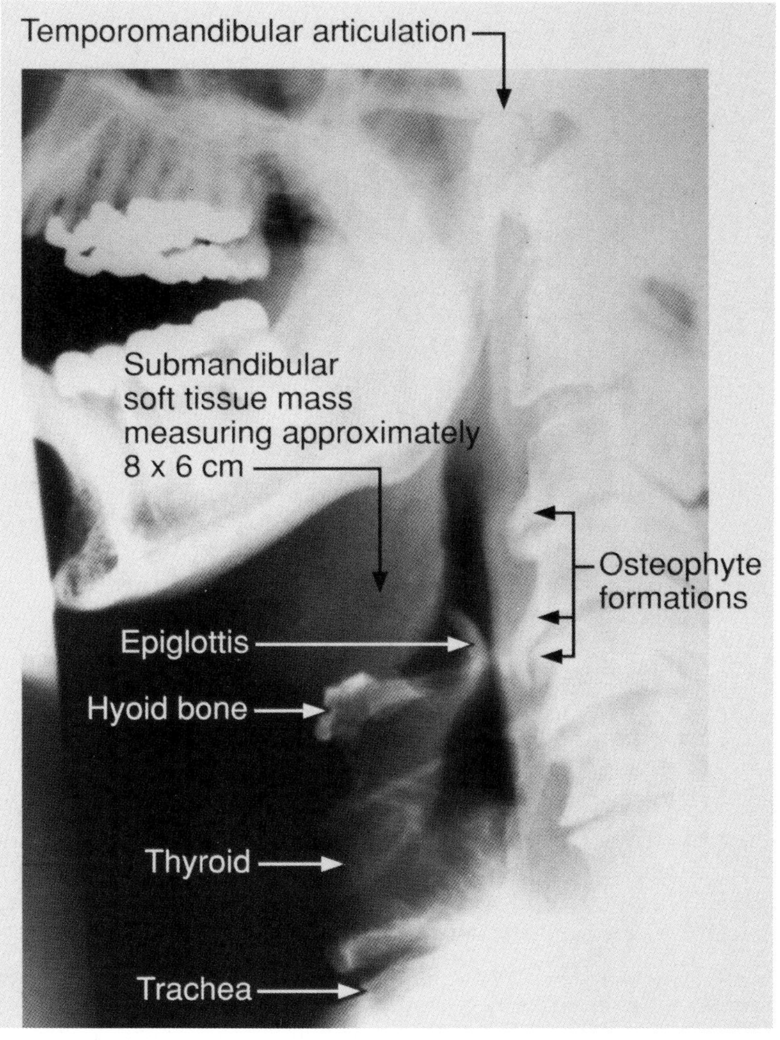

FIG 6–3.
Lateral soft tissue neck plain film.

TABLE 6–2.

Imaging With Plain Films

Temporomandibular joints
    Patient upright 15–30 degrees of angle as
       needed
    Film centered to TMJ
    Aggressive collimation
    Exposure factors
       70 kVp/8–10 mas
       40-in. source-to-image distance (SID)
       Radiation exposure to patient 300 mR
Airway upright
    Patient upright
    Neck in slight extension
    Mouth open
    Tongue out
    Patient's shoulders as low as possible*
    Expose during patient inspiration
    Collimate to the airway
    Center to include the nasopharynx to trachea†
    Exposure factors
       60 kVp/2–5 mas
       40-in. SID
       Radiation exposure to patient 12–20 mR
Imaging the cervical spine with plain films
    Collimate to cervical spine
    Center to C-4 vertebra
    Radiograph in neutral, flexion, and extension
    Exposure factors
       70 kVp/4–8 mas
       40-in. SID
       Radiation exposure to patient 110 mR

*For those patients who are unable to lower their shoulders the centering of the film should be at the level of the vocal folds. Centering higher will project the folds onto the shoulder nearest the film.

†It may be necessary to do a second film for the airway above the shadow of the mandible because of the low exposure factor. In that case, center to the area not visualized on the first film to present as distortion-free image as possible.

Kodak regular cassettes, 40-in. nongridded, source-to-image distance, using Dupont Cromex 6 film.

We have modified this examination to meet our needs for airway studies. Our greatest concern is for viewing airway configuration and not the soft tissue. The traditional method includes an exposure technique that often overpenetrates and burns away the anterior border of the airway. A lower exposure technique yields a radiograph with much greater airway detail. To increase that detail further, we collimate the cervical spine off the film.*

*Collimators are x-ray beam restriction devices built into the x-ray tube housing. Beam restriction is important for two reasons: (1) it will lower the patient's radiation dose; and (2) reducing the total number of x-ray photons will reduce the number of photons that strike the patient, as well as scatter radiation. Scatter radiation is the major cause of the poor definition, or washed-out quality, that is sometimes seen on uncollimated films.

TABLE 6–3.

Anatomic Location of Crucial Structures

Cartilage	Bony Landmark
Hyoid	C-2 to C-3
Thyroid	C-4 to upper border, lateral wing
	C-5 to lower border, lateral wing
Cricoid	C-6
Trachea	C-7 and below;
	10–20 cm long, about $\geq$ 12 mm diameter at approximately sixth ring becomes intrathoracic
Carina	T-5 (sternal angle of Louis; second intercostal space)

When viewing lateral neck films, remember that the hyoid bone appears to transect the epiglottis. Table 6–3 provides a guide to anatomic location of crucial structures.

Plain film exposure should be obtained with the patient's mouth slightly open during inspiration and the head placed in moderate extension. We also recommend direction of the central ray to the level of any suspected problem areas to reduce central ray distortions. An important point that should be considered is the position of the patient during this radiographic examination. There can be a great variation in airway configuration when one changes from the upright to the supine position. Radiographing a patient in only a supine or only an upright position produces a single image that can be misleading.

Because the exposure technique is light (i.e., underexposed) compared with the traditional soft tissue film, it is often necessary to take a second film for the airway above the lower border of the mandible. For this projection, standard exposure technique is used. Aggressive collimation to the region of the airway will increase detail and is strongly recommended. For the anterio-

TABLE 6–4.

Imaging a Dynamic Airway in the Anteroposterior Position

Scout exposure and image with
1. Noise reduction at maximum
2. Image showing the base of the skull superimposed over the mandible
3. Center to the vocal folds
4. Patient's neck in slight extension; image as follows, with noise reduction at a reduced level to prevent smearing of the image.
   a. Normal respiration
   b. Deep respiration (nasal)
   c. Deep respiration (oral, mouth opened wide)
   d. Deep respiration (oral, mouth opened wide, tongue out)
   e. Cough
   f. Phonation (A, E, I, O, U)
   g. Swallowing

posterior airway, plain film, standard AP soft tissue neck techniques are adequate (Table 6–4).

C-ARM FLUOROGRAPHY (Table 6–5)

At the Difficult Airway Clinic we have been using an extraordinarily helpful imaging option, the C-arm portable fluorography unit (Fig 6–4). It consists of an x-ray tube that is directed at an electronic image receptor. The image is viewed with a monitor connected to the C-arm. Imaging options on the monitor cart include snapshots (still pictures) and fluorography with or without pixel (tiny dots that compose the image on the C-arm monitor) averaging. The last fluorographic image taken may be held on the screen after the x-ray beam has been turned off and until it is started again. Most C-arms also have the ability to store still images in their computer data banks for future reference. Permanent images can be obtained by recording the fluoroscopic image with a VCR, transferring still images onto x-ray film with the use of a matrix camera, or photographing the images from the monitor screen with a standard camera. To record fluoroscopic C-arm images, we use the technique outlined in Table 6–5.

It is with dynamic studies that the capabilities of the C-arm are best used. The C-arm can show dynamic changes of the airway during normal respiration, deep respiration, swallowing, and tongue and jaw thrust as well as effects produced when the patient phonates or flexes or extends the neck. Using the C-arm, we can study the mechanics of the patient's disease or condition as

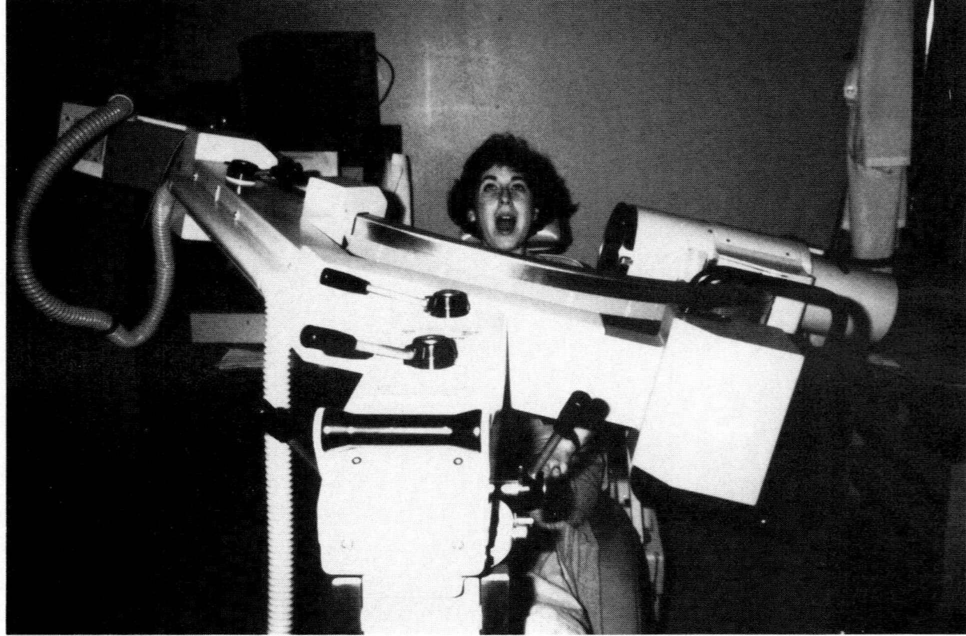

FIG 6–4.
Use of C-arm fluoroscope.

TABLE 6–5.
Steps in C-Arm Fluorographic Imaging Techniques

  I. Temporomandibular joint
   A. Scout exposure image with
     1. Patient in upright position
     2. X-ray beam in lateral position
     3. Maximum noise reduction
   B. Scout exposure to right side of TMJ image with
     1. Maximum noise reduction
     2. Angle of 15–30 degrees as needed to present TMJ free of superimposition
   C. Scout exposure to dynamic, right side of TMJ image by
     1. Decreasing noise reduction as needed to prevent smearing of image with movement
     2. Obtaining 15–30 degrees of angle as needed
     3. Fluorographing at least two cycles of opening and closing of patient's mouth
   D. Repeat exposures B and C for left TMJ
 II. Cervical spine
   A. Scout exposure of cervical spine image with
     1. Patient in upright position
     2. X-ray beam in lateral position
     3. Maximum noise reduction
     4. Patient's shoulders as low as possible
   B. Flexion and extension cervical spine image with
     1. Maximum noise reduction
     2. Noise reduction decreased as needed to prevent smearing of image with movement
     3. Patient's shoulders lowered as much as possible
     4. One complete cycle of flexion-extension fluorographed
III. Nasopharynx
   A. Scout exposure image with
     1. Patient in upright position
     2. X-ray beam in lateral position
     3. Maximum noise reduction
 IV. Oropharynx and laryngopharynx to upper trachea
   A. Scout exposure image with
     1. Patient in upright position
     2. X-ray beam in lateral position
     3. Maximum noise reduction
     4. Patient's neck neutral
     5. Slight inspiration
       NOTE: It may be necessary to do two scout films, one upper (oropharynx) and one lower (laryngopharynx to trachea) because of patient size.
   B. Lateral dynamic airway image with
     1. Patient in upright position
     2. X-ray beam in lateral position
     3. Noise reduction at a reduced level to prevent smearing of the image
     4. X-ray field centered so that bottom of field includes the upper trachea (If this centering does not also demonstrate oropharynx, two sets of dynamic studies should be performed, the first with the trachea at the bottom of the frame and the second with it at the top.)
     5. Patient's neck in neutral position
       a. Normal respiration
       b. Deep respiration (nasal)
       c. Deep respiration (oral, mouth opened wide, tongue in)
       d. Deep respiration (oral, mouth opened wide with tongue out)
       e. Cough
       f. Phonation (A, E, I, O, U)
       g. Swallowing
     6. With patient's neck extended, image under the same dynamics as in IVB5
     7. With the patient's neck flexed, image under the same dynamics as in IVB5.
   C. Lateral dynamic airway study
     1. Follow steps IVB2–7 with the patient supine.

it impacts on the configuration of the airway and is delineated in instanta-
neously generated, dynamic images.

C-arm fluoroscopy is not so valuable for fixed picture representation as is
the soft tissue plain film. One can observe whether the cervical bodies move
and how they move in relation to each other in flexion and extension, including the degree of potential cervical spine mobility at the time of endoscopy or
intubation.

Similarly, TMJ motion can be quickly evaluated. By angling the x-ray beam,
one can observe the left or right side of the TMJs separately as in standard TMJ
studies. One may also view both TMJs simultaneously and thus evaluate bilateral TMJ motion with the assurance of uniform effort. We perform studies with
the patient supine or sitting. We therefore have the ability to quickly evaluate
and compare the effects of patient positioning on airway configurations. Optimum access for intubation can be determined as the patient changes position.
Every position and combination of maneuvers can be quickly evaluated for its
usefulness. By using the C-arm for preintubation evaluation, the anesthesiologist can quickly follow up on questions as they appear, rather than ordering
films, waiting for reports, and perhaps having to order more radiographs to
track down problems or answer questions raised by the first set of films.

This timesaving factor should not be underestimated. Radiation exposure
dosage to patients is an important consideration. We have found that C-arm
studies result in acceptable radiation exposure levels to the patient.* Patient radiation doses under C-arm fluoroscopy range from 300 to 450 mR/min, depending on the structures being imaged. We have also used the C-arm during
endotracheal intubation, and find it a useful aid. When the C-arm is in a lateral
airway position, its image can guide the intubationist to the correct anterior or
posterior maneuver necessary to pass a flexible laryngoscope. In the anteroposterior position the image can help guide its passage in the midline to lateral
plane (Fig 6–5). Because of the C-arm design, switching from anteroposterior
to lateral positions can be accomplished in seconds. In addition, video tapes of
these intubation images are valuable teaching aids.

There are limiting factors involving the use of the C-arm and dynamic eval-
uations of the airway.† The C-arm has a difficult time with body parts that are
small or have a wide range of densities over a small area, for example, fingers

*Population dose recommendation from the Nuclear Regulatory Commission is 500
mR/year. We determine our patient dose two ways: indirect method (calculations
based on exposure factors) and direct method (placing a film badge on the patient's
neck).

†We once had difficulty imaging the airway in a patient who had had a great deal
of soft tissue removed during radical neck surgery. The transverse density of his neck
at the point of the airway was almost the same density as that of air itself. We were
unable to turn down the x-ray beam factors enough to view the airway. Although we
used the lowest setting possible, we were overexposing and burning away the airway.
The solution to this problem was to increase density of the airway and lower the total
amount of x-rays emitted. We did this with the use of Lucite and aluminum filters. A
Lucite wedge filter was placed on the patient, with the thick end of the wedge in an
anterior position. This added "density" to the patient, with that density increasing anteriorly to the point of greatest overexposure. Aluminum filters were placed on the
x-ray tube to reduce the total amount of emitted radiation. With the use of these filters
we produced an acceptable image.

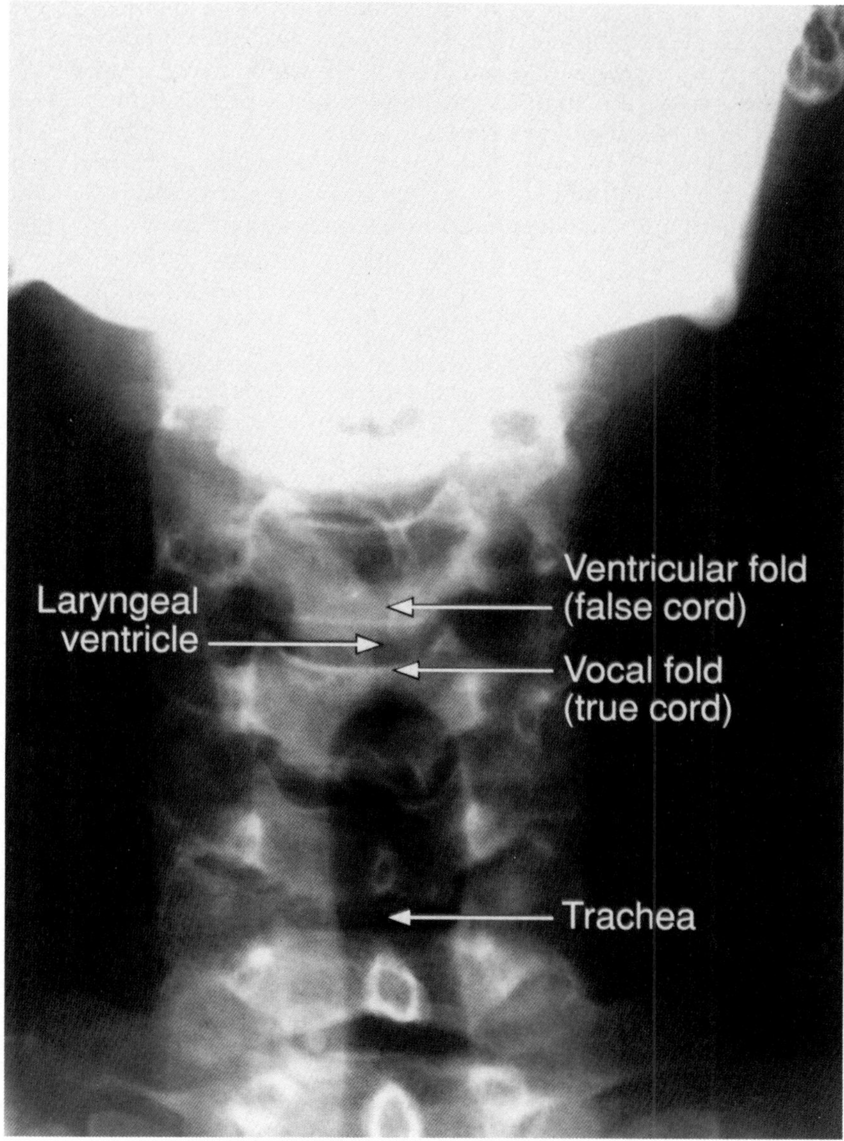

FIG 6–5.
Normal cervical spine, anteroposterior position. Laryngeal "ventricular" structures are synonymous with "vestibular" structures.

or toes. Sometimes the problem manifests itself between the airway (which has very low density) and the cervical spine (which has a medium high density). In such cases a decision must be made about the area of greatest concern, such as the airway configuration. The exposure must be set, realizing that the cervical spine will not be well demonstrated in that individual image. The solution is to evaluate the cervical spine and the airway with separate images.

Another limiting factor of the C-arm is the use of noise reduction. The problem is that the computer is unable to keep up with a dynamic image and still maintain a high degree of noise reduction. The resultant image has a smeared effect. It is therefore necessary to use less noise reduction for the more dynamic portions of the examination. This will create a dropoff in dynamic image quality, but that dropoff does not compromise the value of the C-arm itself. It is, however, noticeable.

The mobility of the C-arm allows for its use in a clinic setting, a preoperative holding area, or in the operating room itself. We strongly recommend its use in assessment and management of upper airway problems.

REFERENCES

1. Lowe AA, Gionhaku N, Takeuchi K, et al: Three-dimensional CT reconstructions of tongue and airway in adult subjects with obstructive sleep apnea. *Am J Orthod Dentofacial Orthop* 1986; 90:364–373.
2. Katsantonis GP, Walsh JK: Somnofluoroscopy: Its role in the selection of candidates for uvulopalatopharyngoplasty. *Otolaryngol Head Neck Surg* 1986; 94:1.
3. Ledley RS: Introduction to computerized tomography. *Comput Biol Med* 1976; 6:239–246.
4. Stark DD, Moss AA, Gansu G, et al: Magnetic resonance imaging of the neck. *Radiology* 1984; 150:447–461.
5. Brember DM, Judelman E: An introduction of xeroradiography. *S Afr Med J* 1974; 48:2289.

Chapter 7

Pulmonary Function Tests for Extrathoracic Obstruction

William L. Eschenbacher

METHODS OF PULMONARY FUNCTION TESTING

The most useful pulmonary function tests for evaluation of extrathoracic airway obstruction are the flow-volume loop and specific airways resistance tests. Other pulmonary function tests for the complete evaluation of pulmonary status include total lung capacity, diffusing capacity (gas transfer), maximal voluntary ventilation, respiratory muscle forces, and cardiopulmonary exercise testing. The application and usefulness of these other tests have been described.[1]

FLOW-VOLUME LOOPS

Flow-volume loops can be obtained with any piece of equipment that measures air flow rate and the volume of air that patients are breathing. Usually they are done with a spirometer that will either measure flow rate by using a pneumotachograph, for example, and integrate the flow signal into a volume, or will measure a volume of air inhaled or exhaled and differentiate the volume signal into a flow rate. The divisions of lung air volumes, including total lung capacity and residual volume, are shown in Figure 7–1. The total amount of air that the patient exhales and inhales as part of this maneuver should be identical. This is the vital capacity.

An example of a normal flow-volume loop is shown in Figure 7–2. The point indicating total lung capacity is at zero on this diagram. The exhalation loop above the horizontal axis then shows the flow rates that can occur when the patient exhales from total lung capacity to residual volume (identified as 4.25 on the horizontal or volume scale). The total volume exhaled is the forced vital capacity (FVC), which in this case is 4.25 L. The inhalation loop shown

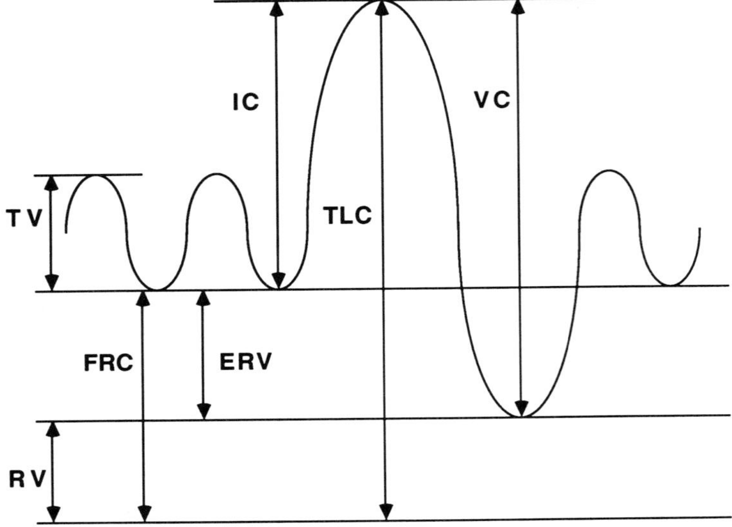

FIG 7–1.
Division of lung volumes as seen with a volume tracing from a spirometer. (*TV* = tidal volume; *IC* = inspiratory capacity; *TLC* = total lung capacity; *VC* = vital capacity; *FRC* = functional residual capacity; *ERV* = expiratory reserve volume; *RV* = residual volume.)

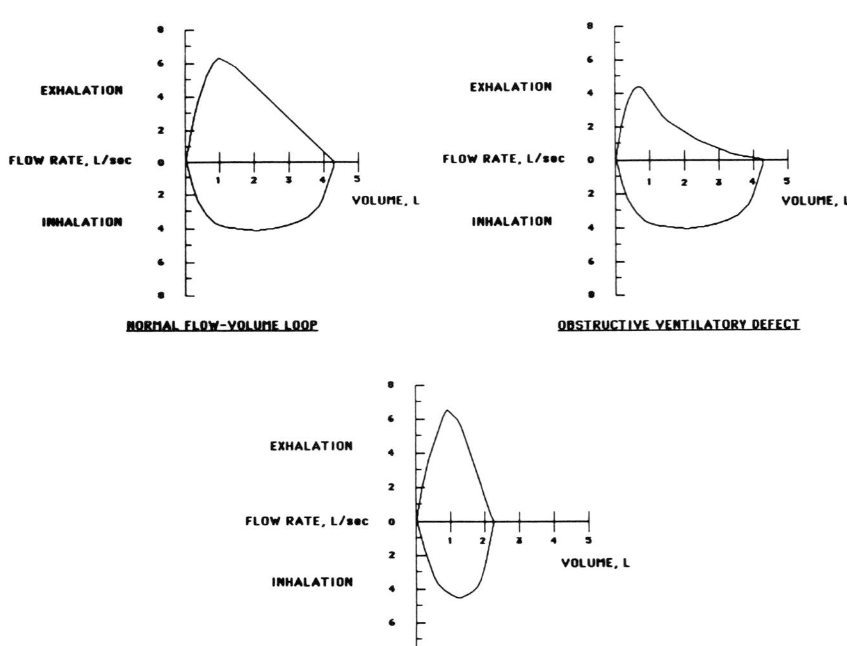

FIG 7–2.
Flow-volume loops from a normal person *(left)*, a patient with obstructive airway disease *(center)*, and a patient with a restrictive lung disease *(right)*.

below the horizontal axis indicates the flow rates that can occur during a maximal inhalation from residual volume back to total lung capacity.

Certain values can be obtained from these flow-volume loops, such as the peak expiratory flow rate (PEFR), which is the highest expiratory flow rate that occurs during the exhalation phase of the maneuver. In this normal example, the PEFR is 6.4 L/sec. The peak inspiratory flow rate (PIFR) can also be determined, and in this case is 4.1 L/sec. Another value commonly used in the evaluation is the volume of air exhaled in the first second of a maximal forced maneuver, or the forced expiratory volume in 1 second (FEV_1). This value cannot be easily determined from the flow-volume loop itself, but is usually reported as part of the spirometric study results.

The shape of flow-volume loops can be of value in the diagnosis and assessment of several common pulmonary diseases. The flow-volume loop in a patient with obstructive lower airways disease such as asthma, chronic bronchitis, or emphysema will have a characteristic appearance, with decreased flow rate especially at the lower lung volumes (closer to residual volume). A typical flow-volume loop from a patient with an obstructive ventilatory defect is also shown in Figure 7–2. In addition, the flow-volume loop of a patient with a restrictive-type lung disease such as diffuse interstitial fibrosis or sarcoidosis may have a characteristic appearance with decreased vital capacity. A typical flow-volume loop from a patient with a restrictive ventilatory defect is also shown in Figure 7–2.

CRITICAL ORIFICES, REDUCED FLOW RATES, AND EXTRATHORACIC OBSTRUCTIONS

The shape of a normal flow-volume loop depends on the force of the respiratory muscles, elastic properties of the lung and chest wall, and resistance to airflow through the airways. The driving force of airflow depends on the pressures that can be generated in the pleural space by the respiratory muscles, which result in a transpulmonary pressure difference that in turn causes the airflow to occur. All other conditions being the same, if a narrowing occurs in the upper airway or at the mouth, the peak air flow rates that can be generated by the individual will be reduced.

Using the insertion of endotracheal tubes as an example, if we plot the flow rates of air that will be generated by increasing driving pressures across different sized openings, we can see that as the diameter of the opening decreases, the flow rate of any given driving pressure will decrease. This effect of different sized openings is shown in Figure 7–3 for the flow rates that will be generated by applying increasing driving pressures to endotracheal tubes of different internal diameters, from 9 to 6 mm inside diameter. As can be seen especially for the 6 mm orifice, after a certain driving pressure is reached the slope of the rate of change of flow rate for the increase in driving pressure is near zero. This means that with further increases in pressure there is little or no increase in flow rate. We refer to such openings as critical orifices.

The presence of a critical orifice in the upper airways will alter the flow-volume loop in a very predictable manner. At first, the highest flow rates will be affected so that, even with increased effort of exhalation or inhalation, no further increase in airflow will occur. Representative flow-volume loops for a

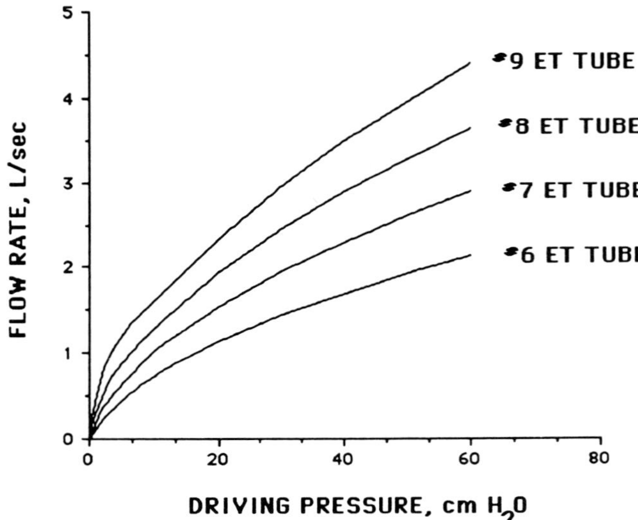

FIG 7–3.
Changes in flow rate of air through different sized endotracheal tubes plotted against the driving pressure through the tubes

normal individual breathing through smaller and smaller orifices is shown in Figure 7–4.

Clinically, this situation would be the same as a fixed extrathoracic or intrathoracic upper airway obstruction that does not change with the respiratory cycle. In this case the decrease in flow rate is seen with both the exhalation and inhalation phases of the flow-volume loop. We can use this information to estimate the size of a fixed upper airway obstruction in a given patient by first identifying such a flow-volume loop with plateauing of both the exhalation and inhalation limbs of the loop and then by noting the maximal flow rates during inhalation and exhalation. For example, if the shape of the flow-volume loop is as seen in Figure 7–4 and the maximal flow rates are approximately 2 L/sec, then the virtual or actual airway diameter at the site of obstruction would be close to 6 mm.

VARIABLE EXTRATHORACIC AND INTRATHORACIC AIRWAY OBSTRUCTION

Having described the characteristic flow-volume loop of a fixed upper airway obstruction, we can also identify lesions that cause obstruction to airflow but that change somewhat with the respiratory cycle. For example, extrathoracic lesions such as bilateral vocal cord paralysis or the narrowed oropharynx in an obese patient will obstruct more during inhalation. This narrowing is caused by the negative intrathoracic pressures generated during inhalation that are transmitted to the upper airways. Such a lesion will have a characteristic flow-volume loop, with flattening of the inhalation limb and a normal exhalation limb. The positive intrathoracic pressures generated during exhalation maintain a patent airway with no evidence of narrowing. A characteristic flow-

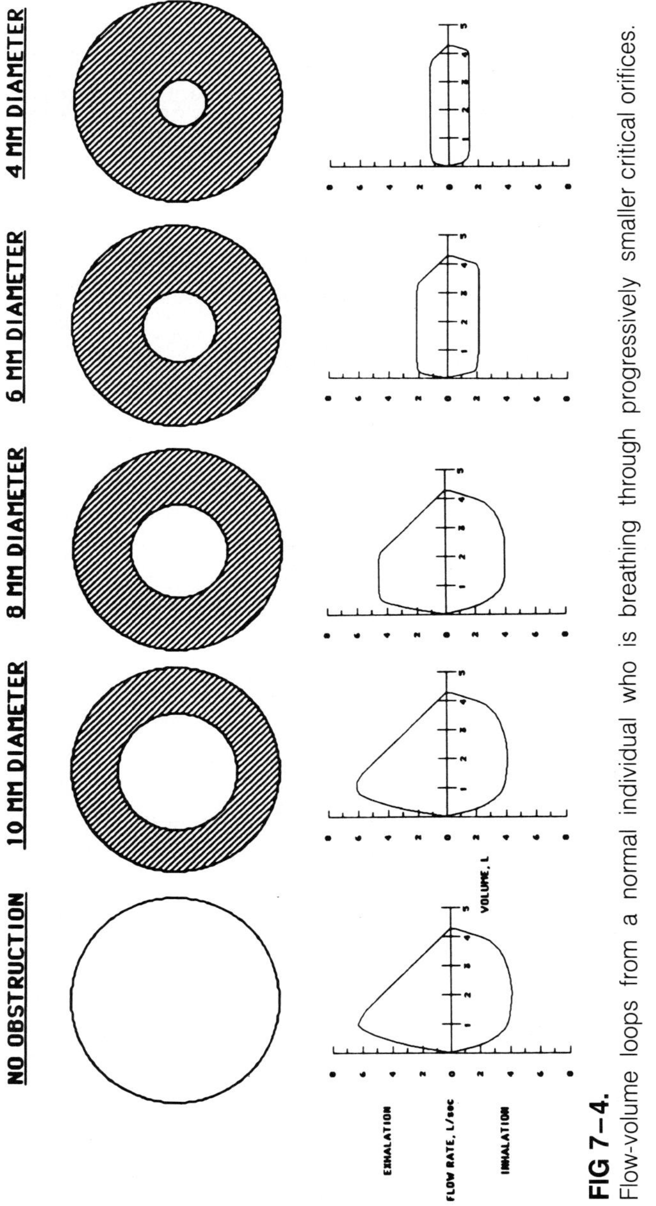

FIG 7–4.
Flow-volume loops from a normal individual who is breathing through progressively smaller critical orifices.

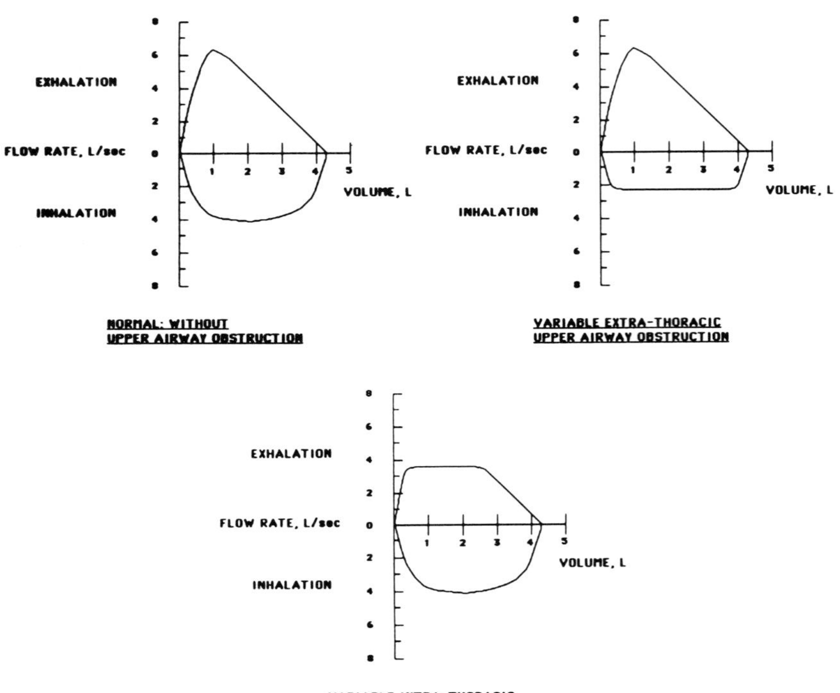

FIG 7–5.
Flow-volume loops from a normal person *(left),* a patient with a variable extrathoracic upper airway obstruction *(center),* and a patient with a variable intrathoracic upper airway obstruction *(right).*

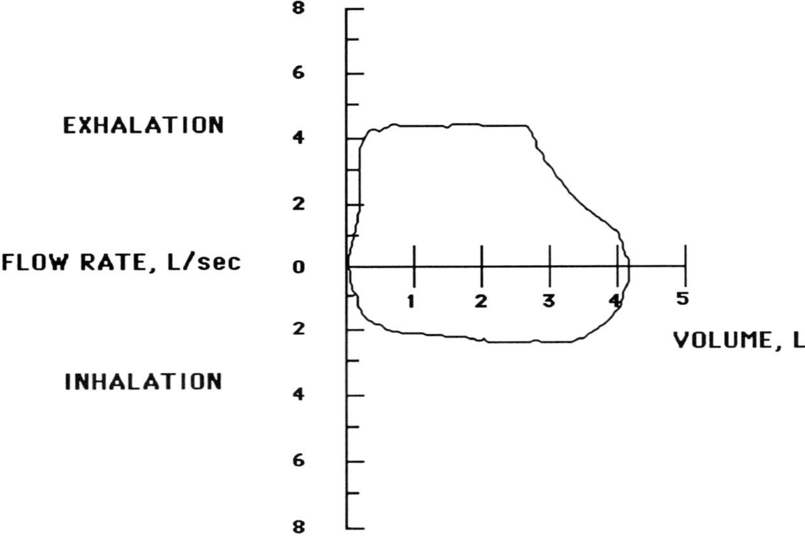

FIG 7–6.
Flow-volume loop from patient with Treacher Collins syndrome with multiple, previous operations on his face and upper airway. Patient has fixed upper airway obstruction with maximal diameter of approximately 8 mm (maximal flow rate 4.2 L/sec). A pharyngeal muscle conus was thought to funnel down to a restricted upper airway. A 5.5 mm endotracheal tube was used for subsequent general anesthesia.

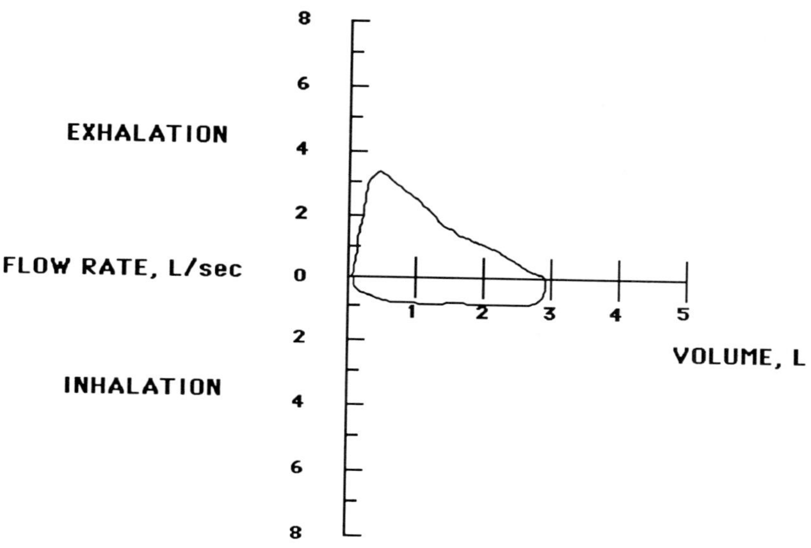

FIG 7–7.
Flow-volume loop from patient with history of rheumatoid arthritis and cervical spinal instability. Loop configuration suggests variable extrathoracic upper airway obstruction with evidence of flaccid pharyngeal walls that collapsed during inhalation. Loop does not suggest fixed upper upper airway obstruction.

volume loop for a variable extrathoracic upper airway obstruction is shown in Figure 7–5.

The opposite situation would exist for an intrathoracic upper airway lesion. Here the susceptible area of the upper airway would be compressed during exhalation, because of the positive pleural pressures that are transmitted to the central airways. The exhalation limb of the flow-volume loop would be altered, with decreased flow rates. During inhalation the transmitted negative pleural pressures would maintain the airway open and result in normal flow rates during inhalation. A characteristic flow-volume loop for a variable intrathoracic upper airway obstruction is also shown in Figure 7–5.

A classic finding in a clinical setting is Treacher Collins syndrome (Fig 7–6). Contrast this with rheumatoid arthritis and cervical spine instability (Fig 7–7).

It should be noted that making the diagnosis of an upper airway obstruction from the characteristic shape of the flow-volume loop can be difficult or impossible when there is underlying lower airways disease, such as chronic bronchitis or emphysema.[2]

REFERENCES

1. Clausen JL: *Pulmonary Function Testing, Guidelines and Controversies: Equipment, Methods and Normal Values.* Philadelphia, WB Saunders Co, 1982.
2. Gelb AF, Tashkin DP, Epstein JD, et al: Nd-YAG laser surgery for severe tracheal stenosis physiologically and clinically masked by severe diffuse obstructive pulmonary disease. *Chest* 1987; 91:166–170.

Chapter 8

Two- and Three-Dimensional Analyses of Tongue, Airway, and Soft Palate Size

Alan A. Lowe

John A. Fleetham

ANATOMIC ABNORMALITIES IN OBSTRUCTIVE SLEEP APNEA

Obstructive sleep apnea (OSA) is defined as a recurrent cessation of respiration associated with an upper airway obstruction during sleep. Since OSA syndrome was first described by Gastaut et al.,[1] knowledge related to the condition has expanded rapidly. However, many unsolved questions remain. Remmers et al.[2] suggested that a patent airway results from a controlled interaction between the anatomy and physiology of the upper airway. In normal subjects during inspiration, although subatmospheric intraluminal pressure develops, airway collapse is prevented by the action of the dilator muscles, especially the genioglossus muscle. This response is not seen in OSA. Several studies have recently suggested that patients with OSA syndrome have craniomandibular and anatomic airway abnormalities.[3-15] Lowe et al.[3] reconstructed tongue and upper airway structures by means of three-dimensional (3D) computed tomographic (CT) scans and calculated volumes and surface areas for these structures. Even though CT has many advantages as a measuring tool for airway size, it is time consuming and expensive for routine clinical use.

Cephalometrics, though having the limitation of any two-dimensional (2D) method, also has several significant advantages, including low cost, easy access, and reduced invasiveness. In this chapter we evaluate cephalometric linear and cross-sectional area variables for tongue, airway, and soft palate size and compare these variables to 3D CT measurements by means of direct visual and linear regression techniques.

CEPHALOMETRIC TECHNIQUES

Patients are seated in an upright position with the Frankfort horizontal plane parallel to the floor and instructed to lightly contact their back teeth.[4] The dorsum of the tongue is coated with Esobar Esophageal Cream (Therapex Inc., Montreal, Quebec, Canada) to enhance the outline of the tongue and pharyngeal soft tissues. Tracings are constructed of traditional contours and points. In addition, a number of pharynx, tongue, and hyoid measurements are identified and digitized (Fig 8–1).

In addition to the traditional linear cephalometric variables used in the evaluation of OSA,[4-7] a number of additional variables have been quantified. These are detailed in Appendix 8–A.

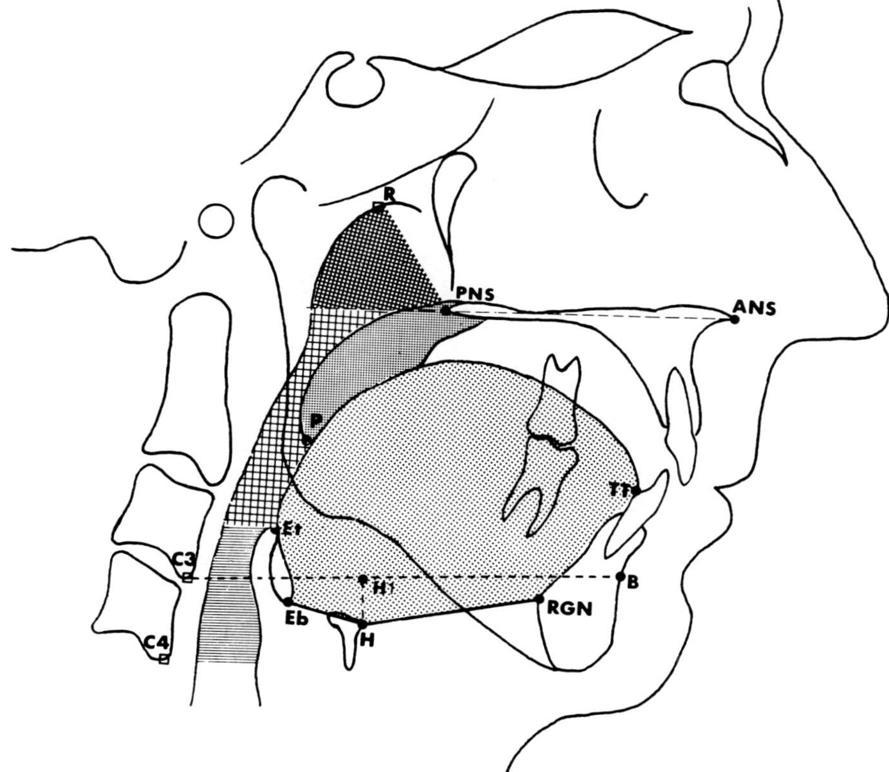

FIG 8–1.
Diagrammatic representation of anatomic points, contours, and planes used to identify tongue, airway, and soft palate on lateral cephalograms. X and Y coordinates of tongue tip, deepest point of epiglottis, most superior and anterior point of epiglottis, and most superior and anterior point on the hyoid bone are identified. Retrognathion *(RGN)* is the most posterior point of mandibular symphysis along a line perpendicular to the Frankfort horizontal plane. In addition, *C-4* is the most anterior and inferior point on the fourth vertebral column. *P* indicates the most inferior point of the soft palate, *R* is the point on the posterior pharyngeal wall at the intersection of the cranial base and lateral pterygoid plate, and *PNS* and *ANS* identify posterior and anterior points on the palatal plane. *(TT =* tongue tip; *H =* hyoid bone; *Eb =* base of epiglottis; *Et =* tip of epiglottis.)

Each patient undergoes a Siemens DR CT scan. Patients are positioned supine on the examination table so that the soft tissue Frankfort plane (tragus of the ear to soft tissue orbitale) is perpendicular to the floor.[3] The patient is instructed to relax (teeth apart) and to continue regular breathing but not to swallow during any one scan. Patients are evaluated while awake. Scans are obtained from the level of the Frankfort plane to a level below the sixth cervical vertebra. After one scan is completed the examination table is shifted 8 mm and the next scan is obtained.

Tracings are made on acetate paper for each of the slices for tongue, airway, soft palate, masseter muscle, and mandible. Boundaries are outlined in the middle of tissue transition zones to take into account partial volume averaging. A data entry program permits digitization of all slices using a Hewlett-Packard (Model 9874) digitizer. A cross-hair cursor is used to enter the contour of each of the structure codes into the computer (Hewlett-Packard 1000E series). Analysis programs determine the cross-sectional area of specific structures. Volume measurements based on known cross-sectional areas of a series of contiguous slices and on the thickness of each slice are also calculated. Details for the calculation methods to determine volume and cross-sectional area have been reported previously.[3]

A sample OSA case assessment summarizes the data for one patient and compares it with data for similar skeletal subtype OSA patients and controls (Plate 1). All patients with OSA who are evaluated as possible candidates for uvulopalatopharyngoplasty (UPPP) undergo cephalometric and CT analysis as part of the routine diagnostic workup. This report is prepared for the attending physician before any therapy decision is made. Lateral and superior views of the tongue and airway are provided (Plate 1). A cephalometric overview provides the values for 21 craniofacial variables and compares them with means obtained for OSA and control subjects matched for sex and skeletal type.

The next segment of the report provides a soft tissue cephalometric analysis. The soft palate cross-sectional area for the patient in Plate 1 is large compared with controls. The narrowest cross-section of the airway is 59.2 mm^2 seen on section 9 in the oropharynx, and the largest cross-sectional area of the tongue is 2162.1 mm^2 observed on the same section. The soft palate is widest at 459.0 mm^2 on section 10. The table accompanying Plate 1 reveals that this patient has a large tongue and soft palate volume compared with control subjects. Furthermore, the partial airway volume is slightly less than the mean for the 50 OSA patients in the data base.

COMPARISON OF CT AND CEPHALOMETRIC DATA

To visually compare the differences between cephalometric and CT data for patients of the same skeletal subtype, we have provided two cephalograms and four 3D graphic plots for each of a matched pair of class I OSA patients in Plate 2. The two patients were compared on the basis of similar craniofacial variables obtained from the lateral cephalograms shown at the top of the figure. The 3D plots on the extreme left are views of the masseter muscle, mandible, and airway as viewed from directly above with the anterior view to the top. In contrast, the 3D plots on the right view the patients from a side posi-

sleep apnea. Correlation of airway size with physiology during sleep and wakefulness. *Am Rev Respir Dis* 1983; 127:221–226.
12. Suratt P, Dee P, Atkinson R, et al: Fluoroscopic and computerized tomographic features of pharyngeal airway in obstructive sleep apnea. *Am Rev Respir Dis* 1983; 127:487–492.
13. Stein M, Gamsu G, DeGeer G, et al: Cine CT in obstructive sleep apnea. *AJR* 1987; 148:1069–1074.
14. D'Urzo A, Lawson V, Vassal K, et al: Airway area by acoustic response measurements and computerized tomography. *Am Rev Respir Dis* 1987; 135:392–395.
15. Sinclair B, Hannam A, Lowe A, et al: Complex contour organization for surface reconstruction. *Comput Graph* 1989; 13:311–319.
16. Liistro G, Stanescu D, Dooms G, et al: Head position modifies upper airway resistance in men. *J Appl Physiol* 1988; 64:1285–1288.
17. Brown I, McClean P, Boucher R, et al: Changes in pharyngeal cross-sectional area with posture and application of CPAP in patients with obstructive sleep apnea. *Am Rev Respir Dis* 1987; 136:628–632.
18. Cartwright R, Samelson C: The effects of a nonsurgical treatment for obstructive sleep apnea—the tongue-retaining device. *JAMA* 1982; 248:705–709.

APPENDIX 8–A

Cephalometric Variables Used to Evaluate Obstructive Sleep Apnea

Tongue

TGL Tongue length: linear distance between TT and Eb

TGH Tongue height: linear distance between a point on the most superior curvature of the tongue dorsum and the base of a line drawn perpendicular to the TT-Eb line

Soft palate

PNS-P Soft palate thickness: linear distance between PNS and P

MPT Soft palate length: maximum thickness of the soft palate measured on a line parallel to the palatal plane

Upper airway

IAS Inferior airway space: thickness of the airway along a line extended through the Go-B point plane

MAS Middle airway space: thickness of the airway along a line parallel to the Go-B point plane through P

SPAS Superior posterior airway space: thickness of the airway behind the soft palate along a line parallel to the Go-B point plane through the midpoint of the line PNS-P

SAAS Superior anterior airway space: thickness of the airway anterior to the soft palate along a line parallel to the Go-B point plane through the midpoint of the line PNS-P

VAL Vertical airway length: linear distance between PNS and Eb

Hyoid bone

MPH Vertical hyoid: linear distance along a perpendicular line from H to the Go-Gn plane

C3H Horizontal hyoid: linear distance between C3 and H

HRGN Horizontal hyoid: linear distance between H and RGN

HH1   Vertical hyoid: linear distance between H and a perpendicular line to the C3–RGN plane

Five cross-sectional areas were evaluated:
Tongue: area outlined by the dorsal configuration of the tongue surface and lines that connect TT, RGN, H, and Eb
Soft palate: area confined by the outline of the soft palate, starting and ending at PNS through P
Nasopharynx: area outlined by a line between R and PNS, an extension of the palatal plane to the posterior pharyngeal wall and the posterior pharyngeal wall.
Oropharynx: area outlined by the inferior border of the nasopharynx, posterior surface of the soft palate, a line from P to the dorsal surface of the tongue (parallel to the palatal plane), the posterior inferior surface of the tongue, a line parallel to the palatal plane through the point Et, and the posterior pharyngeal wall.
Hypopharynx: area outlined by the inferior border of the oropharynx, the posterior surface of the epiglottis, a line parallel to the palatal plane through the point C-4, and the posterior pharyngeal wall.

Chapter 9

Physiology and Variations of the Difficult Airway

Martin L. Norton

Any anatomic obstruction of the upper airway may contribute to the difficult airway syndrome. Conditions such as nasal septal deviation, adenoid or tonsil hypertrophy, craniovertebral anomalies, vocal fold paresis or paralysis, and glottic web have been reported to impede access to the airway.

PHYSIOLOGIC VARIATIONS

Lesser known and less well understood are the physiologic variations. During sleep, and anesthesia as well, the tone of the tongue musculature and velopharyngeal sphincter is reduced. Excellent descriptions of the controlling mechanisms and their related biomechanics are discussed by Fink[1] and Fink and Demarest.[2]

Sukerman and Healy[3] have a somewhat different view. They believe that the patency of the upper airway is partially controlled by the central nervous system and that spontaneous adjustment of the shape and volume of the upper respiratory tract can be demonstrated. Tactile and proprioceptive messages from the pharyngeal mucosa and musculature supply higher centers with information important for involuntary adjustments. Patency of the pharyngeal airway is maintained by adjustment in its muscular tone.

The pharyngeal muscles must increase their tone to overcome the tendency to collapse during inspiration. The forces contributing to upper airway collapse during inspiration include (1) surrounding atmospheric pressure and weight of the nuchal tissue, (2) local compliance of the airway walls, and (3) negative pressure inside the lumen of the airway during inspiration.

ANATOMIC VARIATIONS AND RESULTING BIOMECHANICAL CHANGES

To these we must add other forces and conditions such as anatomic variations and the resulting biomechanical changes they impose and superimposed positioning effects with abnormal biomechanics induced by the use of endo-scopic instruments and approaches, as well as the effects of sedatives, analge-sics, and anesthetics. Similarly, airway wall compliance may be affected by fatty infiltration, fluid from edema and exudates, and localized lesions.

Both Fink and Sukerman and their colleagues discuss the complex relation-ship between air flow and upper airway resistance, noting that airflow varies inversely with the resistance and directly with pressure developed between the alveoli and the airway opening. The greater the resistance to airflow, the greater the driving force needed to maintain a normal tidal volume. Conse-quently, if resistance is high, a larger negative pressure must be created during inspiration. This increased negative pressure is transmitted along the airway and in turn increases the tendency of the airway to collapse.

The Bernoulli effect also contributes to collapse. If the volume of flow is constant, the velocity of air at a constriction will decrease. The lower pressure at the site of narrowing will increase the tendency to collapse (Fig 9–1). Under-standing these phenomena is paramount to an appreciation of the biomechan-ics of upper airway ventilation, but they certainly should not be new concepts to the anesthesiologist, otolaryngologist, pulmonologist, and thoracic surgeon. For example, the Bernoulli principle specifies that flow energy is partitioned into potential energy (pressure) and kinetic energy (velocity). If the total en-ergy is constant, acceleration of streamlined flow at a constriction is indicated by a gain in kinetic energy and a corresponding loss of potential energy. The loss of potential energy, in the context of the airway, results in a dynamic fall in pressure at the glottic constriction, which then tends to constrict further.

During inspiration the glottic aperture increases as the posterior cri-coarytenoid muscle contracts and opens the vocal fold aperture. During expira-tion the activity of this muscle decreases and the vocal folds return to their pas-sive position. The respiratory motion of the vocal folds is important in decreas-ing airway resistance during inspiration and in regulating the rate of airflow during expiration.

The epiglottis, which may occlude the glottic chink, is retracted ventrally by its attachment to the hyoid bone through the hyoepiglottic ligament, thereby opening the hypopharynx. The hyoid bone lies ventral to the genio-glossus muscle and serves as a point of attachment for several muscles, most notably the geniohyoid, the digastric, and the thyrohyoid. Contraction of the first two pulls the hyoid ventrally, thereby pulling the base of the tongue and the epiglottis ventrally.

The main muscle of the tongue is the fan-shaped genioglossus, with its fi-bers inserting laterally on the internal surface of the mandible. When the ge-nioglossus contracts during inspiration, it pulls the ventral wall of the orophar-ynx further ventrally. Thus the tongue enlarges the lumen of the oropharynx, resulting in a collapsible pharynx stemming from the dorsal movement of the ventral pharyngeal wall, whose motion is resisted by contraction of muscles at-tached to the mandible, including the genioglossus, geniohyoid, and digastric.

Early and convincing clinical evidence for this proposition derives from ex-perience with anesthetized humans presented in the landmark paper by Safar and associates.[4]

Closure of the mouth and extension of the neck establishes a patent oropharynx by stretching the muscles attached to the mandible and thereby in-

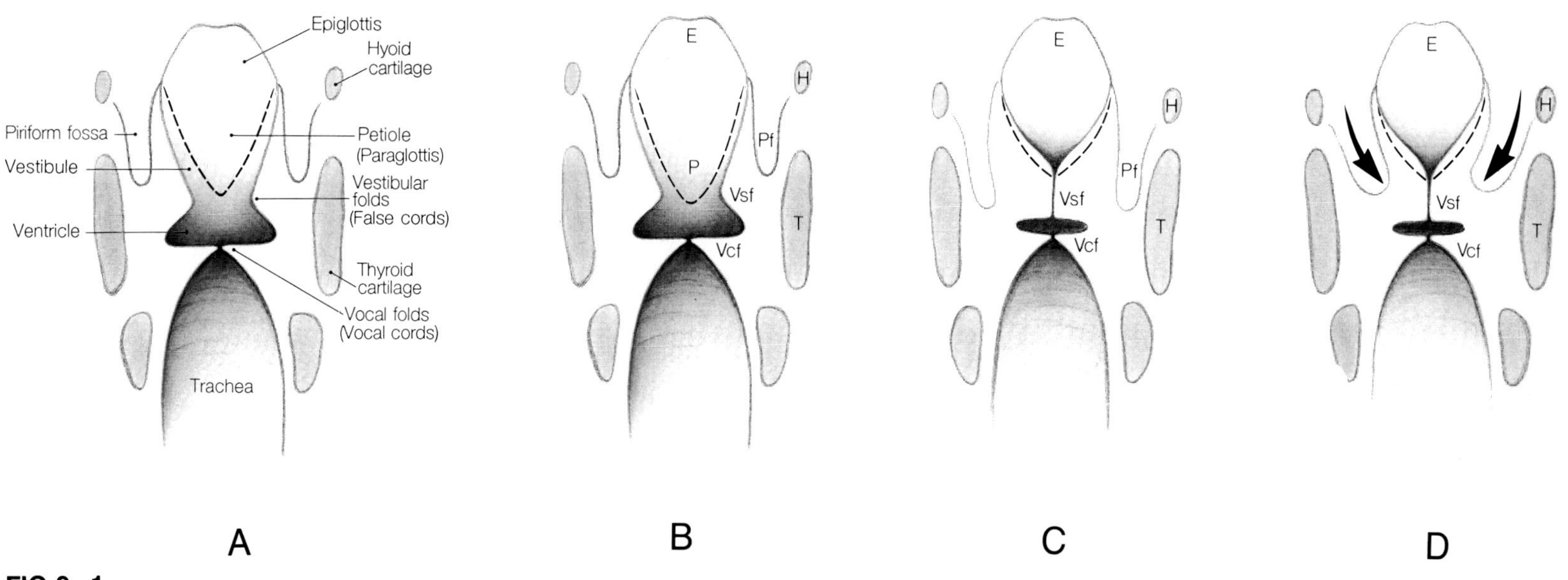

FIG 9–1.
Mechanism of laryngospasm. **A,** coronal section through the larynx viewed from the posterior aspect during normal glottic closure (e.g., phonation). **B,** reflex glottic closure. **C,** laryngospasm. Note shortening of the distance between hyoid and thyroid cartilages, caused by contraction of extrinsic laryngeal muscles. In addition to glottic closure, this obliterates the ventricle and the vestibule, to produce ball valve closure by the paraglottis at the level of the vestibular folds. **D,** positive pressure worsens airway obstruction due to laryngospasm by increasing lateral pressure at the level of the vestibular folds, thus forcing them medial.

creasing the force exerted by the genioglossus, geniohyoid, and digastric muscles. This pulls the ventral wall of the pharynx away from its dorsal wall.[5, 6]

REFERENCES

1. Fink BR: *The Human Larynx*. New York, Raven Press, 1975.
2. Fink BR, Demarest RJ: *Laryngeal Biomechanics*. Cambridge, Mass, Harvard University Press, 1978.
3. Sukerman S, Healy GB: Sleep apnea syndrome associated with upper airway obstruction. *Laryngoscope* 1979; 6:878–884.
4. Safar P, Escarraga LA, Chang F: Upper airway obstruction in the unconscious patient. *J Appl Physiol* 1959; 14:760–764.
5. Sauerland EK, Mitchel SP: Electromyographic activity of intrinsic and extrinsic muscles of the human tongue. *Tex Rep Biol Med* 1975; 33:445–455.
6. Sauerland EK, Mitchel SP: Electromyographic activity of human genioglossus muscle in response to respiration and to positional changes of the head. *Bull Los Angeles Neurol Soc* 1970; 35:69–73.

PART III

> Order and simplification are the first steps toward the mastery of a subject—the
> actual enemy is the unknown.
>
> *The Magic Mountain*
> Thomas Mann, 1924

This section examines specific problems that can result in a difficult airway. Chapters 10 and 11 are devoted to the discussion of bony abnormalities and soft tissue deformities or excess that can complicate the anesthetic management during surgery. The problems described under soft tissue considerations tend to be underestimated because they are not easily quantified and are rarely as obvious as a bony deformity.

Chapters 12 through 14 examine the problems posed in groups of patients who have specific types of associated problems, such as obesity and sleep apnea, burns, and oral surgery, and finally, in children. Missing from this final section is discussion of the iatrogenic airway posing difficulty for future anesthetic management. A future edition may devote a chapter to this complication. Included in this group of patients would be congenitally deformed children who even a decade ago would not have survived beyond the perinatal period. Now many of these children are surviving with potentially fatal deformities to be dealt with in later childhood. Also remarkable is the increased number of elderly patients who are surviving radical resection of head and neck cancer and then returning for repeated procedures for plastic repairs or disease recurrence. The challenges posed to the anesthesiologist in managing these patients will prove to be one of the mixed blessings of medical advance in the last decade of the 20th century.

Chapters 14 and 15 deal with techniques of management in general terms for both children and adults. The argument presented tries to persuade the intubationists to group techniques in terms of the problems to be overcome rather than relying on a complex decision tree that is all too easily forgotten in an emergency. The use of simple "tricks" and equipment is emphasized in the first instance. The general approach to selecting techniques as part of an anesthetic plan is simplified into overcoming problems of access to the airway, visualization of the larynx, and the nature of the glottic intubation target itself. Thus selection of management techniques may be tied into the individual cases described in similar terms throughout this atlas.

Chapter 10

Micrognathia, Cervical Spine, and Other Bony Considerations in the Difficult Airway

Martin L. Norton

Bony areas such as the temporomandibular joint, as discussed by Dr. Upton in Chapter 13, and problems such as craniofacial dysostoses, which involve disproportions or impose mechanical limitations to airway access, must be taken into account by the endoscopist. *Micrognathia* (small jaws) is the most striking feature in the spectrum of bony anomalies, but maxillofacial and nasal malformations also contribute to the difficulty of establishing and maintaining an effective airway. Micrognathia is the term most frequently used to describe this anomaly of the mandible, although other terms that have appeared in the literature include hypoplasia of the mandible, mandibular hypotrophy, congenital mandibular atresia, brachygnathia, ateliosis of the mandible, and hypomicrognathia.[1]

Retrognathia (posterior displacement of the chin), a more accurate and inclusive term, refers to several conditions that can lead to backward chin displacement without an abnormally small jaw. Retroposition of the chin is a finding common to many types of jaw deformities.

Appendix A–2 suggests the types of the various malformations contributing to a difficult airway.

MICROGNATHIA

Micrognathia (sometimes called retrognathia) is the prime, constant bony finding that signals trouble for access to the airway. It is the most difficult problem to deal with, primarily because of the attachment of the root of the tongue and the effects this and other tendinomuscular structures have on suspension of the larynx. These latter structures lie more superior in relation to the mandible (often described by the practicing endoscopist as anterior) and are thereby drawn closer to the base of the tongue.

The result is that the rigid laryngoscope blade, whether curved or straight, cannot readily deflect the soft tissues of the laryngopharynx. Thus visualization of the additus laryngis and positioning of soft tissue are extremely difficult, if not impossible.

If the horizontal ramus (extension) of the mandible is small relative to the maxilla, as in micrognathia, it will also be reduced relative to the length of the genioglossus and geniohyoid muscles. Therefore these muscles must actively contract to a length much shorter than their passive length to maintain a normal sized pharyngeal lumen.

Another point to consider when opening the mouth is the effect of Bernouilli's principle in maintaining the airway. This exposes the tongue and soft palate to atmospheric pressure. The anterior portion of the tongue relaxes, producing a dorsal motion of the belly of the genioglossus muscle and thereby decreasing the size of the posterior pharyngeal lumen. The entire transmural pressure of the pharynx is now exerted across the soft palate, moving it dorsally and narrowing the lumen of the oropharyngeal space. Classic examples are shown in Treacher Collins (Fig 10–1), Goldenhar's (Fig 10–2), Hallermann-Streiff-François (Fig 10–3), and arthrogryposis multiplex (Fig 10–4; Plate 5) syndromes.

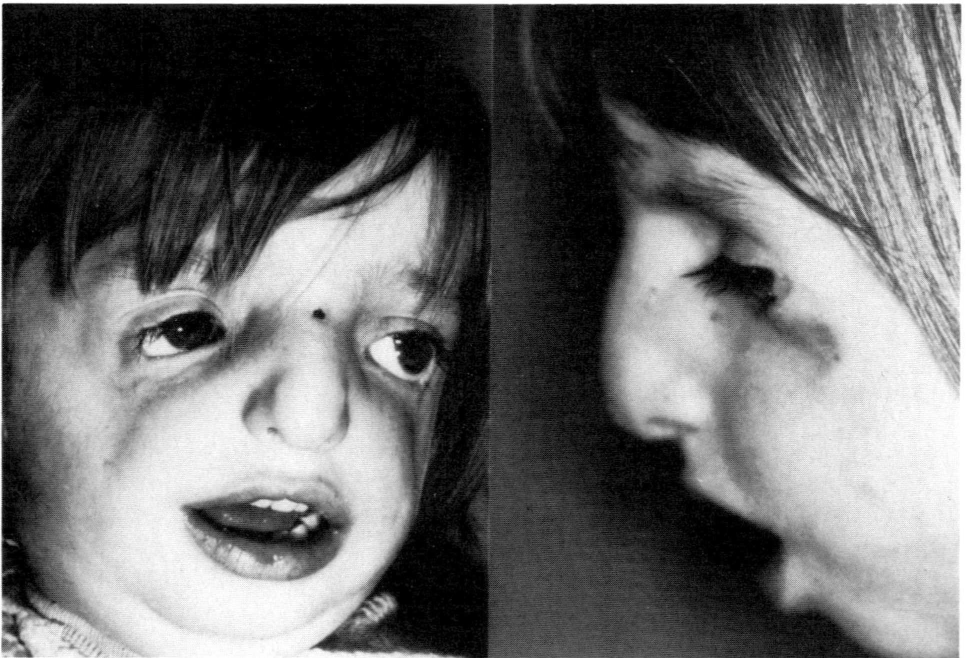

FIG 10–1.
Treacher Collins syndrome.

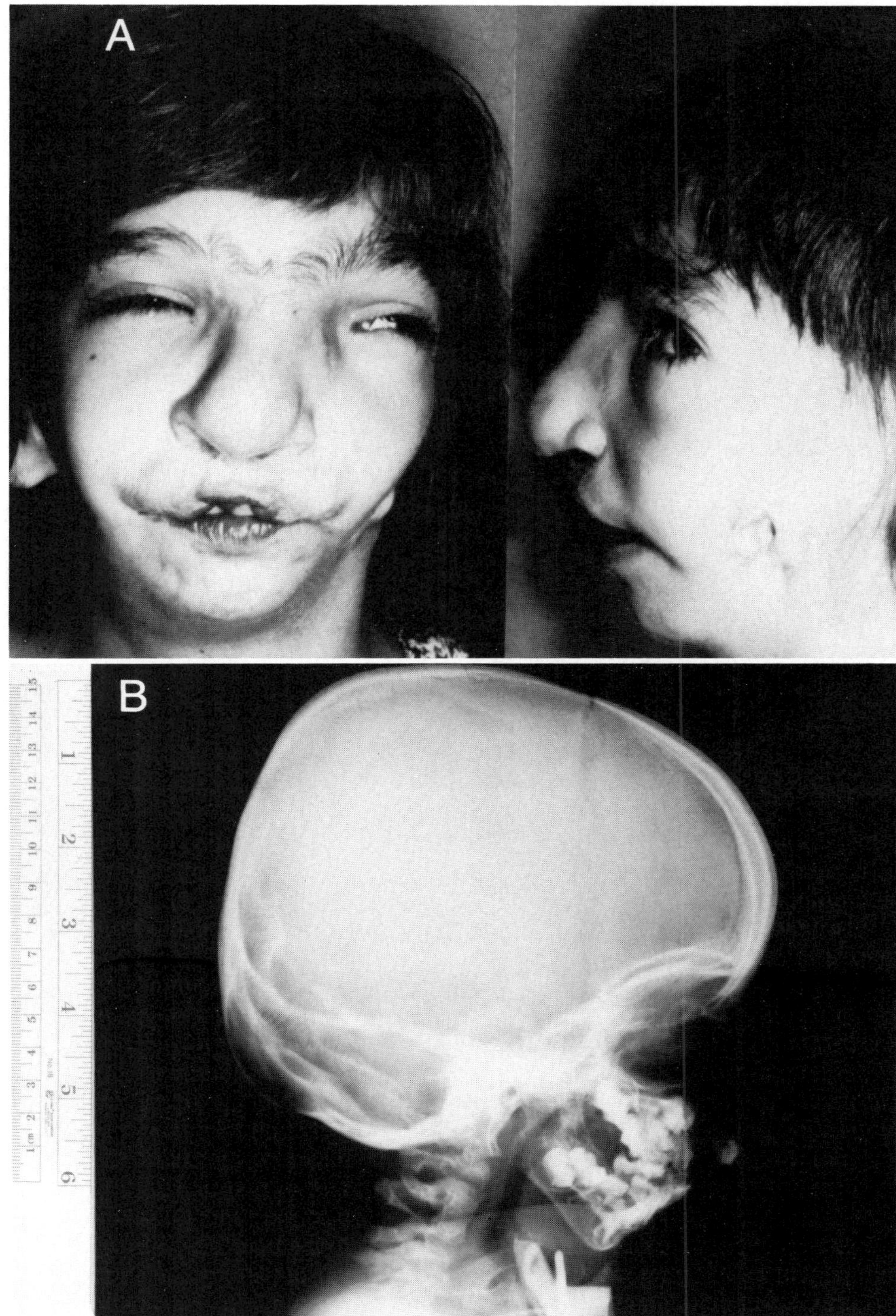

FIG 10–2.
Goldenhar's syndrome. **A,** frontal and lateral views; **B,** x-ray view.

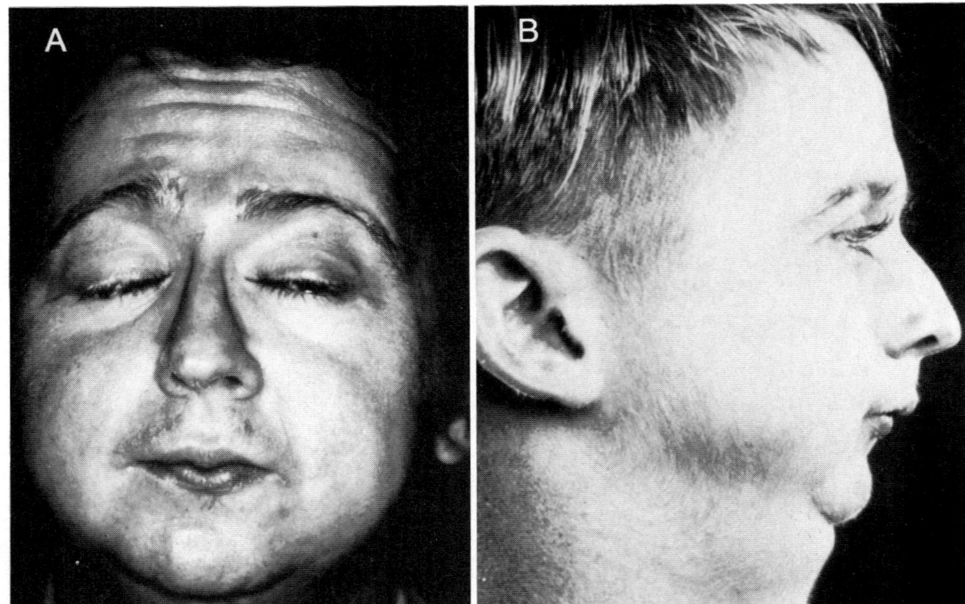

FIG 10–3.
Hallermann-Streiff-François syndrome. **A,** frontal view; **B,** profile; **C,** underlying pathologic condition.

C

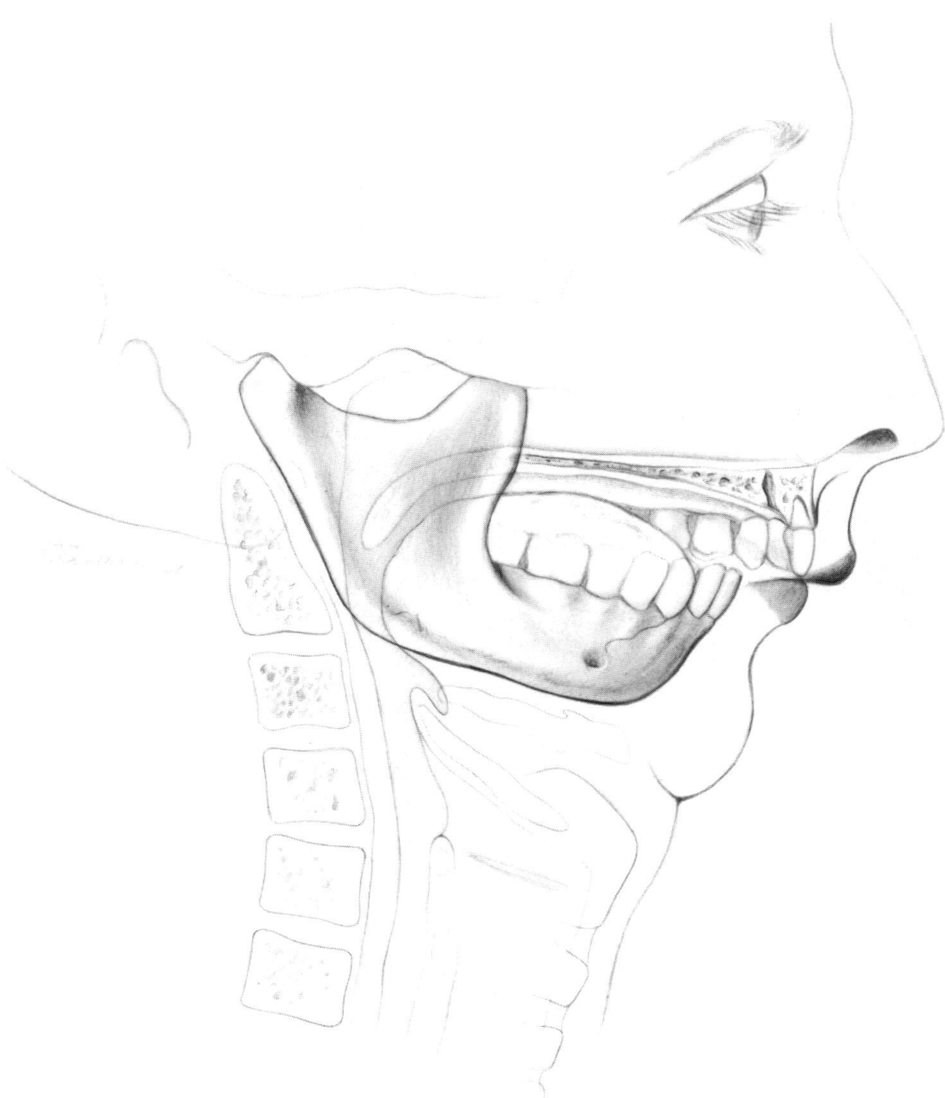

FIG 10–3   (cont.).

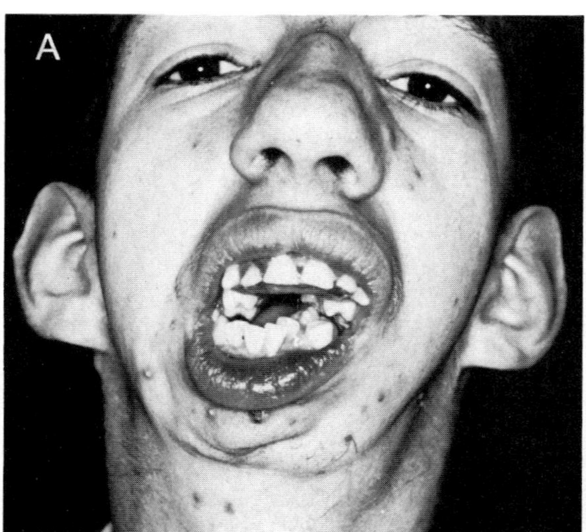
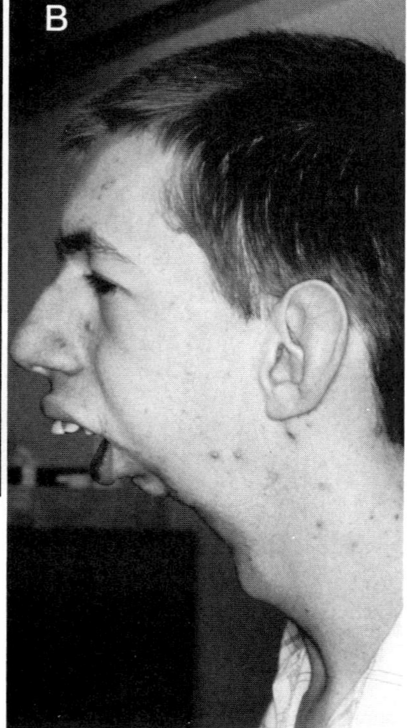

FIG 10–4.
Arthrogryposis multiplex. **A,** frontal view; **B,** profile, **C,** underlying pathologic condition. *See also* Plate 5.

C

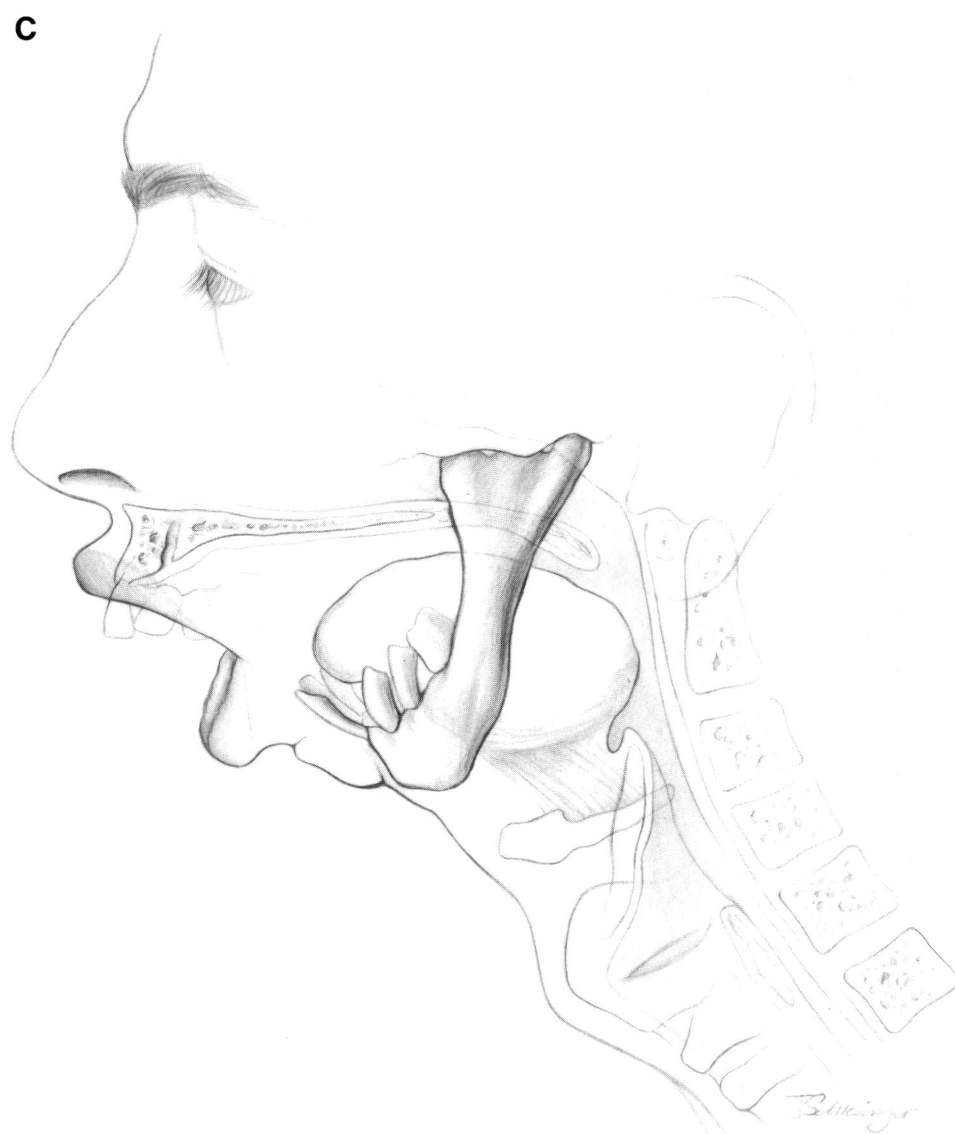

FIG 10–4 (cont.).

On initial frontal viewing of the patient with Hallermann-Streiff-François syndrome (see Fig 10–3), the most striking feature is microstomia. However, the lateral view clearly demonstrates the micrognathia and a strong indication of hyoid-to-thyroid limitation. Crouzon's syndrome (Fig 10–5) may or may not represent true micrognathia, inasmuch as this cranial malformation may occasionally give the appearance of micrognathia without its actual presence.

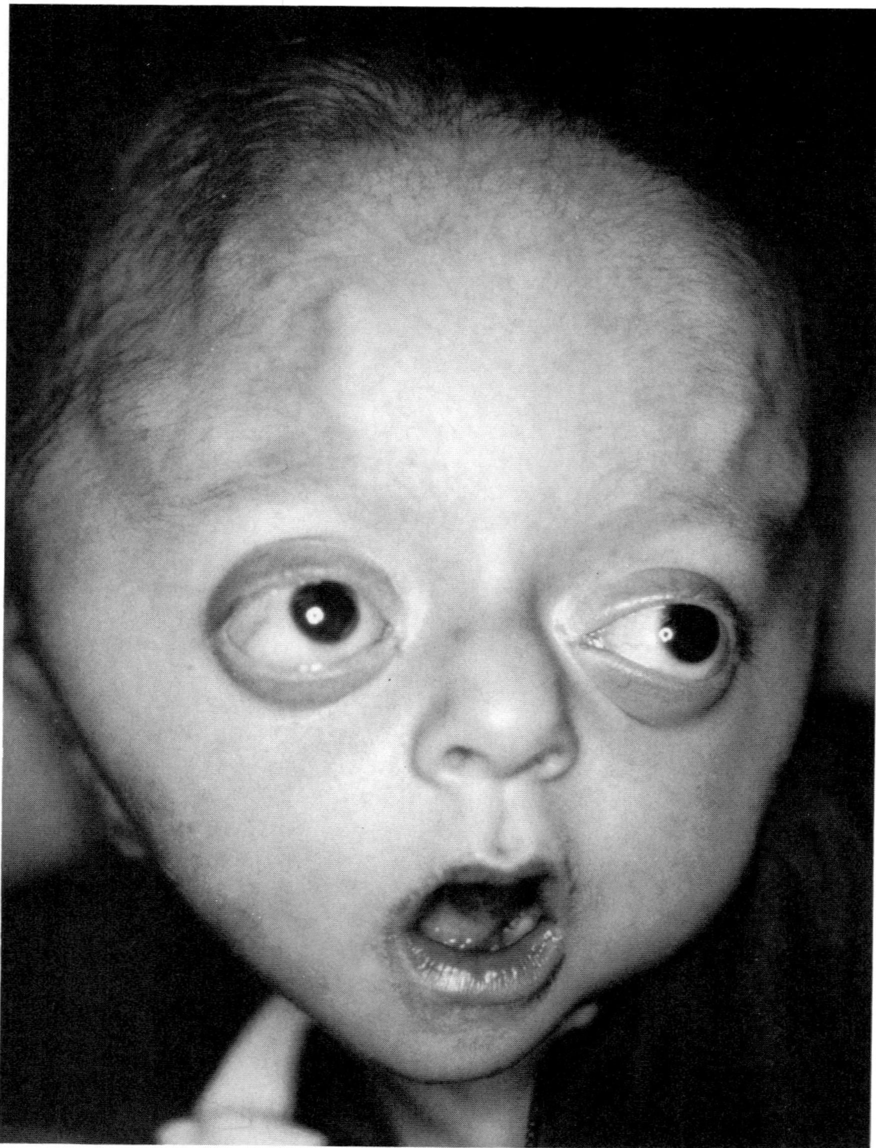

FIG 10–5.
Crouzon's syndrome.

CERVICAL SPINE

The range of mobility of the cervical spine is a major factor in the ease of endoscopy and intubation, and the successful endoscopist requires a significant understanding of its biomechanics. The complexity of this area is emphasized by the fact that there are at least 23 joints or points of contact at which motion occurs, from the occiput down to the first thoracic vertebra. All have incongruous surfaces that combine sliding and rotation with some degree of flexion.

There is more mobility at the upper and lower ends of the neck than in the midcervical region; this makes the unit concept of motion inapplicable to the cervical vertebrae. Motion in the sagittal plane is called flexion or extension, depending on the direction of movement. Motion in the transverse plane is called rotation, and motion in the frontal plane lateral bending. Average ranges are reported as flexion, 70 degrees ± 10 degrees; extension, 75 degrees ± 10 degrees; rotation, right or left, 75 degrees ± 10 degrees; and lateral bending, right or left, 45 degrees ± 10 degrees.[2] However, these studies were done in

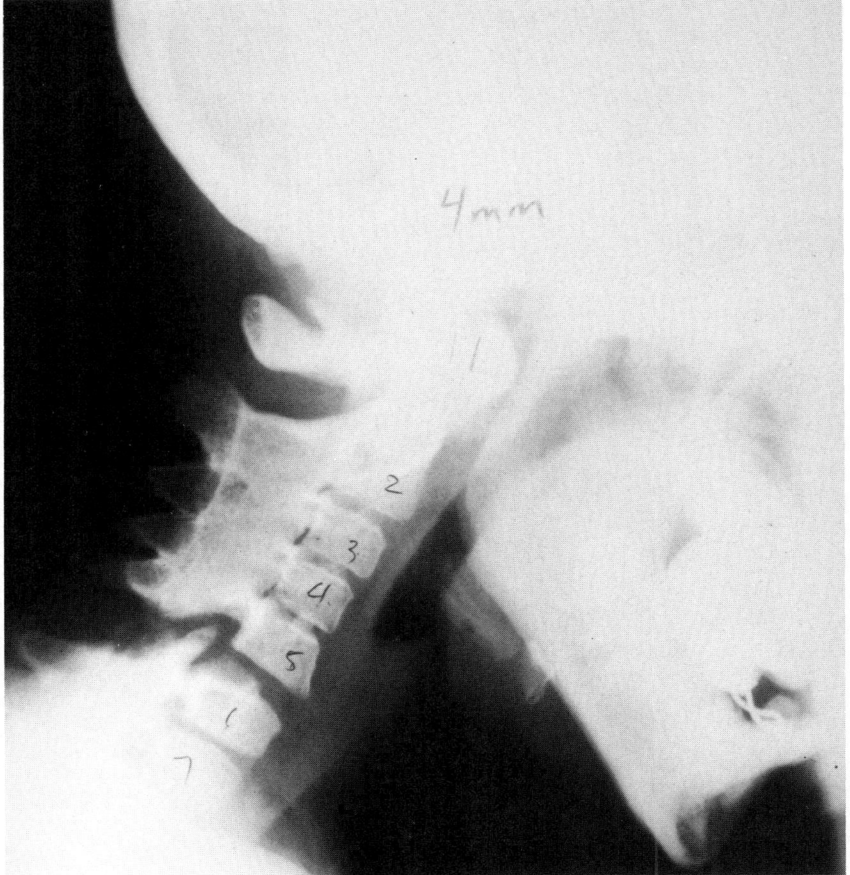

FIG 10–6.
Patient with positional movement risk caused by hypermobility at interspace C5-6.

young persons without disability. In older people mobility is gradually lost, starting perhaps as early as age 25 to 29 years.

The greatest amount of flexion-extension occurs in the interspace between the fifth and sixth cervical vertebrae, plus or minus one vertebra. In flexion each vertebra below the axis shifts anteriorly on the subjacent vertebra. In extension the vertebrae shift posteriorly. This produces a diagonal inclination. The atlantoaxial atlas can rotate on the axis approximately 45 degrees in either direction. The remaining 30 degrees of rotation occurs between the lower cervical vertebrae.[3] Nonradiologic measurements of this motion suggest that a gravity goniometer or protractor is the most convenient instrument, although certainly not the most exacting, for estimating the flexion-extension position of the relatively spherical head.

The positional movement of the atlantoaxial axis must be considered when the patient is prepared for endoscopy, especially in the supine position.

A particularly striking example of positional movement risk is presented in one of our patients (Fig 10–6).[4] This patient was referred to us for management of a proposed total hip replacement, with the notation that he could not open his mouth very widely. However, when we reviewed his radiographs we noted that the C-1 and C-2 vertebrae were fused, C-2 and C-3 moved relatively normally, the transverse processes of C3 to C5 were totally fused, and there was marked laxity of ligaments in the C5-6 interspace. There was serious hypermobility at C5-6, which presented the hazard of trauma to the spinal cord on movement of the head to the traditional position for endotracheal intubation. This case demonstrates the need to comprehensively examine any patient with any of the indications of airway access problems.

Striking cervical spinal problems are found in osteoarthritis (ankylosing spondylitis, Fig 10–7), juvenile rheumatoid arthritis (Fig 10–8), and Klippel-Feil syndrome (Fig 10–9). Atlantoaxial instability (Fig 10–10) represents another problem in the cervical area. This problem is primarily, but not solely,

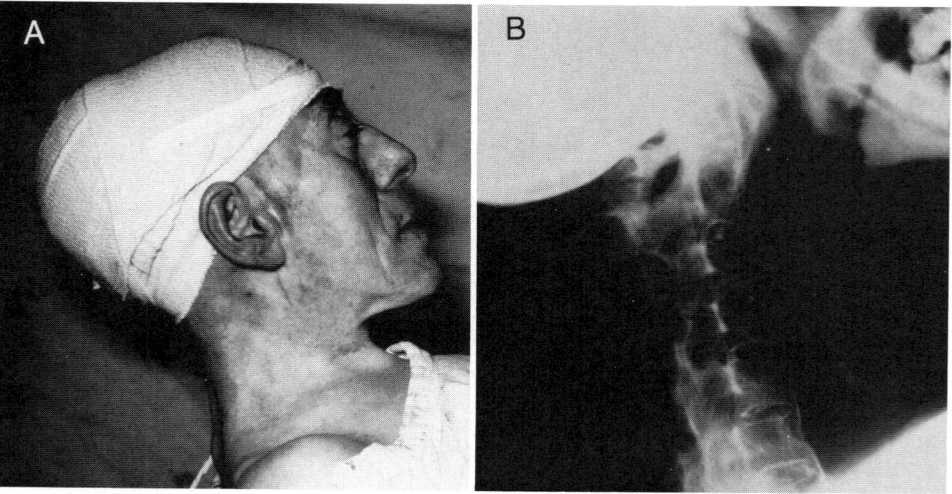

FIG 10–7.
Ankylosing spondylitis. **A,** note fixation of cervical spine with the patient supine. **B,** x-ray view.

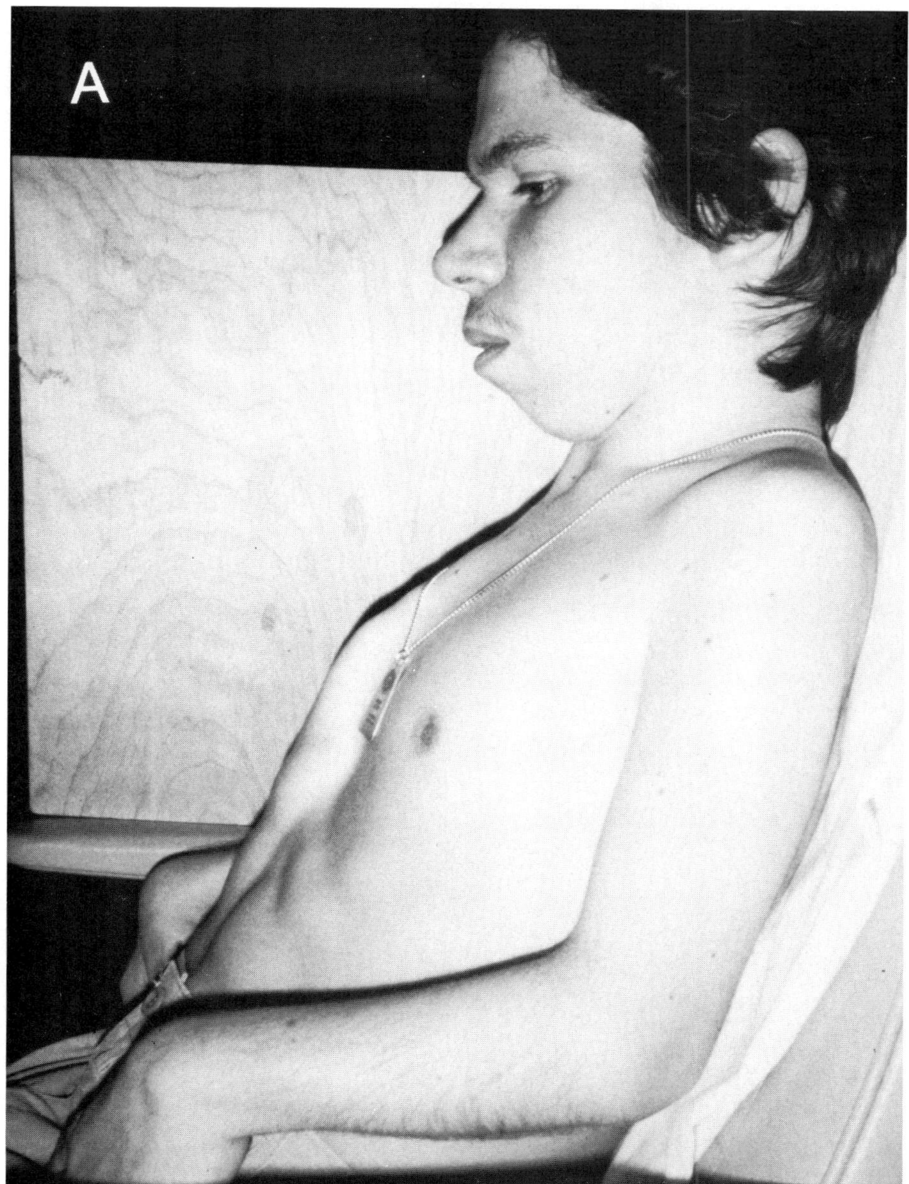

FIG 10–8.
Juvenile rheumatoid arthritis. **A,** Photograph of patient; **B,** underlying pathologic condition; **C,** x-ray view.

B

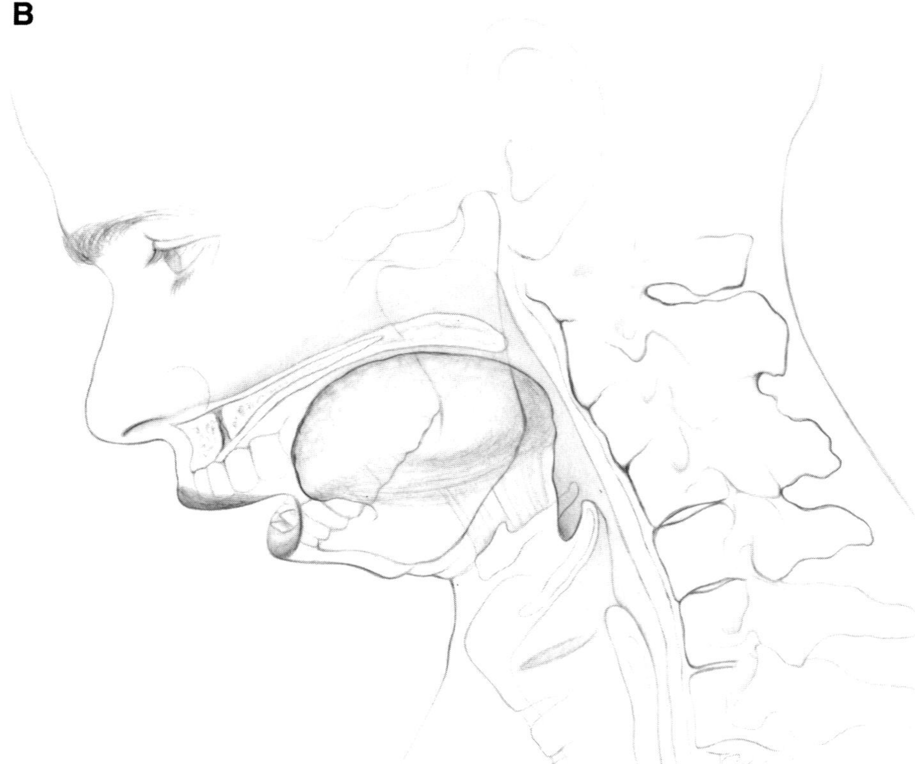

FIG 10−8 **(cont.).**

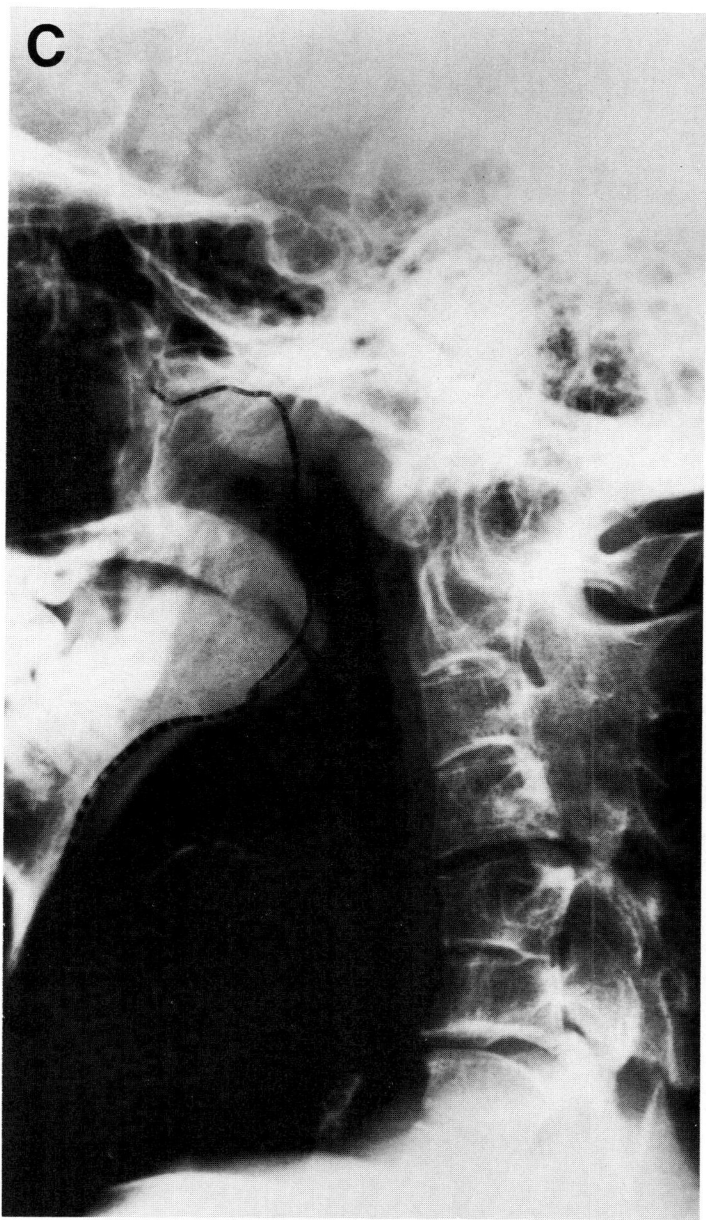

FIG 10–8 **(cont.).**

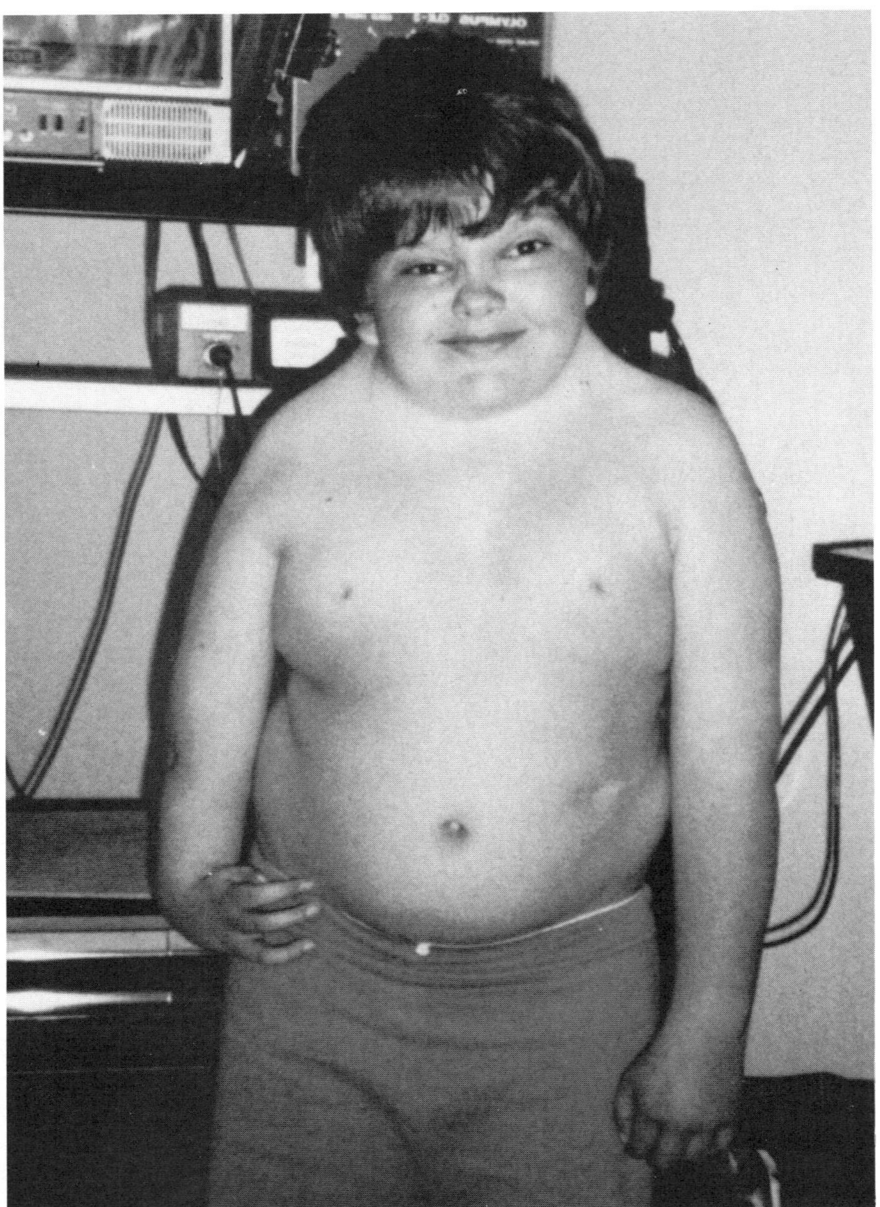

FIG 10–9.
Klippel-Feil syndrome.

found in women more than 40 years of age who have rheumatoid arthritis and have been receiving corticosteroid therapy for a long time.[4] A serious complication is subluxation of the atlantoaxial joint, which may lead to compression of the spinal cord by the odontoid process.

This joint should also be considered in patients with varying types of dwarfism, because of the high incidence of cervical spine maldevelopment. Another odontoid process problem is found in patients with osteoporosis, spe-

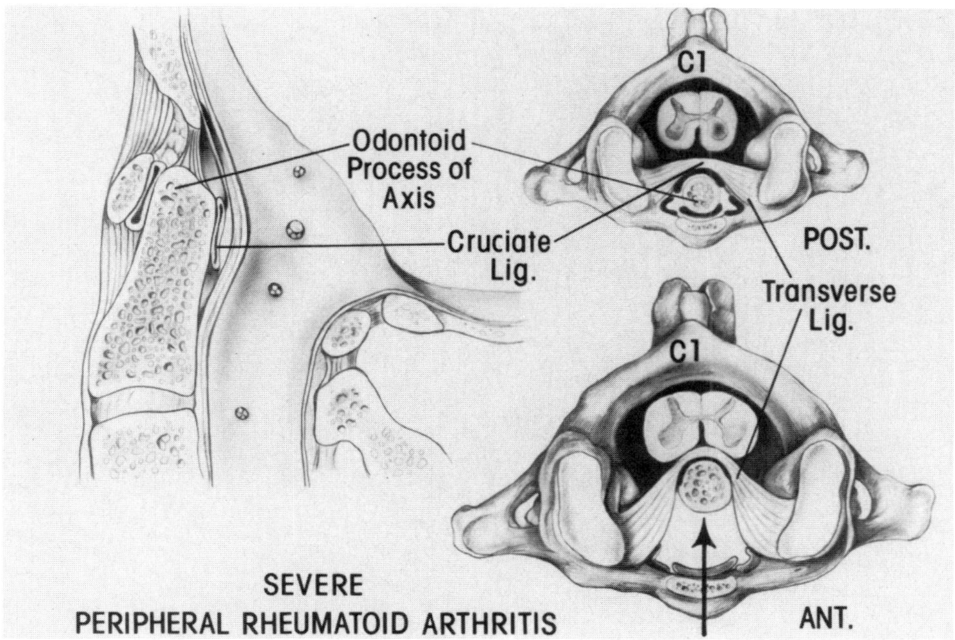

FIG 10–10.
Atlantoaxial instability.

cifically Paget's disease. With osteoporotic concerns and changes caused by Paget's disease in the odontoid process, hyperextension can produce fractures of the odontoid and subsequent cervical cord trauma during extension. The common practice of manually manipulating the head to maximal hyperextension for endoscopy is particularly risky.

REFERENCES

1. Randall P: The Robin sequence: Micrognathia and glossoptosis with airway obstruction, in *Plastic Surgery*, vol 4. *Cleft Lip and Palate and Craniofacial Abnormalities.* Philadelphia, WB Saunders Co, 1990, pp 3123–3125.
2. Kottke FJ, Mundale MO: Range of mobility of the cervical spine. *Arch Phys Med* 1959; 40:379–382.
3. Fielding JW: Cineroentgenography of the normal cervical spine. *J Bone Joint Surg* 1957; 39A:1280.
4. Norton ML, Ghanma NA: Atlantoaxial instability revisited: An alert for endoscopists. *Ann Otol Rhinol Laryngol* 1978; 87:554–557.

Chapter 11

Soft Tissue Considerations in the Difficult Airway

Martin L. Norton

The discussion of soft tissue concerns during airway intubation includes conditions that both directly and indirectly assert influences on the airway. In addition to lesions that are well-known causes of difficult intubations, those that may not usually be associated with difficult airway problems are examined.

MACROGLOSSIA AND GLOSSOPTOSIS

Macroglossia and glossoptosis are two syndromes that have a major influence on our ability to visualize the larynx as well as other structures of the oropharynx, esophagopharynx, and laryngopharynx. Macroglossia refers to enlargement of the tongue; glossoptosis is downward and backward displacement of the tongue to the point of close approximation of the basal tongue to the posterior pharyngeal wall. Among many diseases or syndromes that manifest this feature are dwarfism, hemangiopericytoma (Plate 6), Down syndrome, lymphangioma, cretinism, and amyloidosis.

It is important to note that these syndromes may take many forms; the tongue in amyloidosis may be enlarged, and it may also become stiffened and firm to palpation as well as being equally obstructive. In all of these we are obligated to conceptualize the function of the tongue in relation to the oropharyngeal structures and mechanisms of swallowing and respiration (See descriptions in Chapters 8, 12, and 13.) Similarly, an achondroplastic dwarf may appear perfectly normal externally and indeed esthetically beautiful of face, but a complete examination will reveal glossoptosis in most of these patients.

OTHER SOFT TISSUE PROBLEMS

Two other examples of specific soft tissue problems encroaching on the airway are best visualized from a computed tomography (CT) scan of the airway. The first (Fig 11–1) is a postsurgical problem. A carcinoma of the floor of the mouth had been excised widely, with the tongue sutured to the floor of the mouth over the defect. When I saw the patient she was unable to advance her tongue, and the basal portion lay quite posterior. The consequences included fixation of the epiglottis, an obvious consequence in view of the anatomic relationship of the epiglottis and the tongue.

The extent of the problem was more clearly elucidated after review of the lateral view of a flat plate of the airway (see Fig 11–2). The base of the tongue was clearly delineated with the wings of the hyoid in direct and close approximation to the base of the tongue. This produced a situation most anesthesiologists call "anterior larynx" but that is more correctly called "superior larynx." My view differs from that of Sivardjan and Fink, who find the hyoid bone and epiglottis shifted anteriorly.[1] However, the patients they cited were all in the supine position with extended necks. Our dynamic fluoroscopic studies show a shift cephalad (superiorly) with change in position from the upright (sitting) position to the supine position. I submit that the differences observed by

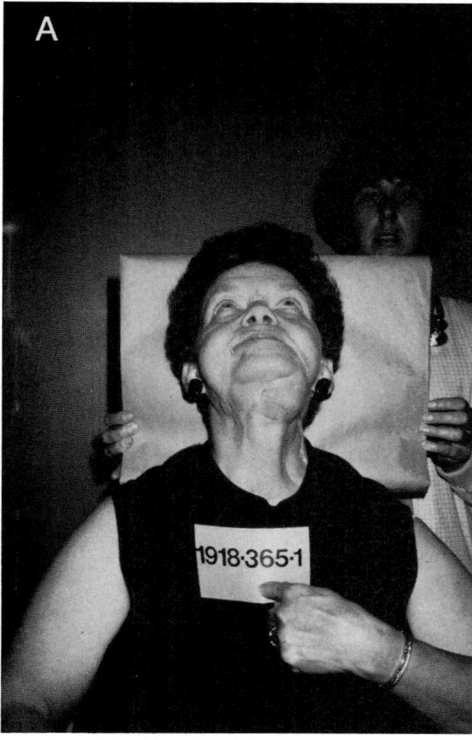

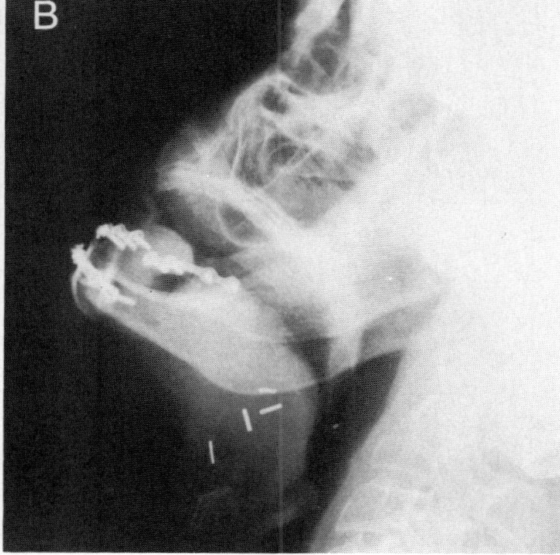

FIG 11–1.
A, postsurgical patient with carcinoma of the floor of the mouth. **B,** lateral flat plate radiograph of the patient in **A** (note clips).

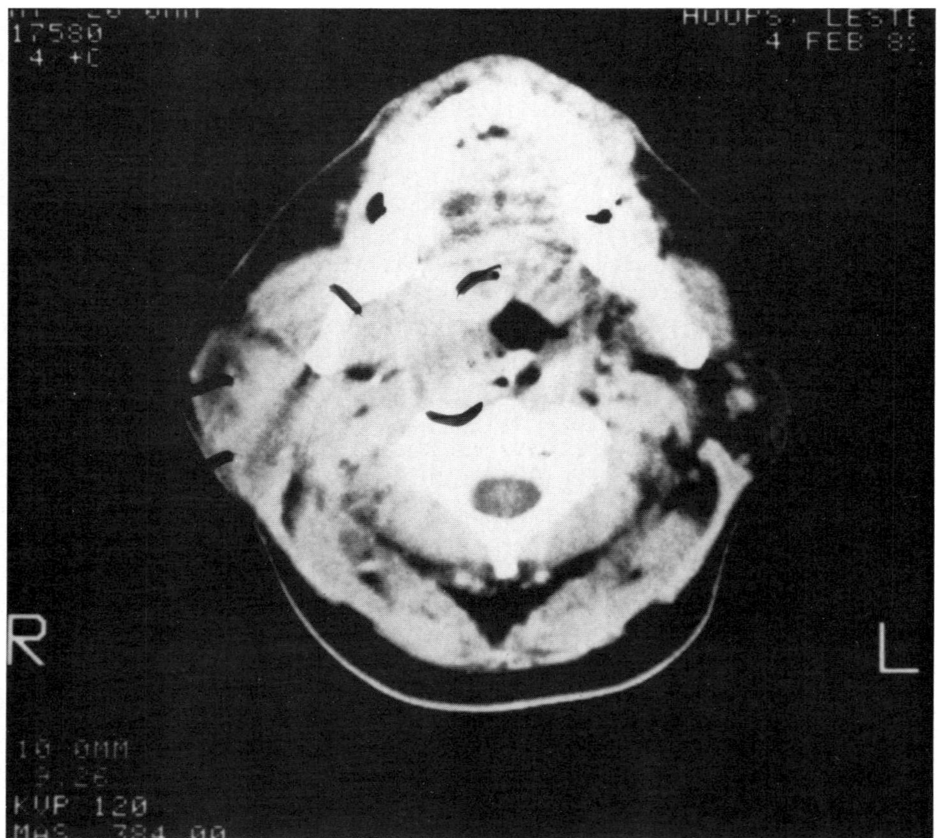

FIG 11–2.
CT scan of a neck mass under the right angle of the ramus of the mandible.

Sivardjan and Fink were more related to collapse of the ventral (anterior) structures because of loss of the suspensory mechanism secondary to general anesthesia and muscle relaxation.

Further review of the pathway that the endotracheal tube would have to traverse demonstrated a Z-shaped channel. This patient also had keloids of the neck, which to some extent limited head motion.

After fiberoptic transnasal intubation I noted a very strong reflex pattern with a Müller 4 test (see Chapter 12 for a discussion of Müller's test). This response was so severe that at times it was not possible to advance the fiberscope or the nasotracheal tube. Transit was accomplished by synchronizing the advance while encouraging the awake patient to exert deep respiratory efforts.

Another patient had a mass of the neck under the right angle of the ramus of the mandible. On further examination I noted that the mass encroached on the airway at the level of the pharynx. Digital palpation indicated that there was an extension behind the last molar and in the posterior pharynx to the midline and down the pharynx along the midline to the point that I was able to touch the epiglottis. It was interesting to note that the patient had no gag reflex on palpation over this area. The left side of the midline was totally free of the mass to palpation, and there was a very active gag reflex. Review of the CT scan (Fig 11–2) confirmed my clinical impression and provided support for the conclusion that access to the airway by the oral route was possible using a left-handed Macintosh blade with an intubation guide (Norton Teflon or Eschmann woven) for insertion of the endotracheal tube.

NEUROFIBROMATOSIS AND MUMPS

Figure 11–3 shows a case of extensive neurofibromatosis in a child. The problem in this case is merely soft tissue in a space-occupying context.

Following this is a depiction of parotitis, or mumps (Fig 11–4), which be-

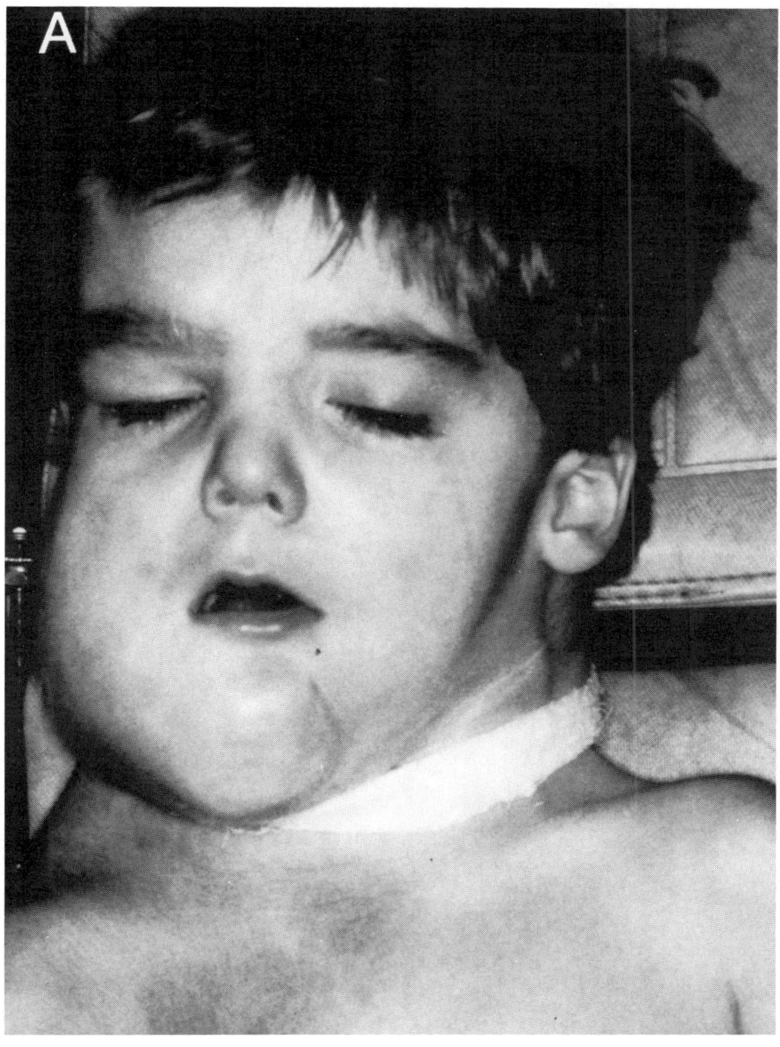

FIG 11–3.
A, patient with neurofibromatosis; **B,** underlying pathologic condition.

B

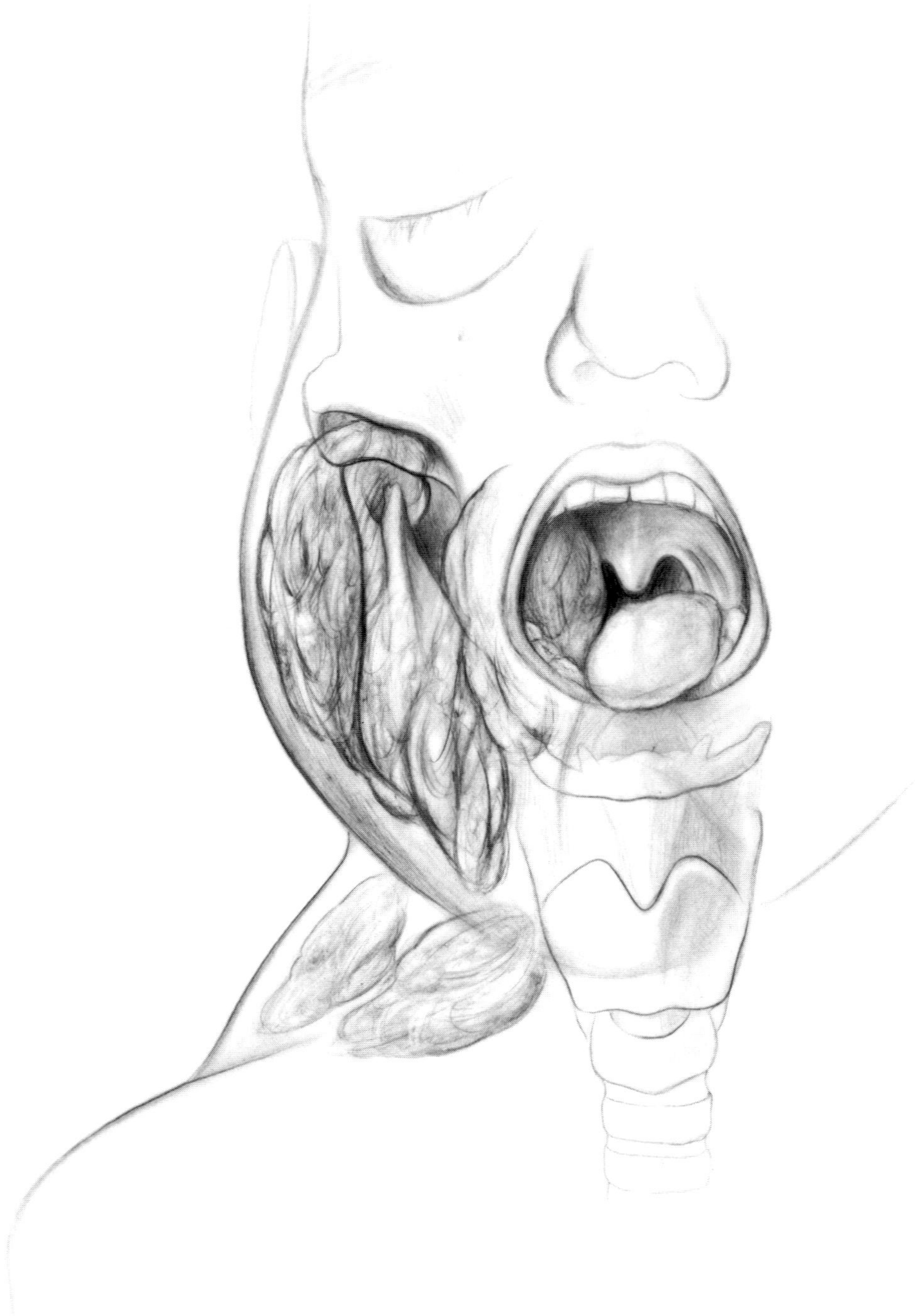

FIG 11–3   **(cont.).**

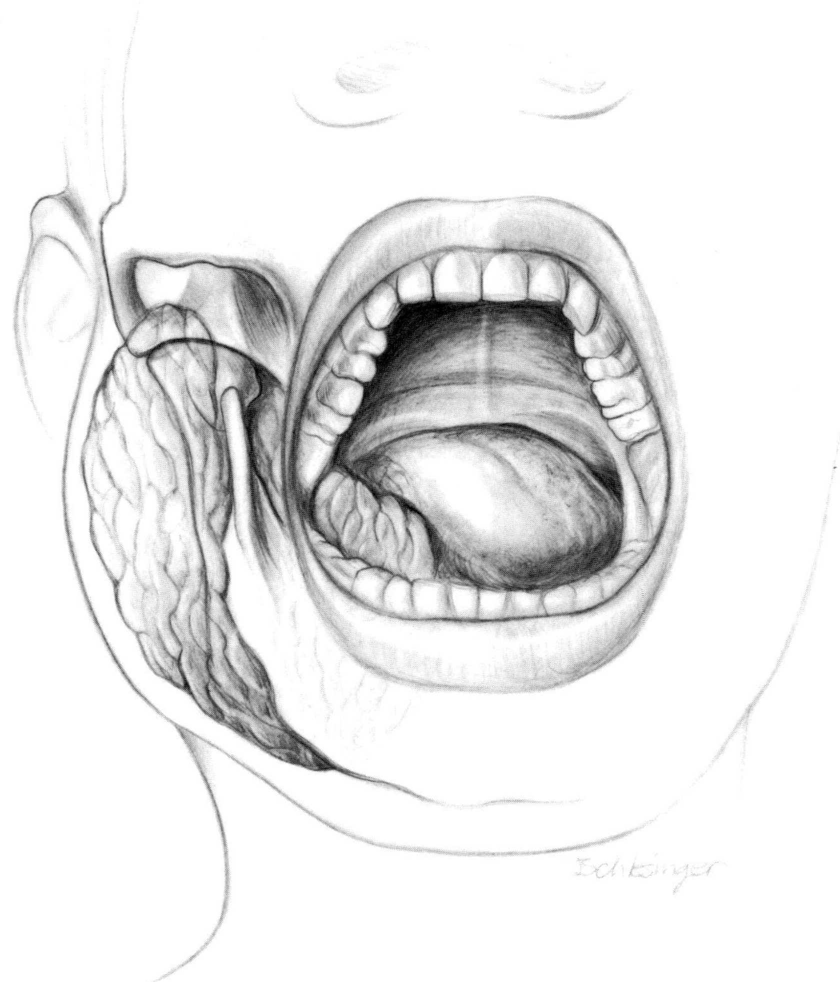

FIG 11–4.
Mumps (parotitis).

sides its soft tissue–occupying component produces pain referred to the temporomandibular joint (TMJ) and ear canal with trismus.

NEUROMUSCULAR DISORDERS

Occasionally other disease processes will present airway considerations. Figure 11–5 demonstrates central core myopathy with continuous hyperlordosis. It underlines the fact that late diagnosis of neurologic and myopathic disorders may have far-reaching effects on bony development, which in this case radically affects access to the airway.

In another representative case access to the airway was obtained by a ret-

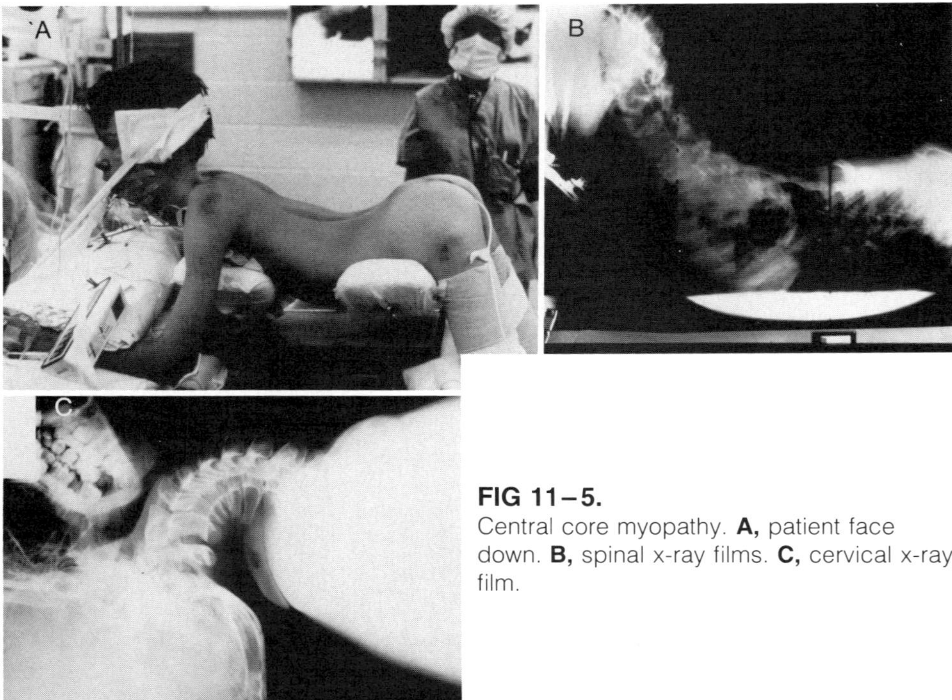

FIG 11–5.
Central core myopathy. **A,** patient face down. **B,** spinal x-ray films. **C,** cervical x-ray film.

rograde wire technique. The wire was passed through the membrane between the cricoid and first tracheal cartilage. It was visualized through the mouth, and partially pulled out through the mouth to enable the fiberoptic endoscope (on which a suitable endotracheal tube had been threaded) to be itself threaded onto the wire. Then, with the wire used as a guide (not a stylet), the fiberoptic endoscope was advanced visually into the trachea and the endotracheal tube was moved into position.

MISCELLANEOUS SOFT TISSUE PROBLEMS

The endoscopist is often faced with soft tissue problems not immediately related to the airway. Examples of these are lesions affecting movement of the neck. This patient had pain in the neck, positioning of the head as in torticollis, and tingling sensation in the hands on rotation of the head but not on flexion-extension. A review of her CT scan (Fig 11–6) at the level of C-1 and C-2 demonstrated an extrinsic mass eroding the ramus of the body of the C-1 vertebra and extending into the epidural space. Based on visual examination, the endoscopist could not have suspected the hazard of standard rigid blade endoscopy merely by the external appearance of the patient. The maneuver used by many endoscopists, placing one hand under the chin with the other pushing downward on the top of the head, risked driving the odontoid process up into the medulla oblongata because of the weakening of the structural integrity of the C-1 vertebra.

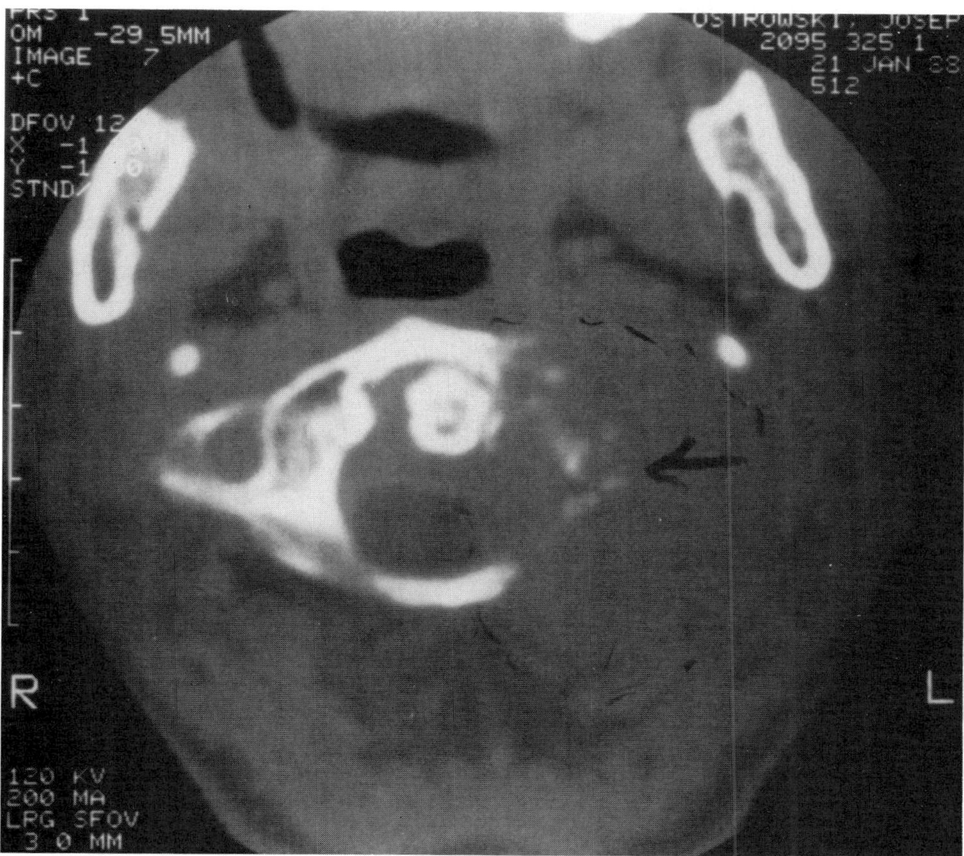

FIG 11–6.
CT scan of an extrinsic mass eroding the ramus of body of C-1 vertebra, extending into the epidural space.

This particular problem may also occur with other pathologic processes involving the dens, such as fractures, Paget's disease, extreme osteoporosis, and most frequently in patients with platybasia, softening of the skull bones, resulting in the floor of the posterior cranial fossa bulging upward in the region of the foramen magnum.

Therefore it is incumbent on the endoscopist not to use this maneuver routinely for positioning the patient for rigid blade laryngoscopy. Habits in and of themselves can sometimes lead to disaster!

A rare condition, fibrofascial myositis ossificans progressiva (Fig 11–7), presented an unusual problem. This disease of unknown origin consists of bone formation within muscles. It starts as an interstitial fibromyositis, and ultimately osteoid and cartilage formations develop in the connective tissue, enclosing intact muscle fibers. With progression, limitation of movement, contractures, deformities, scoliosis, rigidity of the spine, abnormal posture, and limited expansion of the thorax occur. (This condition should be differentiated from calcinosis universalis, in which calcium deposits in the skin, subcutaneous tissues, and connective tissue sheaths around muscles usually occur in re-

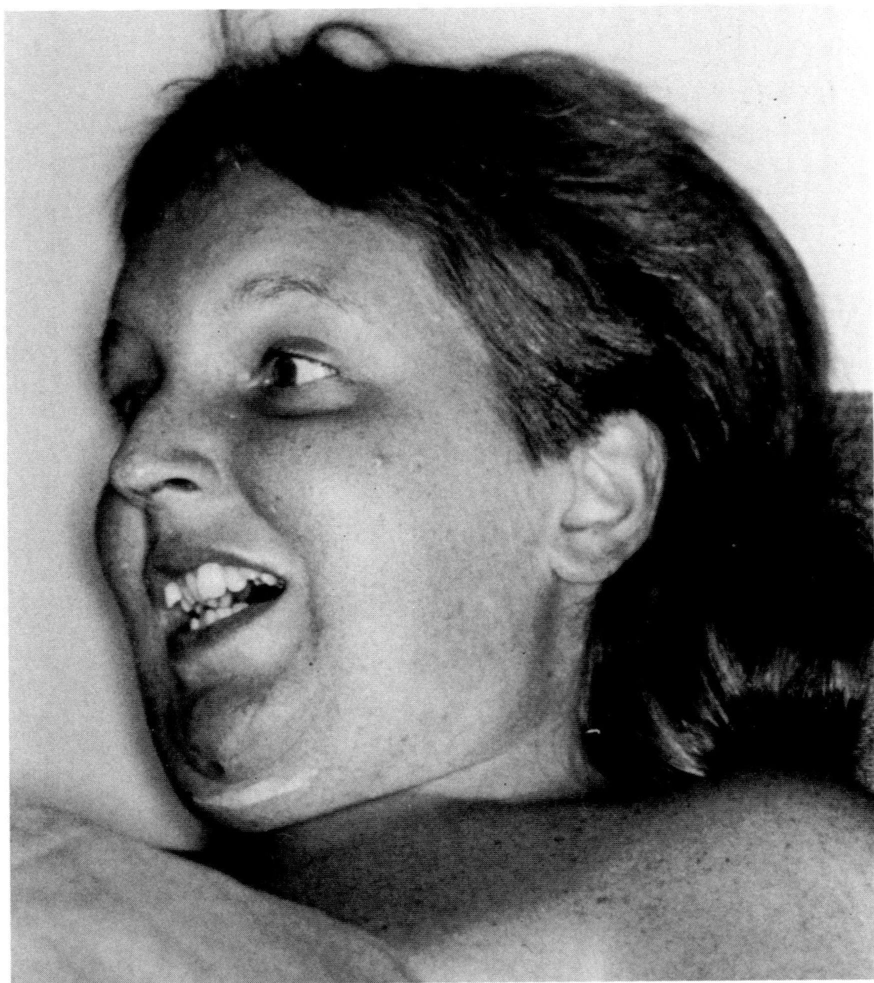

FIG 11–7.
Patient with fibrofascial myositis ossificans progressiva. Note maximal mouth opening with cervical spinal fixation.

lation to scleroderma or polymyositis. However, this differentiation is by no means clear-cut.)

This patient had no movement of skeletal musculature. She could move only her fingers, lips, and eyelids and had limited function of the tongue. Her pharyngeal musculature was progressively weakening, although it still was possible for her to suck nutritive fluids through a straw. She was referred for consideration of airway access to allow teeth to be removed for placement of that straw. She had very limited motion at the TMJ, and her masseter muscles were significantly invaded and rigid. Still, she could communicate, working from an adapted electrically controlled wheelchair, and she was mentally alert and functioning at a high intellectual level, although obviously euphoric.

Airway access through the oropharynx was almost impossible, and the route available was determined to be through the nasotracheal pathway. It is important to note that she had a Müller 2 test result, which confirmed the limitation of pharyngeal muscle activity.

An analogous patient with a diagnosis of dermatomyositis and calcinosis universalis (Fig 11–8; Plate 7) had similar signs and symptoms, but because of the added problem of dermatomyositis, intravenous access was extremely difficult. However, this patient showed no sign of bony cervical limitation, only hardening of the cervical soft tissues, caused by the calcinosis, and the nasotracheal access route was patent.

A major factor to be addressed is the postglossectomy, post–radical neck surgery, postradiation situation, particularly where there is a degree of induration, fixation of the tongue, and approximation of the hyoid to the base of the tongue or plastic flap substituting as the floor of the mouth (Fig 11–9). Access

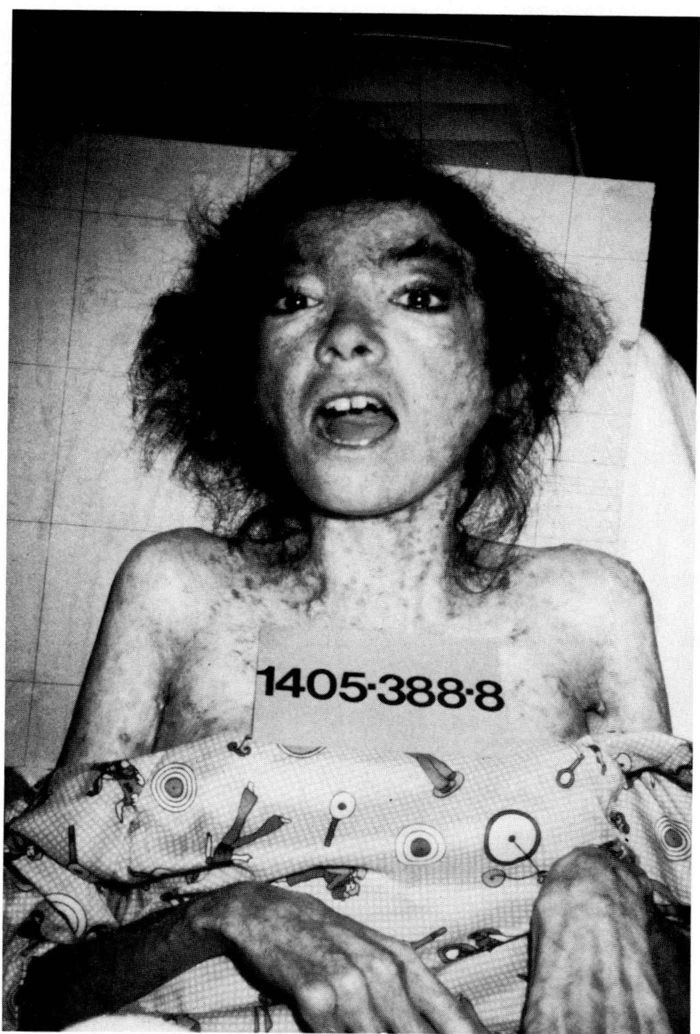

FIG 11–8.
Patient with dermatomyositis and calcinosis universalis.

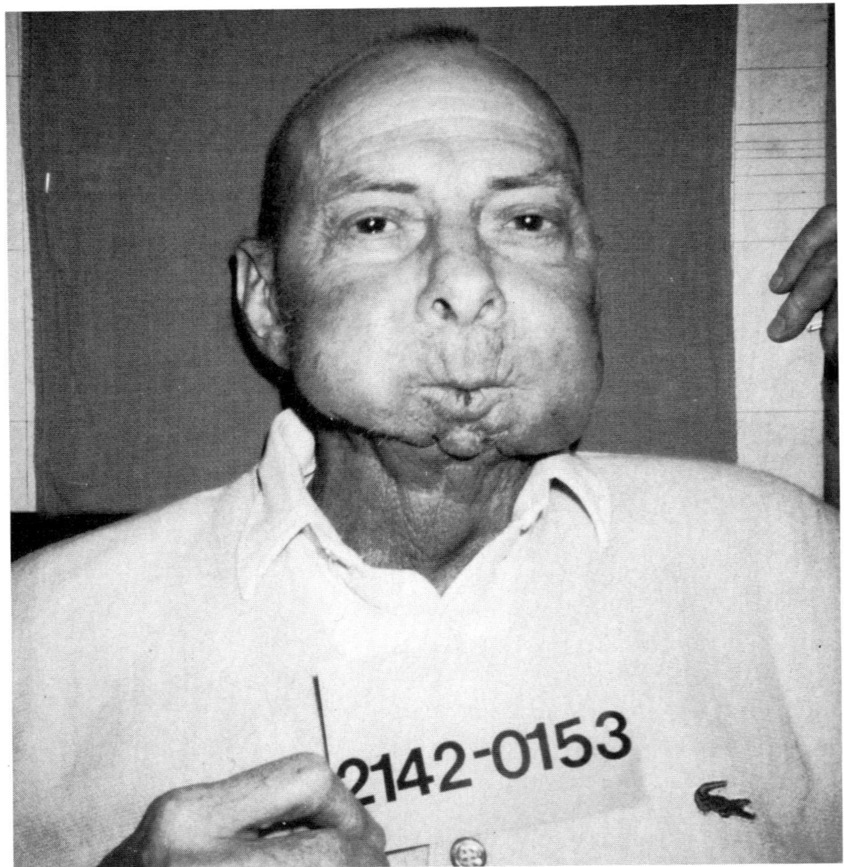

FIG 11–9.
Patient after glossectomy, mandibulectomy, radical neck surgery, and radiation.

to the airway will be limited by the lack of compressibility of the tongue, extreme angulation required in the posterior pharyngeal area to approach the additus laryngis, and potential edema after endoscopy or intubation causing further obstruction. This will be the case even though radiographs taken with the patient awake and sitting demonstrate a patent airway.

Oral access will be extremely limited, and nasofiberoptic access may prove to be the only "noninvasive" approach. The degree of postradiation induration, concomitant inflammation with submucosal fibrositis, and distortion of the normal anatomy can be extreme, even leading to total airway obstruction. Failure to do a complete evaluation, which includes fiberoptic visualization of all structures (including the trachea and dynamic C-arm fluoroscopic studies in the sitting as well as supine positions with deep breathing and swallowing maneuvers), can lead to dangerously erroneous conclusions regarding management.

Of equal if not greater consequence is the postsurgical situation (e.g., after biopsy of the base of tongue, manipulation of the pharyngeal tissues for rigid blade access or other purposes, and postintubation laryngeal edema). The better part of valor is often to recommend an awake tracheostomy or, at most,

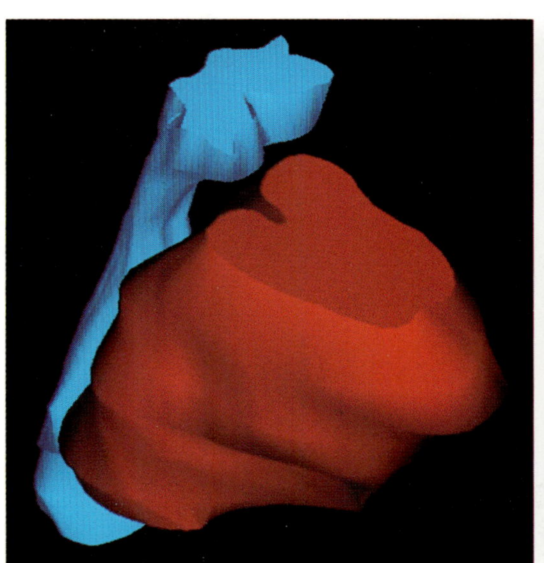 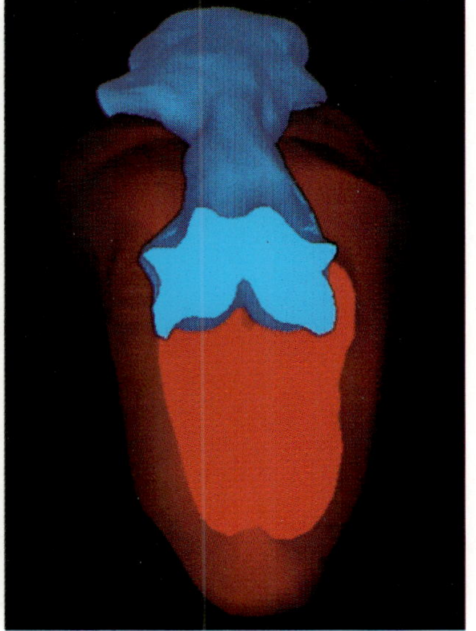

LATERAL VIEW   SUPERIOR VIEW

	Patient	OSA (N = 50)		Control (N = 4)	
		MEAN	S.D.	MEAN	S.D.
Volume (cc)					
Tongue Volume	96.86	94.54	17.56	84.57	6.29
Total Airway Volume	37.37	38.61	9.83	41.79	5.02
Partial Airway Volume	17.35	19.78	5.16	17.91	6.15
Soft Palate Volume	11.21	9.64	2.60	7.64	3.10
Ratio					
Partial Airway to Tongue Volume	0.18	0.21	0.07	0.21	0.08
Soft Palate to Tongue Volume	0.12	0.13	0.18	0.09	0.04
Soft Palate to Partial Airway	0.65	0.52	0.18	0.46	0.22

PLATE 1.

Obstructive sleep apnea case assessment. Patient has retruded maxilla and mandible and high total face height.

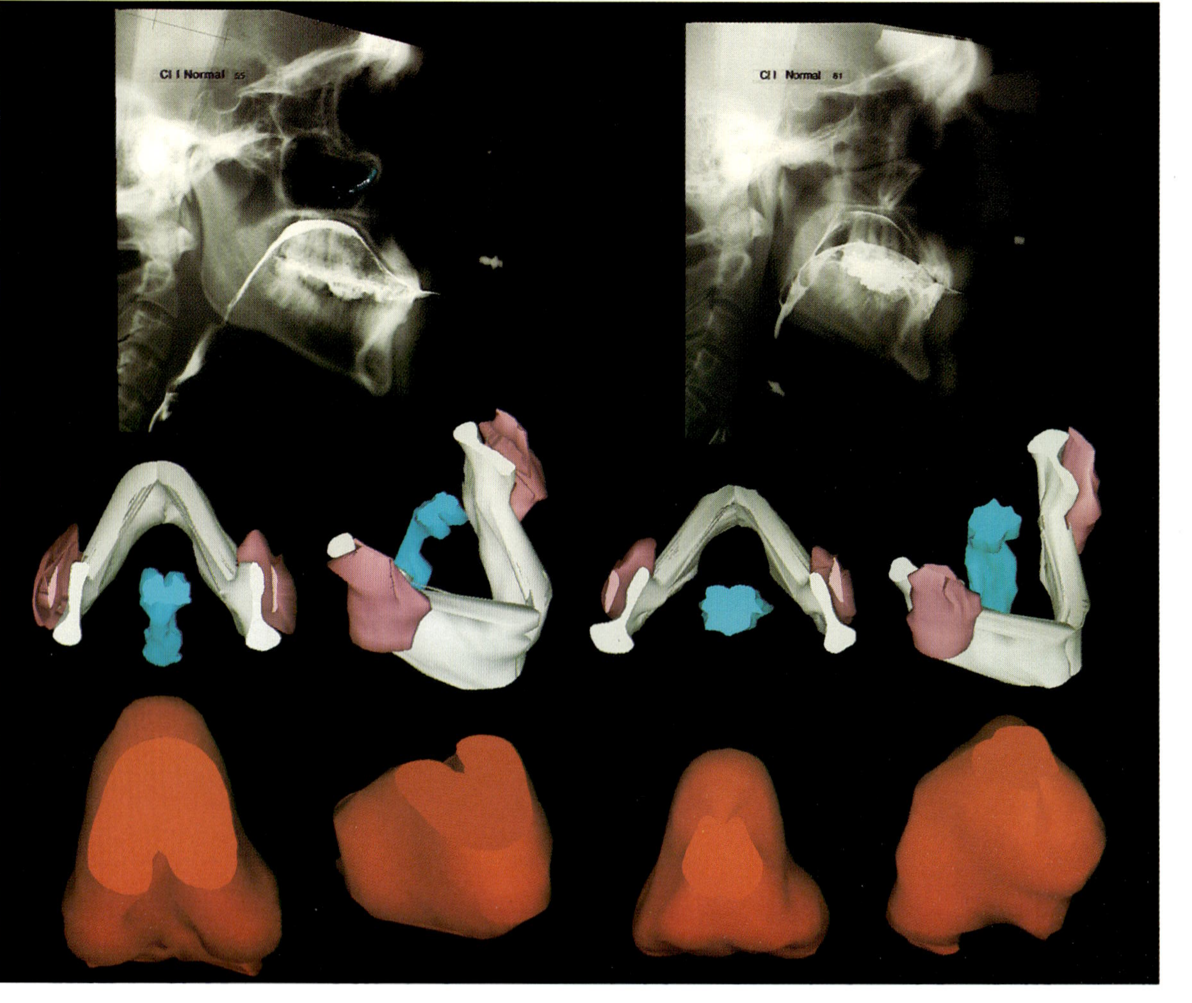

PLATE 2.
Lateral cephalograms and superior and lateral 3D views of two skeletally matched OSA patients with cephalometric values within normal range for class I.

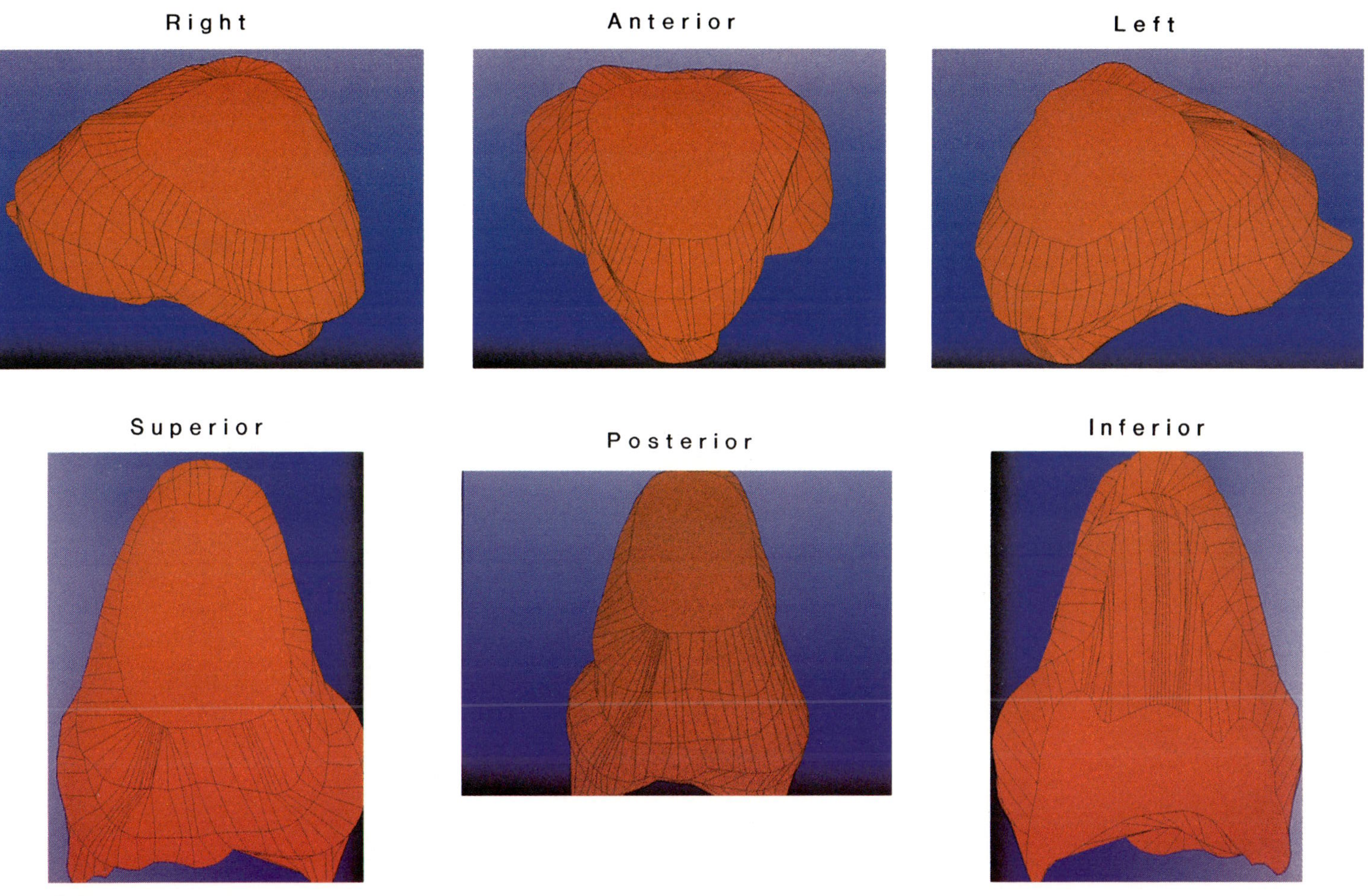

PLATE 3.
Three-dimensional color surface reconstructions of the tongue.

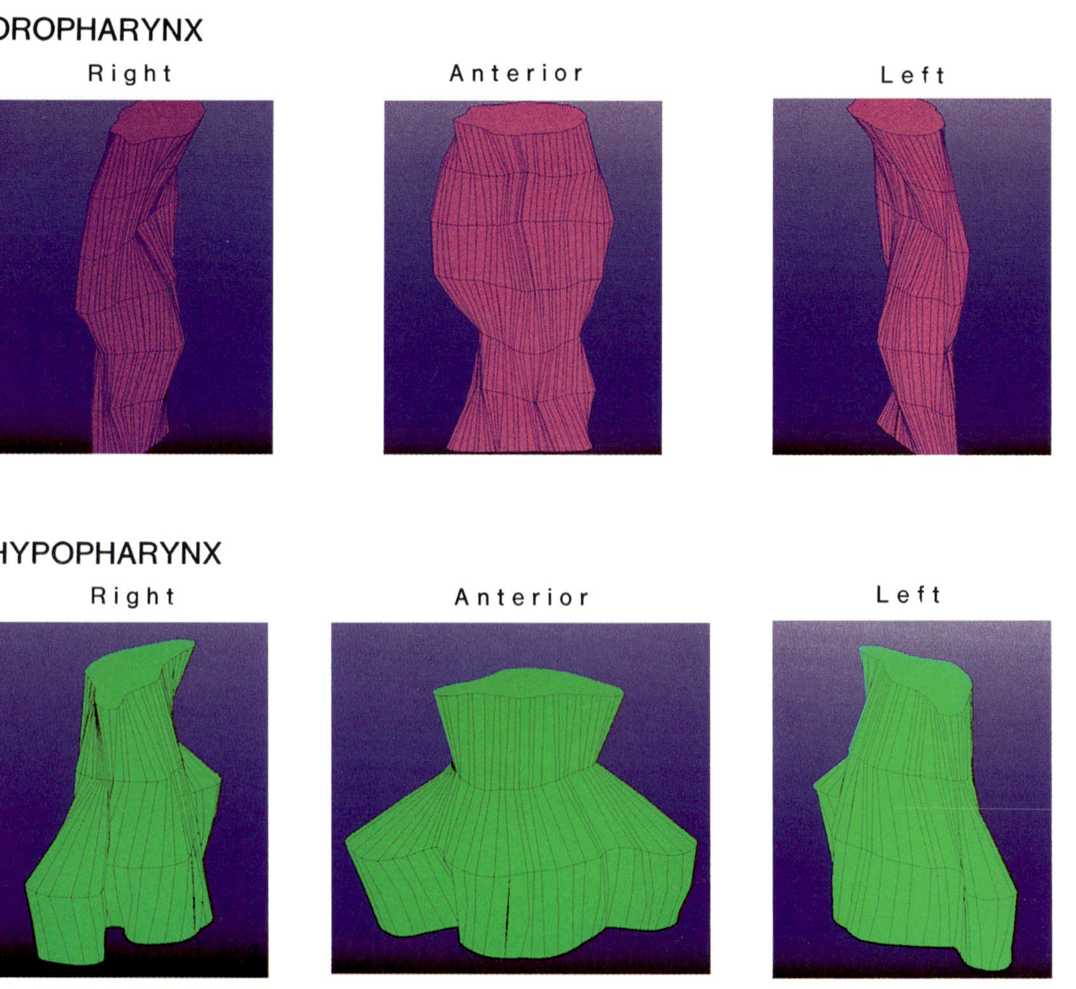

PLATE 4.
Three-dimensional color surface reconstructions of oropharynx *(top)* and hypopharynx *(bottom)*.

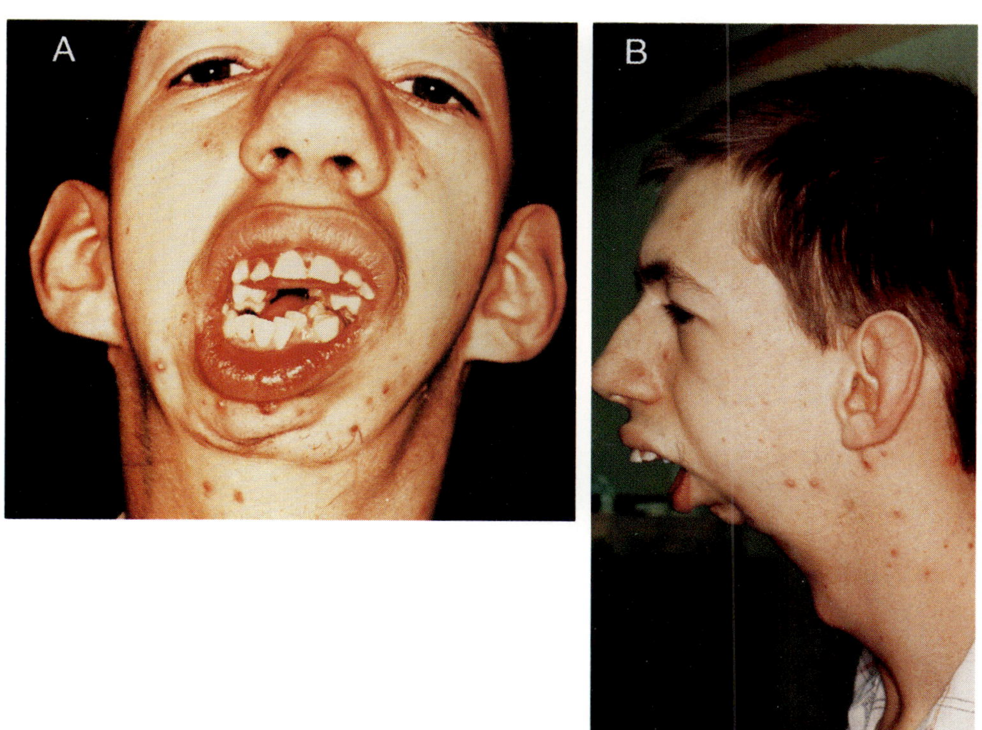

PLATE 5.
Arthrogryposis multiplex. **A,** frontal view. **B,** profile. *See also* Fig 10–4, C.

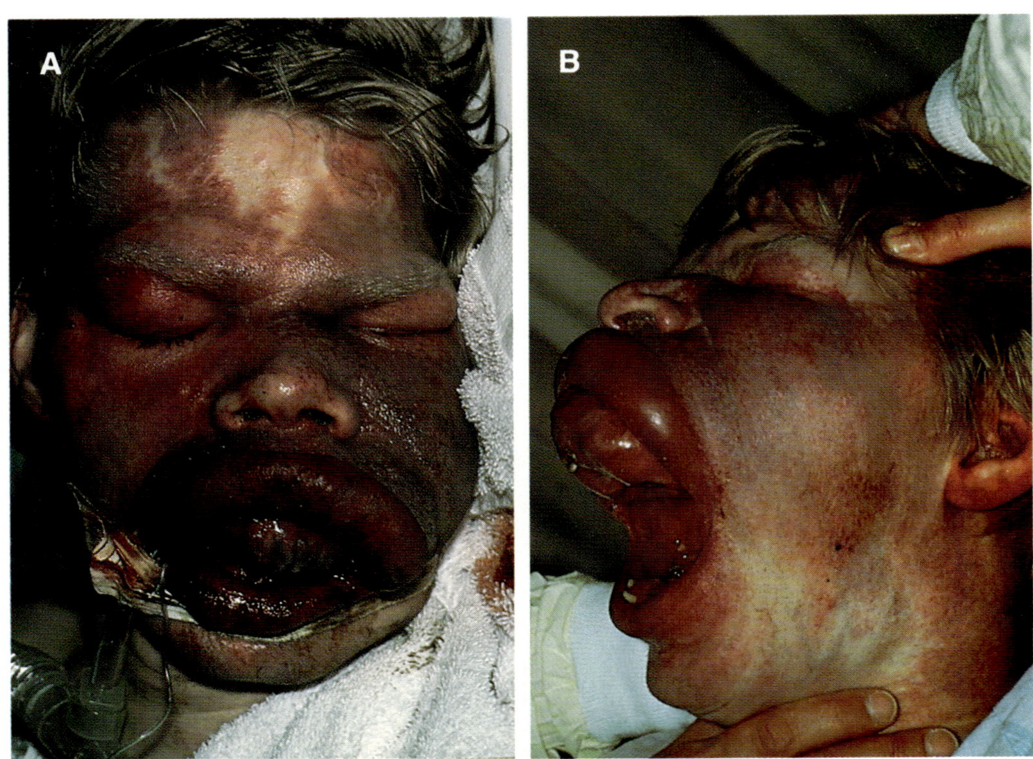
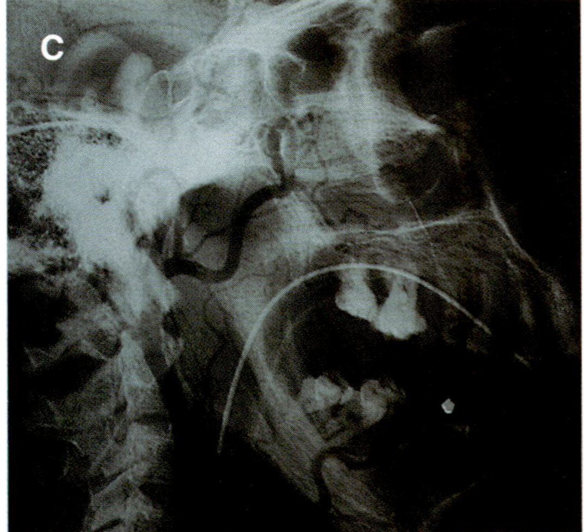

PLATE 6.
Hemangiopericytoma. **A** and **B,** Sturge-Weber syndrome with phenytoin (Dilantin) effect.
C, composite at time of thromboembolization.

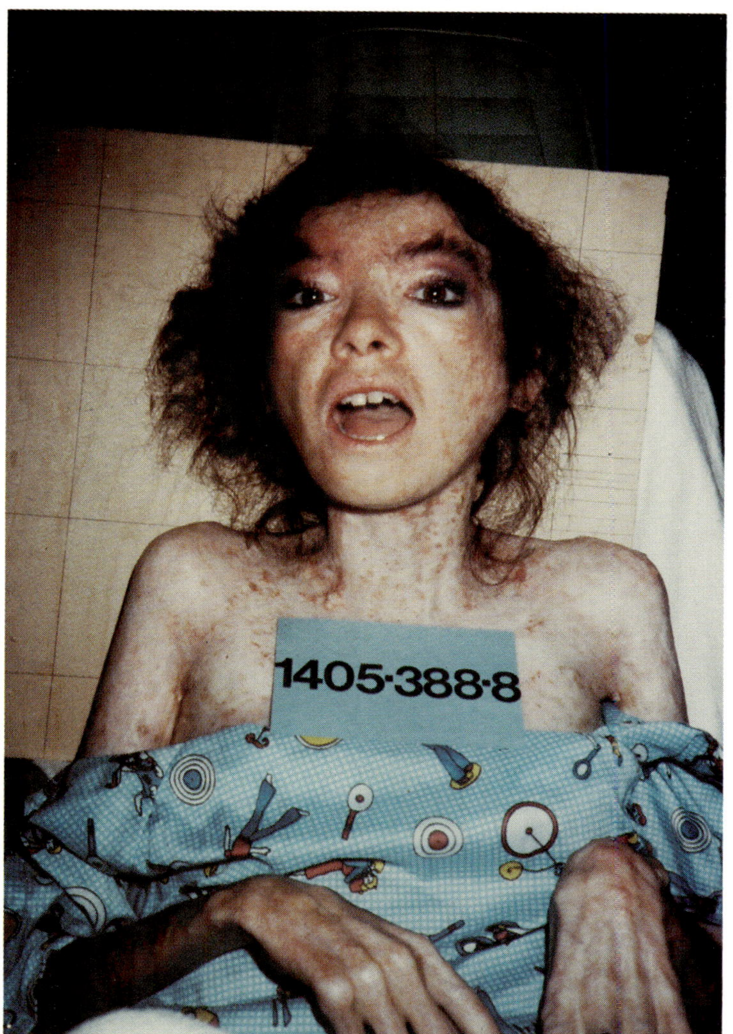

PLATE 7.
Patient with dermatomyositis and calcinosis universalis.

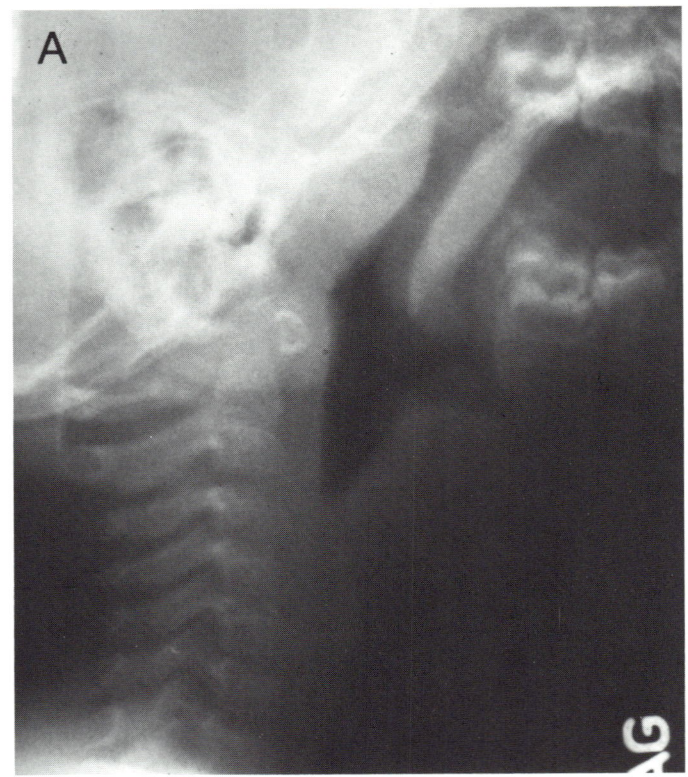

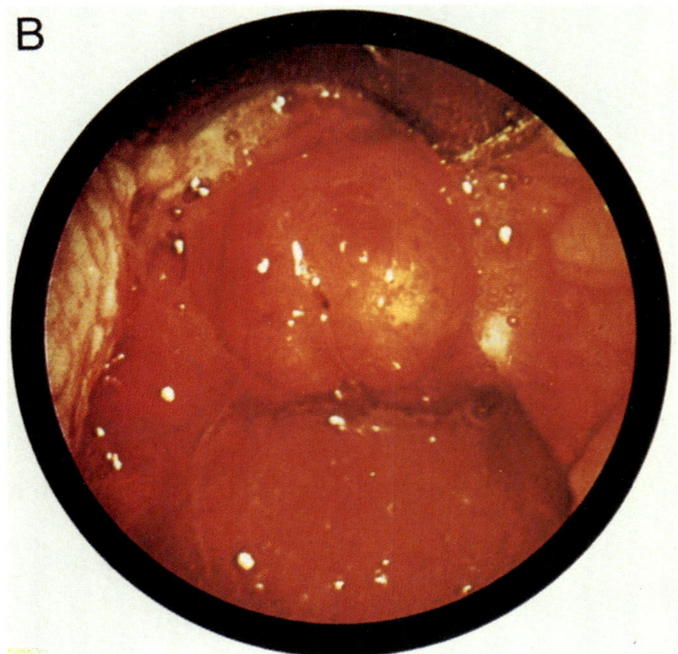

PLATE 8.
A, lateral neck roentgenogram of epiglottitis. Note swelling of the epiglottis, thickening of aryepiglottic folds, loss of vallecular space, and dilated hypopharynx. **B,** epiglottitis. Note markedly inflamed and edematous epiglottis. The airway is almost occluded by inflamed epiglottis, but small dimple shows position of what remains of the patent airway.

monitored, light sedation anesthesia. This, however, does not obviate the need for thorough examination, including soft tissue radiology, and direct fiberoptic observation of tissues of the pharynx and larynx, to support the clinical decision.

Appearances, however, can be deceiving. Disastrous-appearing massive

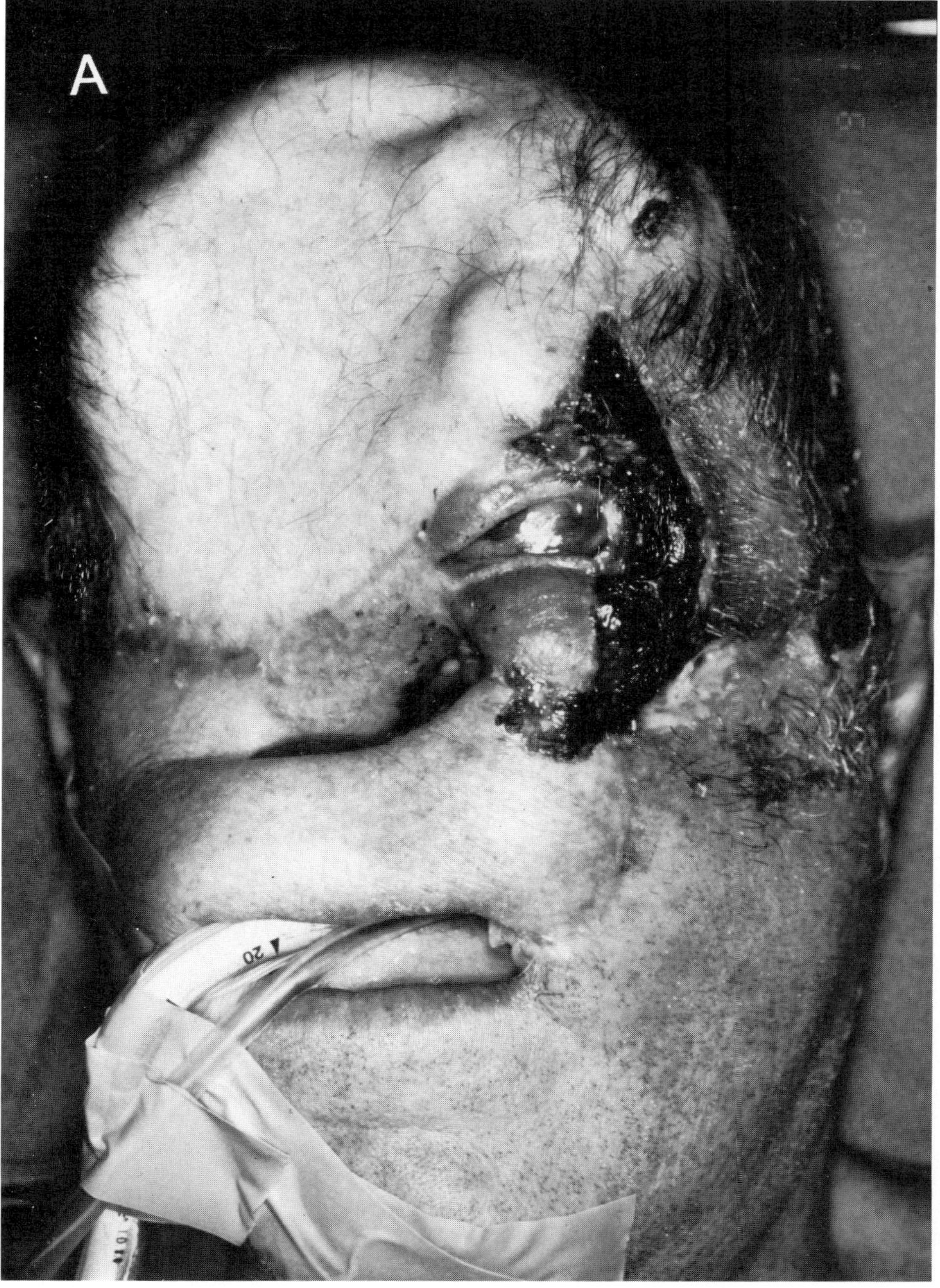

FIG 11–10.
A, patient with basal cell carcinomatosis; **B,** underlying destruction.

B

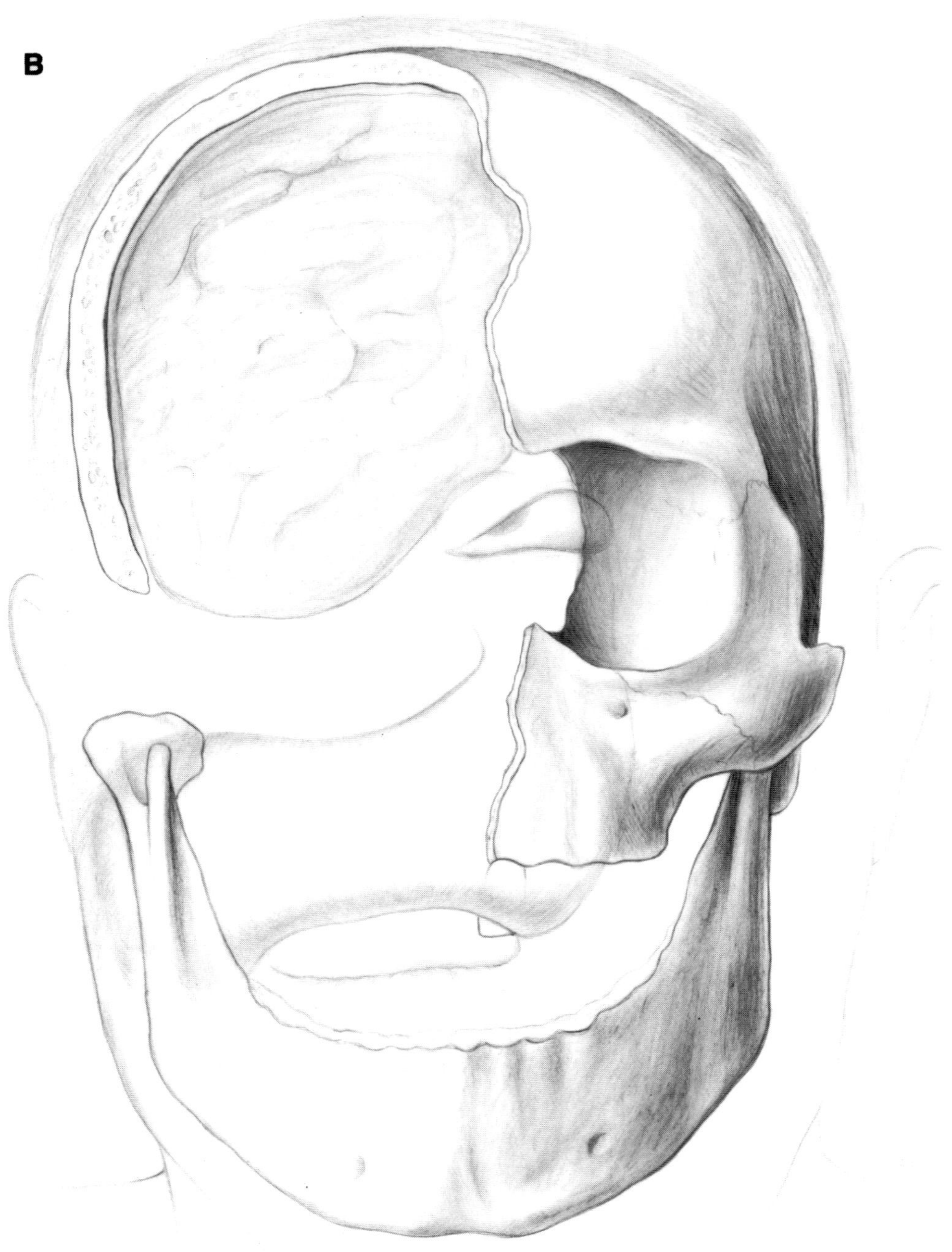

FIG 11–10   **(cont.).**

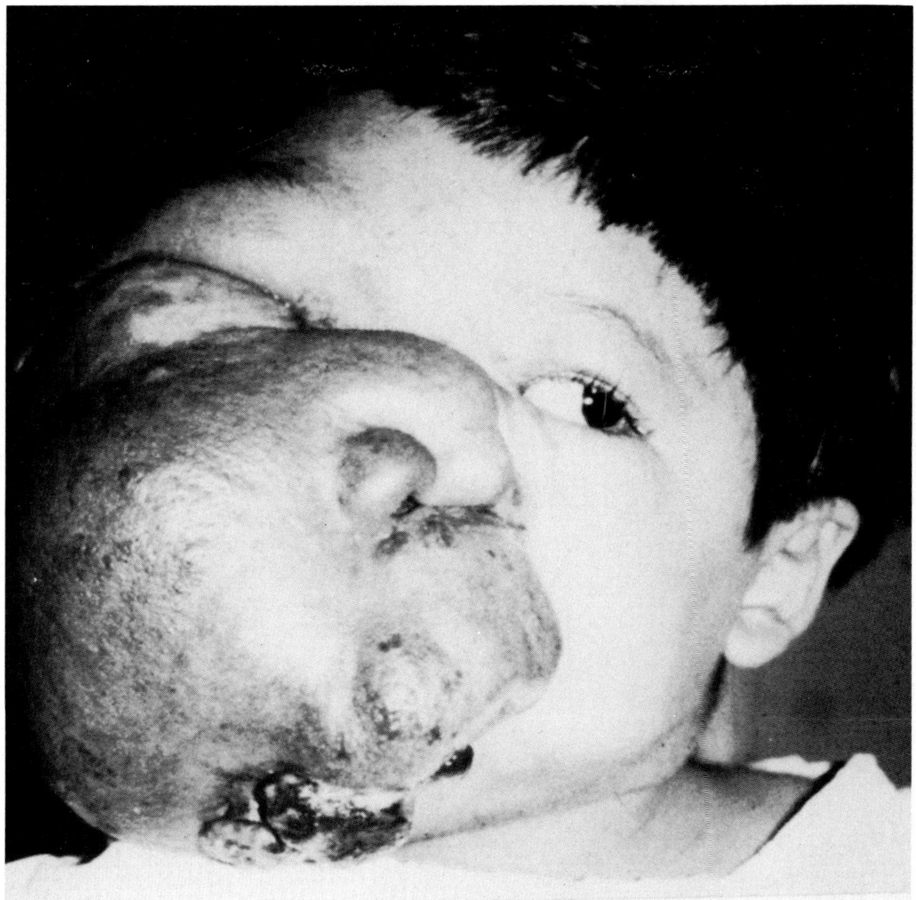

FIG 11–11.
Kasabach-Merritt syndrome (thrombopenia-hemangioma syndrome). (Courtesy of Dr. P. Sirivanasandha, Ramathibodi Hospital, Bangkok, Thailand.)

soft and hard tissue destruction secondary to basal cell carcinomatosis is shown in Figure 11–10. This was in fact only an apparent airway access situation, because the tissue destruction and concomitant plastic surgical amelioration permitted easy access by pushing soft tissue aside.

The patient with Kasabach-Merritt syndrome (thrombopenia hemangioma syndrome, Fig 11–11) demonstrates spectacularly the level of complication presented for airway access in this pediatric patient.

REFERENCE

1. Sivardjan M, Fink BR: The position and the state of the larynx during general anesthesia and muscle paralysis. *Anesthesiology* 1990; 72:439–442.

Chapter 12

Key Medical Considerations in the Difficult Airway: Sleep Apnea, Obesity, and Burns

Martin L. Norton

Jeffrey Kyff

SLEEP APNEA

A clear understanding of the different classes of apnea is essential when one is treating apnea patients. *Central apnea* refers to cessation of nasal and oral airflow with concomitant cessation of respiratory effort. The source of this disorder lies in the pathophysiology of the central nervous system. *Obstructive apnea* is defined as absence of nasal and oral airflow despite continuing respiratory effort, caused generally by anatomic abnormalities in the upper respiratory tract. *Mixed apnea* has both central and obstructive components, with the obstructive part usually following the central.

Originally this syndrome was believed to occur only in obese patients, most vividly represented by the famous character in the Dickens novel after whom the Pickwick syndrome was named. We now know that a number of other types manifest airway obstruction. The mechanism itself is caused by backward movement of the tongue and collapse of the pharyngeal walls (glossoptosis, Fig 12–1), attributable to interference with the dynamic phasic contraction of the pharyngeal and hypopharyngeal muscles. This in turn may be caused by greatly enlarged tonsils or adenoids, macroglossia, or assorted other factors, including the anesthetic sleep state.

The syndrome can be diagnosed from signs and symptoms of chronic sleep deprivation, daytime somnolence, chronic fatigue, loud snoring, morning headache, and often, personality disturbances.

Prudence dictates that we not call all sleep disturbances sleep apnea. There must be diagnostic signs and symptoms, confirmed visually and then by classic techniques in the sleep laboratory. A respiratory pause indicates a cessation of air flow of less than 10 seconds duration. A sleep apneic episode involves a cessation of air flow of more than 10 seconds duration. Sleep apnea syndrome

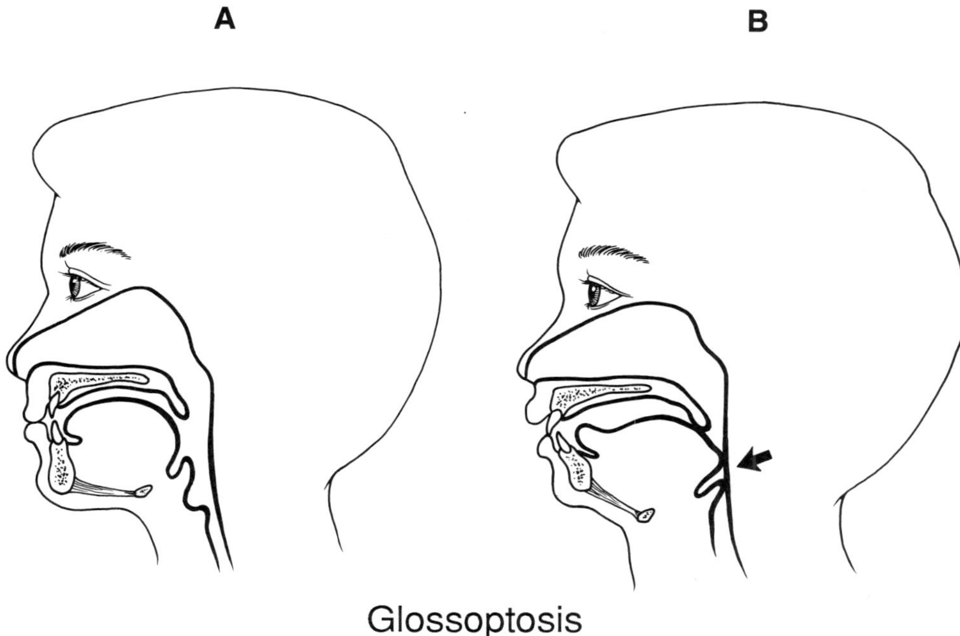

FIG 12–1.
Glossoptosis. **A,** normal tongue placement; **B,** glossoptotic placement *(arrow).*

is diagnosed by at least 30 episodes of true apnea over 7 hours, although apnea patients may have as many as several hundred episodes during the night. The apnea index is the mean number of apneic episodes per hour of sleep as calculated for each individual patient being observed. This is particularly important if active intervention is contemplated to correct the syndrome.

Sleep apnea is interesting because it can illuminate some of the airway problems we encounter in sleeping patients. First, we must remember that this is a syndrome rather than a specific disease. Sorting out the etiologic factors is crucial to an understanding and logical plan for management. Etiologic factors may include neurologic, anatomic, or pathofunctional soft tissue (i.e., mechanical) considerations.

A cause of breathing disturbance not often recognized is related to nasal obstruction. Exactly why oropharyngeal airway obstruction occurs when the nose is occluded is postulated by reports by Blakely and Mahowald[1] and Cole and Haight.[2] It appears possible that nasal obstruction causes a reflex change in the tone of the pharyngeal musculature. Pharyngeal constriction then may represent a compensatory attempt to increase total airway resistance when the nasal passage is limited. This constriction may be caused by loss of abductor tone, increased adductor tone, or hypotonia of all pharyngeal muscles. We must also recognize that mouth breathing appears to be a learned, or at least a later, developmental progression. Newborn infants are nose breathers, and neonates who have obstructions to the nasal passages (choanal atresia) may die. (This is the basic reason for inserting a catheter through the nares of newborn infants at birth to check for any obstruction and to suck out thick mucoid and meconium collections functionally obstructing the nasal passages.)

Similar obstructions have been demonstrated in patients with micrognathia, often complicated by glossoptosis (as in the Pierre Robin anomalad).

Patterns of hypoventilation accentuated by sleep can also develop during the course of disorders of the brain stem as well as in patients with chronic muscular or neuromuscular diseases. They represent a potential cause of asphyxial coma in susceptible subjects.

These patients have potential risks for airway obstruction, frequently unexpected and often catastrophic, during the induction and recovery phases of anesthesia. Induction and recovery should be accomplished with the patient in the sitting position whenever possible, to minimize collapse of pharyngeal wall soft tissue and to take advantage of the suspensory support of the laryngotrachea. Perhaps the safer and more conservative approach is to anticipate sudden airway obstruction in all of these patients and to opt for elective, sedated, but spontaneously ventilating endotracheal intubation in the sitting position. One must also be alert to the rarer abnormalities occurring in association with subacute medullary disease or after surgical damage to the respiratory reticulospinal projection during the course of ventrolateral upper cervical cord section designed to interrupt afferent spinothalamic projections.

An excellent review of mortality in obstructive sleep apnea patients by Jiang et al.[3] suggests the potential risk factors to be faced with anesthesia-induced sleep apnea. Other studies from sleep apnea clinics include the works of Thorpy's group.[4] The obvious reason for our not having documented mortality figures for the anesthesia situation is that the anesthesiologist pays specific attention to early establishment of the airway. However, while sedating the patient to that anesthesia level compatible with inserting one or another form of artificial airway, we tend to superimpose the obstructive component of apnea on the central form. The anesthesiologist's propensity for rapid induction and immediate endotracheal intubation (often more for convenience than patient need) can produce problems in the recovery period or whenever the endotracheal tube is removed, because of any of the earlier observed tissue changes. In other situations the sedated patient has obstructive ventilatory manifestations after premedication or on anesthesia induction.

A particularly revealing diagnostic procedure is the Müller maneuver with fiberoptic endoscopy on the awake patient, as described by Borowiecki et al.[5] This consists of forced inspiratory effort with the mouth and nose closed, and may be extended to describe a variety of mechanisms of pharyngeal collapse involving different portions of the pharynx in patients with craniofacial anomalies.

We have modified this technique for patients who are unable to cooperate readily by doing the procedure with the patient in the sitting, then reclining position and observing the motion of the airway with both a Müller maneuver and with swallowing at different levels. We insert the fiberscope to the level of viewing the epiglottis, exercise the maneuver, withdraw the fiberscope to the base of the tongue, where papillae may be visualized, then repeat the series of steps. Noting the distance of the tip of the epiglottis from the posterior pharynx and the motion of the pharyngeal walls is an intrinsic part of this procedure to reveal the site of pharyngeal collapse. This can be repeated at several levels, as indicated. Conventional grading is recorded:

1+ Minimal movement of the components of the pharynx toward the
center
2+ Movement toward the center decreasing cross-sectional area by 50%
3+ Movement toward the center decreasing cross-sectional area by 75%
4+ Inward movement totally obstructing the airway

OBESITY

Perhaps the most frequently observed airway problem is that in obese patients. A weight of 20% over ideal or twice the predicted weight for age, sex, body build, and height is considered morbid obesity. All physicians recognize that the morbidly obese patient presents ventilatory risks. Not as many are aware of similar hazards in the "relatively" obese. Endomorphism even without morbid obesity (abdominal mass overshadowing thoracic bulk, all anatomic regions notable for softness and roundness, hands and feet relatively small) can signal trouble.

Quite frequently the patient with a short, thick neck and large tongue presents an intubation and endoscopic challenge. The bulk weight of soft tissues and tongue can themselves cause supraglottic obstruction during sleep and induction of anesthesia. During preoperative examination of the patient the mobility of the neck and its range of motion should be carefully delineated. One must be alert to complicating etiologic conditions such as Cushing's syndrome, myxedema, hyperinsulinism, suprasellar hypothalamic lesions, Stein-Leventhal syndrome, and the classic pickwickian syndrome. Similarly, we all are aware of the mechanical instrumentation difficulties experienced during endoscopy in a patient with a massive chest, particularly endomorphic female patients. Many endoscopists consider it mandatory that the obese patient be awake during intubation. Certainly, as discussed, the sitting position is preferable from many viewpoints.

Less often recognized is the relationship of a high arched palate, narrow posterior dentition (intermaxillary space), and narrow anterior central dental arch to endoscopic access and airway patency. This, coupled with the fact that hypotonus of the muscle of the floor of the mouth occurs unusually fast during anesthetic induction in obese patients, explains the frequency of soft tissue obstruction in some patients during the induction phase of anesthetic management. Of particular note, Safar et al.[6] found a significantly high prevalence of airway obstruction in obese patients when their necks were extended.[6]

A phenomenon of polyarthritis with migratory arthralgia that can involve all joints, and particularly the neck, is often observed.

In addition, we must recognize the problem of hypoventilation manifest in all pathologically overweight patients. Tracheotomy has been shown to restore normal arterial CO_2 pressure, as have nasopharyngeal airways.

The major importance of postural changes on lung function should be noted. Functional residual capacity (FRC) decreases as the patient changes position from erect to the Trendelenburg position. This results in hypoxemia, marked reduction in expiratory reserve volume, and maximum volume ventilation and FRC despite only a slight reduction in vital capacity. These are associated with a progressive rapid increase in the work of breathing and compensatory decrease of tidal volume, and the respiratory rate increases. This results in a worsening of ventilation to the already underventilated, dependent portions of the lungs, which then become atelectatic (thus increasing the shunting of arteriovenous blood), and early peripheral airway closure. Add to this the commonly observed thoracolumbar lordosis, limitation of rib movement, inability to raise the lower sternum, and preexistent upper airway mechanical obstructive processes, and we have the all too often seen ventilatory and respiratory catastrophe in the obese patient.

These combined hazards explain the tendency of anesthesiologists to do awake intubations in an obese patient. Here again, use of the flexible fiberoptic endoscope has contributed to patient safety. Another aid is the ventilating laryngoscope using Venturi (jet) principles to enrich the gas at the additus laryngis during intubation attempts and thus extend the time the anesthesiologist needs to locate and intubate the larynx. The concept is also based on a premise, not fully demonstrated, that with proper application the jet gas can be insufflated into the laryngotracheal route by bouncing off the posterior pharynx. This may result in gas being propelled into the esophagus and down to the stomach. However, inadvertent gastric dilatation can readily be remedied by prompt insertion of a nasogastric or orogastric tube as soon as airway control has been assured. One must always keep in mind the risk of regurgitation; consequently, the semi-Fowler position will be of assistance, as will ready availability of adequate suction devices.

Multiple symmetric lipomatosis falls into a slightly different category of obesity syndromes. This unusual disease is characterized by the formation of multiple, nonencapsulated lipomas with a predilection for the nape of the neck, the supraclavicular region, and the deltoid region and produces an extraordinary bull-necked appearance (Madelung collar or neck; Fig 12–2). The danger in this situation is that the lipomas tend to infiltrate along fascial planes and can cause life-threatening tracheal, laryngeal, and particularly mediastinal compression. The supine position, even moderate sedation, and certainly general anesthesia in the supine position before splinting of the upper airway can add to the danger.

Access to the airway is crucial! Positioning of the patient for either diagnostic or surgical intervention requires serious thought. In addition, consideration must be given to debulking the lipomas around the airway and in the mediastinum to avert compression of vital structures. When dealing with these patients, hypertriglyceridemia, hyperuricemia, hyperinsulinemia, and renal tubular acidosis must also be ruled out. Remember, these lipomas can develop anywhere, similar to von Recklinghausen's neurofibromatosis (see Fig 10–5).

Sleep Apnea Case History*

A 10-year-old boy referred to an otolaryngologist had a history of heroic snoring and daytime hypersomnolence. He denied problems with nasal obstruction and had no previous episodes of tonsilitis. He was noted on physical examination to be

*Courtesy of Dr. Henry T. Hoffman, Assistant Adjunct Professor, Division of Head and Neck Surgery, University of California, San Diego.

morbidly obese, standing 136 cm tall and weighing 101 kg. He had a short, thick neck and tonsils large enough to obscure view of the posterior pharyngeal wall. Chest x-ray, electrocardiographic, and pulmonary function studies all were normal. A polysomnogram demonstrated obstructive sleep apnea with arterial desaturations less than 70% on 267 occasions during 426 minutes of testing. The lowest saturation recorded during this study was 16%.

A tracheostomy was believed necessary to treat this severe obstructive sleep apnea until the patient was able to lose enough weight to allow other treatment (tonsillectomy and uvulopalatoplasty). After administration of the preanesthetic medication (ranitidine [Zantac] 150 mg and metoclopramide [Reglan] 10 mg) the patient was transported to the operating room without sedation. In the controlled environment of the operating room 3 mg midazolam was slowly administered, and topical cocaine intranasally. While awake, the patient then underwent nasotracheal intubation with a 6.5 mm nasotracheal tube over a pediatric bronchoscope. The tracheostomy was performed with the patient under general anesthesia, without incident.

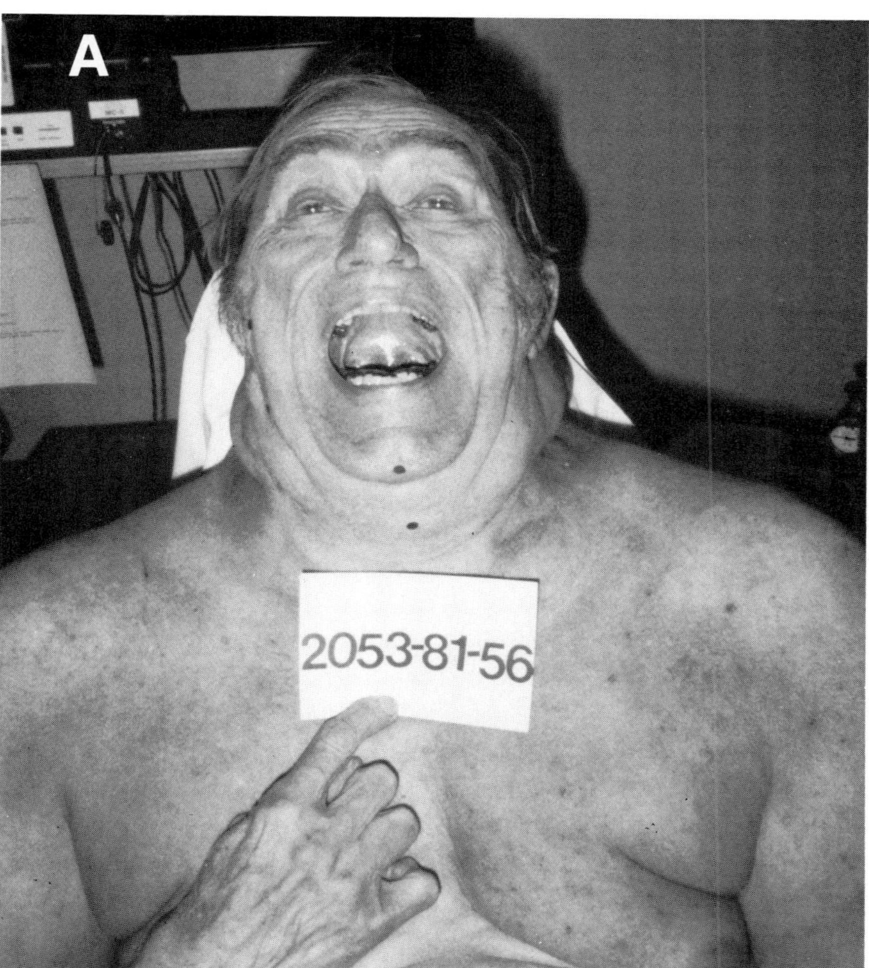

FIG 12–2.
Multiple symmetric lipomatosis.

B

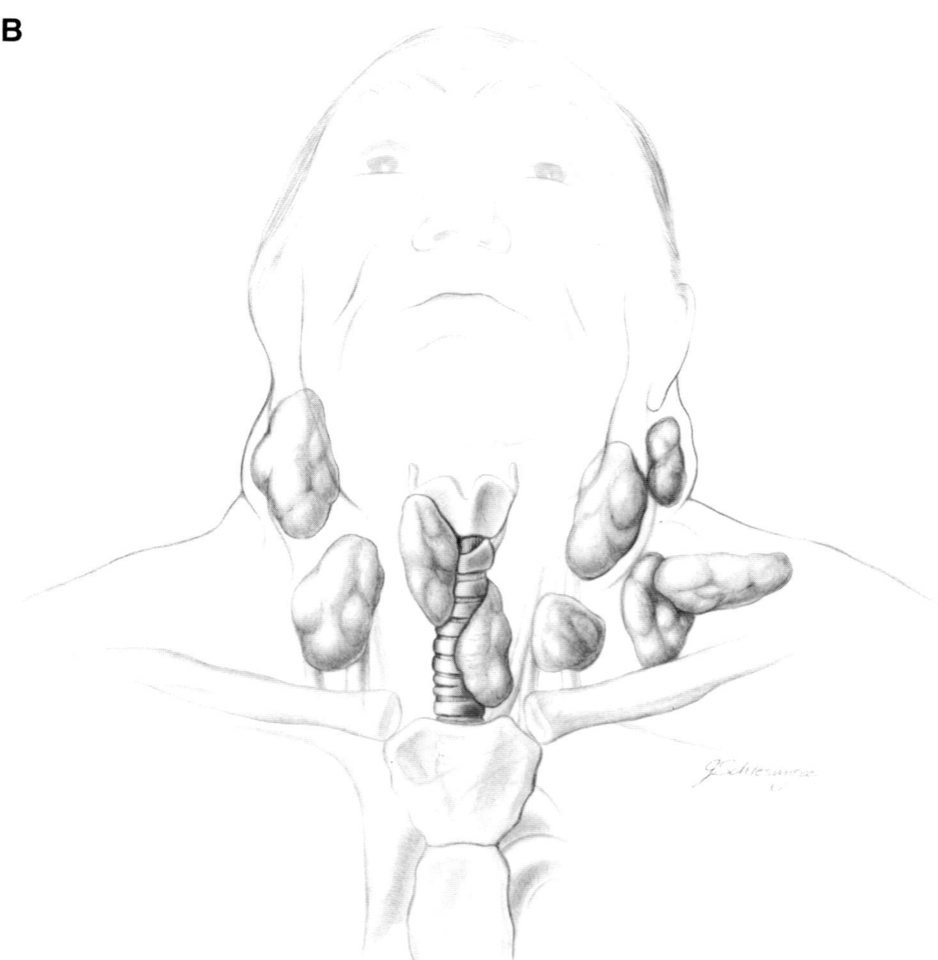

FIG 12-2   (cont.).

Discussion

Airway management is particularly difficult in obese patients with sleep apnea. Most adults with a similar body habitus and obstructed oropharynx are best treated with a tracheostomy under local anesthesia. Tracheostomy in a short, thick neck may be difficult, and under local anesthesia requires patient cooperation. Although this 10-year-old boy was able to tolerate nasotracheal intubation, it is unlikely that he would have cooperated during an awake tracheostomy.

This case is presented to highlight one of several options the anesthesiologist has in securing difficult airways. Awake intubation allows for safe induction of general anesthesia by permitting the patient to maintain a patent pharynx and spontaneous respirations. Control of the airway by positive pressure mask breathing would be difficult in this very obese patient if he were anesthetized before intubation. As the level of anesthesia deepened with resultant loss of muscle tone and collapse of excessive oropharyngeal and pharyngeal soft tissue, complete airway obstruction would result, requiring emergent intubation. The added safety of an intubation in this awake patient compensated for the small amount of discomfort he experienced. Although the patient did recall struggling with the anesthestiologist, who was "jamming something in my nose," he stated that he would not mind going through the procedure a second time if it were important for his health.

Mention is made of the preanesthetic medication used in this case to note the significant absence of any sedating drugs. Even mild sleeping pills should be avoided in patients with sleep apnea to avoid further depression of already compromised respirations.

THE BURNED PATIENT

Airway management in the burned patient requires skill and experience in intubation as well as knowledge of the natural history and course of burn injury.[7] The airways of many patients are prematurely intubated because they have soot on their faces. Other patients are at risk for airway obstruction because of swelling of soft tissues during the resuscitation phase of their injury. Because of physician inexperience, the airways of some patients may not be intubated until after intubation is no longer possible.

Carbonaceous sputum has been used as a sign of inhalation injury in the burned patient. This is a very weak sign. The most definite thing that can be said about this finding is that the patient has inhaled carbonaceous air, which may occur as the result of a great many causes. Of much more concern are findings of facial burns, pharyngeal burns, or singed nasal hairs. Hoarseness and stridor are particularly ominous signs and indicate the need for immediate therapy.

People who have inhaled steam have extremely difficult airway access because of massive edema. This is manifested primarily in the nasal and oropharyngeal tissues as well as the neck and facial soft tissues.

On the other hand, lye and other caustic chemical burns are usually limited to the oropharynx and pharyngoesophagus, although areas such as the pyriform sinuses and vestibular folds of the larynx may be affected. Adhesion of a swollen tongue to the posterior pharynx is also a real danger. Farther down the tracheobronchial tract, casts may form as a result of dehydration and mouth breathing or secondary to nonhumidified endotracheal tube ventilation and poor tracheobronchial toilet. This may be aggravated by suppression of surfactant and lysosomes.

Regularly scheduled inhalation of nebulized racemic epinephrine may reduce upper airway swelling sufficiently to avoid endotracheal intubation, but such patients must be watched closely and their airways intubated promptly if signs of impending airway obstruction do not quickly abate or if they worsen. Methods of intubation may include direct laryngoscopic visualization, blind nasal, flexible fiberoptic visualization of the vocal folds and trachea (via oral or nasal routes), and rigid bronchoscopy. Adequate suction is critical for all forms of intubation, but particularly when fiberoptic endoscopes are used. Secretions tend to be thick and tinged by the inhaled products of combustion. They easily obscure visualization and are frequently difficult to remove through the endoscope.

Another important consideration is tissue edema. Edema caused by direct tissue injury to face, pharynx, and lungs as well as generalized edema is of significance. Properly resuscitated burned patients also develop edema in any tissues that are still viable, that is, areas of superficial (partial thickness) burns or in areas underneath more completely burned tissues. Edema may develop in tissues distant from burned areas, such as the face, pharynx, and larynx. Inhalation injury to the pulmonary interstitium frequently does not manifest itself until the third postburn day, when soft tissue edema may be at its worst and intubation most difficult. Compromise of the upper airway by edema may result in a totally inaccessible airway. The edema may become so intense that an expeditious tracheostomy may be technically impossible. This is a particularly important consideration in patients with burns involving greater than 20% of their total body surface area, where fluid requirements begin at 4.2 L/day in the mythical 70 kg patient and increase with the patient's weight and percentage of body area burned.

Frequently a judgment about intubation must be made early in the course of treatment, while the airway is still asymptomatic (Table 12–1). Failure to intubate within the first 24 hours of burn injury may preclude intubation later. During the first 24 hours, soft tissue swelling may become so extensive that range of motion of the cervical spine and temporomandibular joints may be limited by the surrounding tissues. This is usually accompanied by soft tissue edema about the face and neck and can prove a deadly combination. Edema about the head and neck may be minimized by placing the patient in a 30-degree, head-up position, if possible, to facilitate lymphatic and venous drainage.

TABLE 12–1.

Indications for Endotracheal Intubation in Burn Patients*

Absolute	Relative (Requires Physician Judgment)	Unlikely
Hoarseness and stridor (not responding promptly to racemic epinephrine aerosol treatment)	Singed nasal hairs Facial burns	No hoarseness or stridor
Oral burns	Injury occurred in closed space	No singed nasal hairs No facial or oral burns
Arterial blood gas levels inappropriate for FiO_2	Large burn for age and previous medical history	Arterial blood gas levels appropriate for FiO_2
Depressed level of consciousness such that patient is unable to protect airway		Injury did not occur in closed space
Carboxyhemoglobin >10 in presence of depressed level of consciousness		Carboxyhemoglobin normal for smoking history
		Patient alert and responding appropriately

*All criteria are relative, and physician judgment must always supersede any published list of criteria. "Absolute" criteria should always take precedence over "relative" or "unlikely" criteria. Similarly, "relative" criteria should supersede "unlikely" criteria.

Another consideration is the seriousness of the overall injury. Burns involving greater than 50% body surface area, even in otherwise healthy patients, very often require endotracheal intubation during the first week after injury, when intubation may be difficult or impossible. It is therefore essential to anticipate the need for endotracheal intubation before this time. Causes of respiratory failure may include sepsis, resulting in increased metabolic demands and alterations in level of consciousness, inhalation injury, or inability to compensate for the increased metabolic demands of the burn injury itself. *The most common time for pulmonary inhalation injury to be manifest is on the third postinjury day, when tissue edema is maximal.* Surgery for escharotomy (Fig 12–3) or wound debridement is frequently performed during this time, and intubation becomes necessary because of competition with surgeons for the airway, intraoperative positioning (e.g., prone, extreme lateral), and the technical demands of massive transfusion or managing hemodynamic instability.

In addition, very young patients (<2 years), elderly patients, or patients with underlying medical diseases suffer increased morbidity and mortality from burns of lesser severity and frequently develop respiratory failure soon after injury, even when the upper airway is not directly involved.

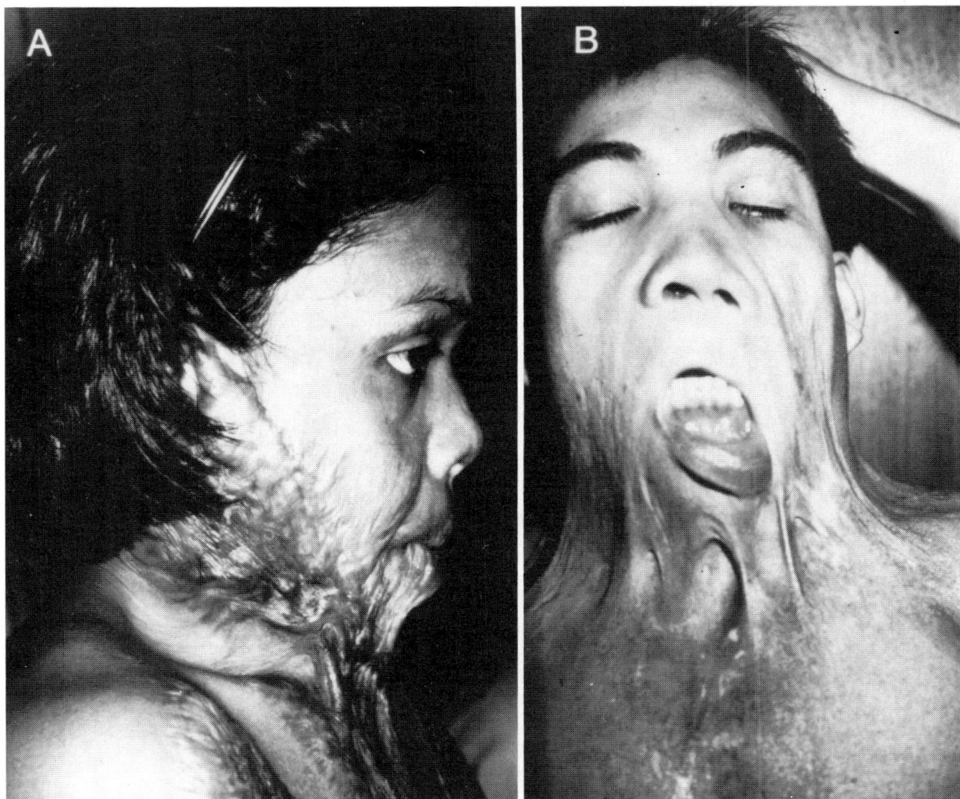

FIG 12–3.
Cicatrix. Two extreme examples limiting cervical motion and airway access. (Courtesy of Dr. Chinda Youngchaiyudh, Royal Thai Hospital, Bangkok.)

Intubation is generally accomplished in a routine fashion, through the oral route with a laryngoscope. However, several things about burned patients warrant discussion. First are the psychologic aspects of disfigurment and the smell of burned tissue, both of which must be ignored. Second, these patients frequently have a significant quantity of oral secretions. Third, the various topical agents used for wound treatment make the skin very slippery.

Securing endotracheal tubes should routinely be done with ties of either cloth or intravenous extension tubing. These may be secured over the ears, taking care to leave sufficient slack that tissue necrosis is not induced and that venous drainage from the head through the internal and external jugular veins is not occluded, thus avoiding cerebral edema. Endotracheal tubes should not be secured to anything else, such as nasogastric tubes, so that a confused patient cannot remove all tubes by catching hold of one. Frequent adjustments in the securing ties are necessary to accommodate changes in soft tissue edema.

The use of fiberoptic equipment in either nasal or oral intubation is a necessary skill for those managing the airways in burned patients. The adage that says to use this method when needed, before laryngoscopy or blind instrumentation, is particularly true in this setting. Secretions, burned nasopharyngeal tissue, and edema make endoscopy difficult, and the addition of laryngoscope-induced bleeding will further reduce the chances of successful intubation.

The instrument has particular application after smoke inhalation. It has been established that patients with severe laryngeal edema due to smoke inhalation will eventually require intubation.[8] Proper endoscopic evaluation will assist in choosing between endotracheal intubation and tracheostomy.

REFERENCES

1. Blakely BW, Mahowald MW: Nasal resistance and sleep apnea. *Laryngoscope* 1987; 97:752–754.
2. Cole P, Haight JSJ: Mechanisms of nasal obstruction in sleep. *Laryngoscopy* 1984; 94:1557–1559.
3. Jiang HE, Kryger MH, Zorick GJ, et al: Mortality and apnea index in obstructive sleep apnea. *Chest* 1988; 94:9–14.
4. Thorpy MJ, et al: *Sleep Res* 1989; 18:316.
5. Borowiecki B, Pollak CP, Weitzman ED, et al: Fibro-optic study of pharyngeal airway during sleep in patients with hypersomnia obstructive sleep-apnea syndrome. *Laryngoscope* 1978; 88:1310–1313.
6. Safar P, Escarraga LS, Chang F: Upper airway obstruction in the unconscious patient. *J Appl Physiol* 1959; 14:760–764.
7. Roi LD, Flora JD Jr, Davis TM, et al: A severity grading chart for the burned patient. *Ann Emerg Med* 1981; 10:161–163.
8. Wanner A, Cutchavaree A: Early recognition of upper airway obstruction following smoke inhalation. *Am Rev Respir Dis* 1973; 108:1421–1428.

Chapter 13

Oral and Maxillofacial Surgical Considerations in the Difficult Airway

L. George Upton

Establishment or maintenance of an adequate airway is often an important component in the management of diseases, injuries, or developmental deformities of the oral and maxillofacial region.

EMERGENT CONSIDERATIONS

The patient with maxillofacial trauma often represents a challenge in establishing or maintaining an adequate airway.[1] Fractures of the midface and mandible, as well as soft tissue lacerations, may create significant bleeding into the nasal and oral pharynx, thus compromising the patient's ability to adequately exchange air, and also present significant visualization problems during attempts to pass an endotracheal tube. This may be further complicated by the loss of normal laryngeal suspension with bilateral subcondylar fracture dislocations.

Loss of tongue support is another potential threat to airway maintenance. This may be secondary to bilateral parasymphyseal fractures (Fig 13–1) or avulsion injury of the symphysis secondary to self-inflicted gunshot wounds (Fig 13–2). These patients may have no other injury or illness and are in a conscious state. They frequently demonstrate the ability to maintain an airway in a sitting position, with loss of the airway occurring when they assume a supine position. Support of the anterior symphyseal segment with interdental wires or arch bars usually eliminates the airway difficulty. Loss of a bone segment with

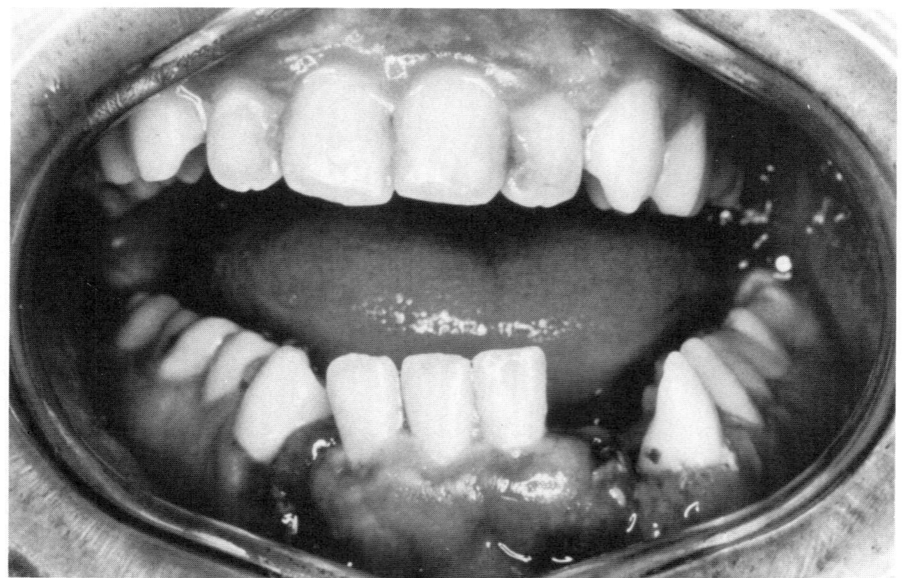

FIG 13–1.
Bilateral parasymphyseal fracture with resultant loss of anterior support of genioglossus muscle. Such injury may result in loss of airway when patient is in the supine position.

gunshot injuries generally requires mechanical airway support and subsequent intubation or tracheostomy in the acute phase.

Decisions regarding airway establishment must be based on the expected treatment outcomes for such patients. For example, patients with combined nasoethmoidal and maxillomandibular injuries requiring bilateral nasal packs and intermaxillary fixation should, in most instances, have a tracheostomy at the outset of the procedure because their nasal and oral apertures will ultimately be closed to endotracheal tubes (Fig 13–3).

Regarding patients in intermaxillary fixation, additional considerations include the use of the nasoendotracheal tube functioning as a nasopharyngeal airway following extubation by allowing the tube to remain in the posterior pharynx for a period of time. Normally if extubation is done while the patient is awake, he or she must be spontaneously breathing and swallowing appropriately before extubation. Additional measures to facilitate airway protection include using intrasurgical corticosteroids, using nasal decongestants, having wire cutters at the bedside, removing gastric contents before the patient leaves the operating room, and using nasal airways as indicated.

Infection may also be an acute airway challenge. Masticator space infections are associated with acute trismus in which a patient may be unable to open his or her mouth widely on preoperative examination. In such instances, a muscle-relaxing anesthetic will generally, but not always, allow adequate opening to occur.

A more severe problem is associated with Ludwig's angina (Fig 13–4), which is an extensive, multispace infection of the floor of the mouth[2, 3]

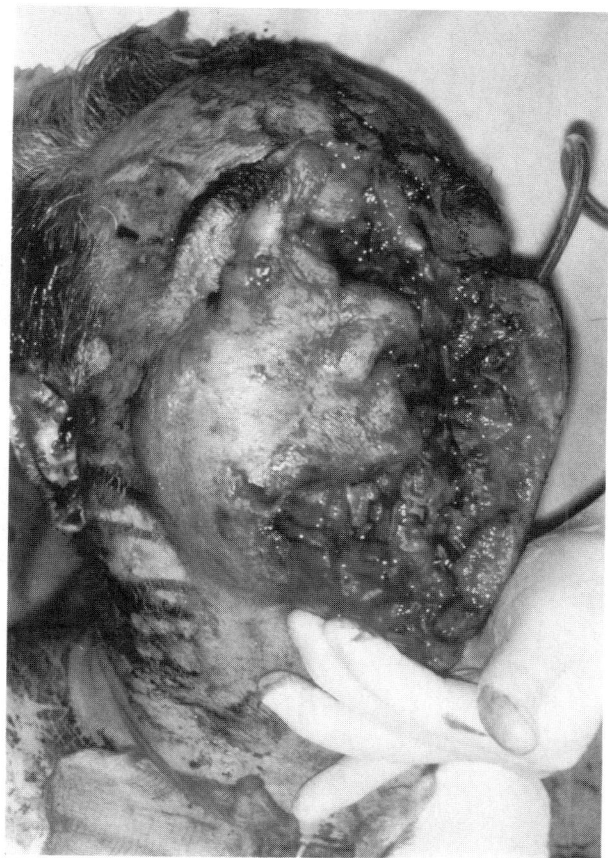

FIG 13–2.
Loss of tongue support secondary to avulsive injury from self-inflicted gunshot wound. Massive edema and significant hemorrhage compound airway management in this patient.

classically associated with infected mandibular first, second, or third molars. The infection spreads into the sublingual, submental, and bilateral submandibular spaces, producing severe elevation and posterior displacement of the tongue. Threat to life occurs with upper airway obstruction secondary to tongue displacement and obstruction, with additional risk associated with spontaneous rupture of the abscess into the hypopharynx during intubation attempts.[4] These patients can also maintain an adequate airway in a sitting position but demonstrate obstruction in a supine position. Such cases are best treated through elective tracheostomy before incision and drainage attempts.[5, 6]

This approach is important not only because it reduces the risk of spontaneous rupture of the abscess during laryngoscopy with potential resultant pulmonary abscesses but also because it reduces the risk of postoperative obstruction secondary to the intense swelling that occurs following exploration of infected anatomic spaces in the operating room (Fig 13–5).

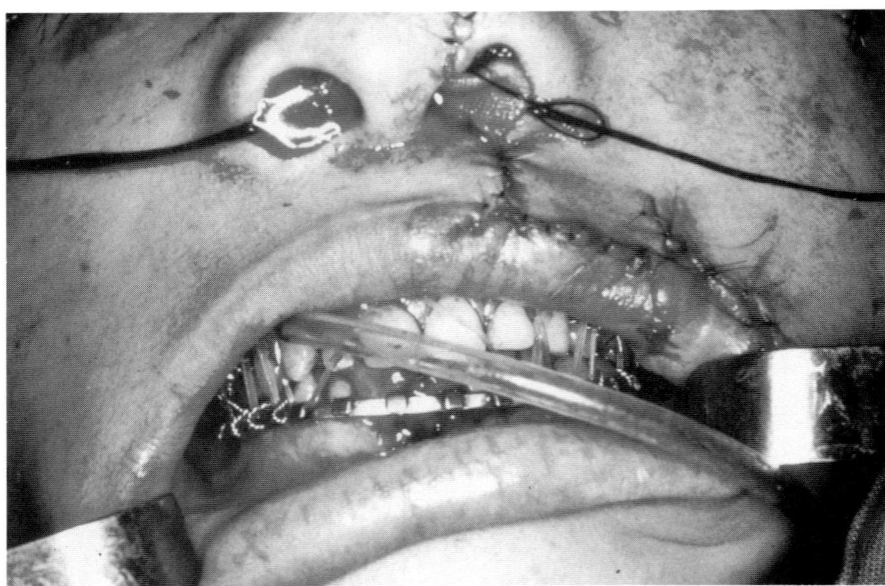

FIG 13–3.
Postoperative appearance of patient with multiple facial fractures. Note both nares, as well as the oral cavity, are compromised as part of treatment of injuries. Decisions regarding sources of airway management should take into account the final treatment result before induction of anesthesia.

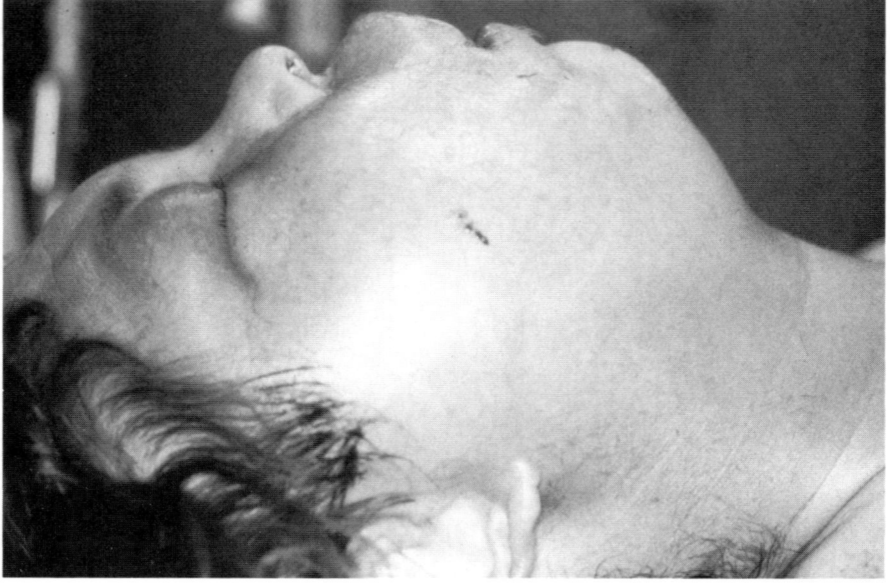

FIG 13–4.
Massive swelling associated with submandibular, submental, masticator, and buccal spaces in association with Ludwig's angina.

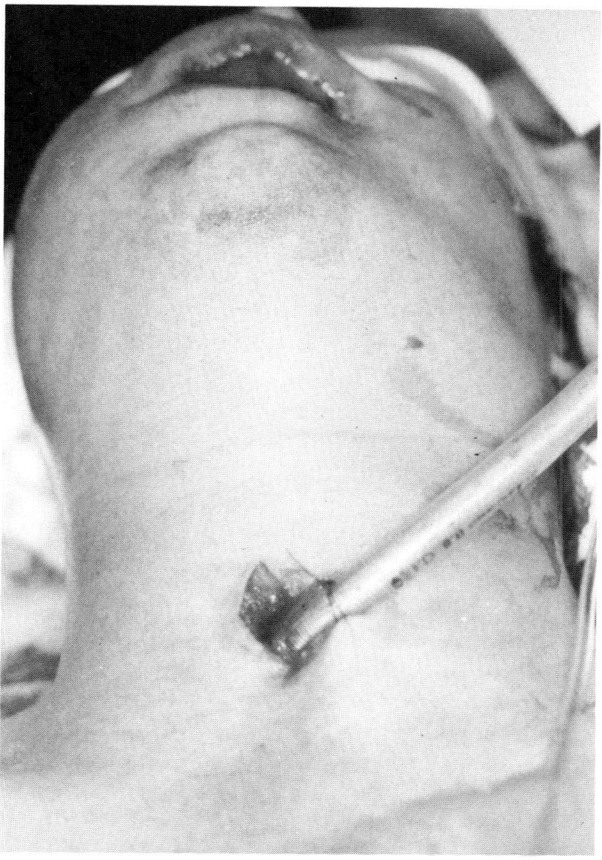

FIG 13–5.
Preinduction establishment of airway avoids potential aspiration from the ruptured abscess during laryngoscopy and prevents postmanipulation obstruction secondary to edema from the incision and drainage process.

ANESTHESIA INDUCTION CONSIDERATIONS

The inability to adequately open a patient's mouth to pass a laryngoscope is a real concern for the anesthesiologist. Patients who have a limitation in mouth opening include those with ankylosis (Fig 13–6), internal derangements of the temporomandibular joint (TMJ), and trismus. Regarding ankylosis, the condition may be caused by a limitation within the joint itself (true ankylosis) or outside the joint space (false ankylosis). True ankylosis may be from bony fusion or fibrous adhesions (Fig 13–7). This may be related to trauma or temporomandibular surgery or infection.[7] The problem may be complicated in children because the ankylosed joint will also produce a significant mandibular deformity by interfering with the growth centers of the mandible (Fig 13–8).[8] If TMJ ankylosis is diagnosed, the best approach is intubation using the fiberoptic nasal endoscope. The other alternative is tracheostomy. In the hands of those skilled in the approach, blind nasal intubation is an option. These techniques are also appropriate for false ankylosis.

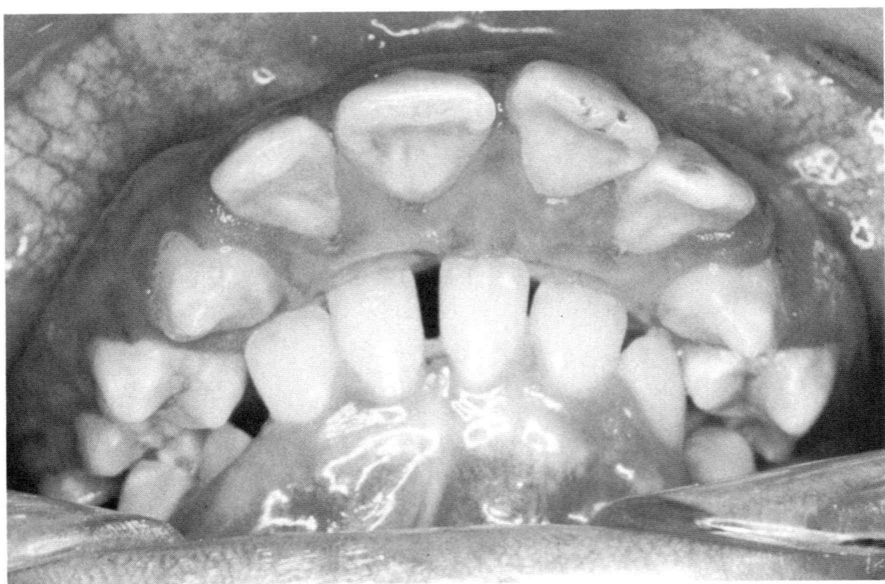

FIG 13–6.
Severe degree of limited opening in a patient with bilateral ankylosis in early childhood.

The interincisal distance in patients with TMJ internal derangements[9] is often limited to 25 mm or less. These internal derangements are the result of a displacement of the fibrous articular disk to a position that may no longer allow adequate forward movement of the condyle (Fig 13–9). Such patients usually have a past history of jaw joint clicking, popping, and episodes of "catch-

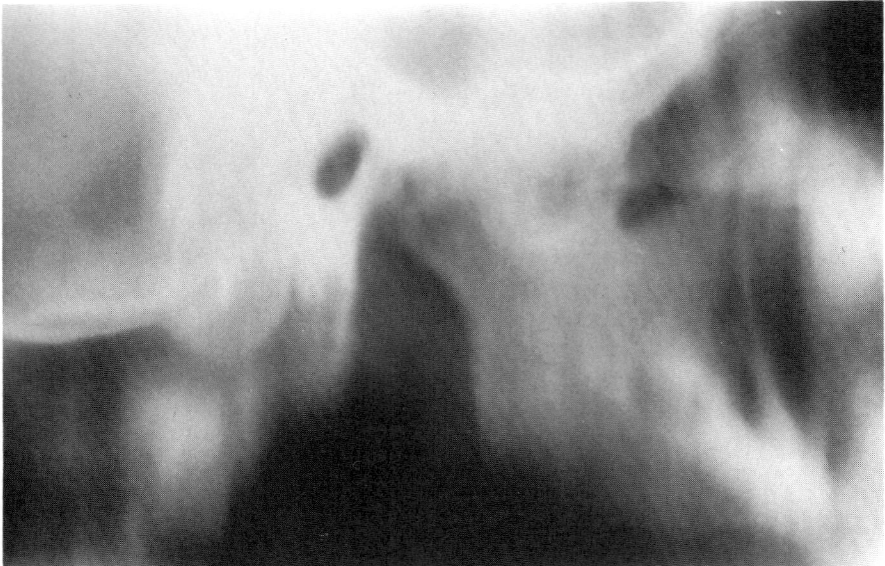

FIG 13–7.
Massive bony ankylosis of the TMJ.

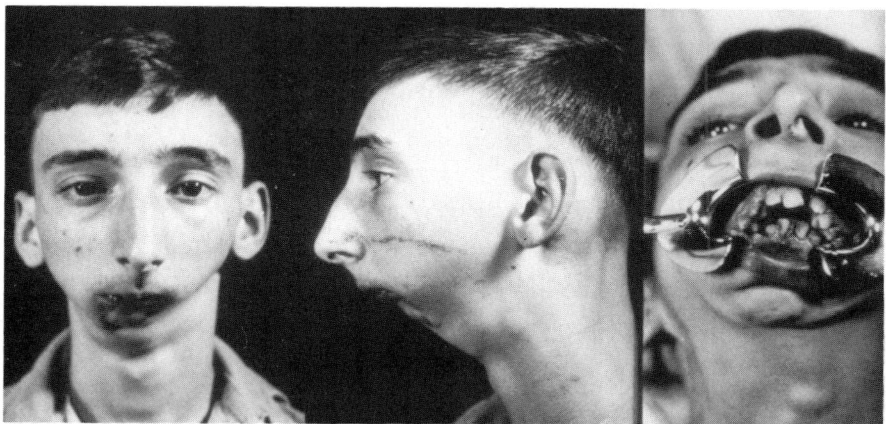

FIG 13–8.
Degree of skeletal deformity associated with bilateral ankylosis.

ing" before TMJ locking. However, they may not have difficulties in jaw opening once they are asleep because a dimension adequate for direct laryngoscopy and intubation may then be achieved, assuming there are no other coexistent conditions to limit opening and laryngeal exposure. Trismus is another condition that may manifest itself in limited jaw opening. It may be associated with infection, muscle injury, or a reflex protective mechanism from joint injury.[10] However, anesthesia induction and adequate mouth opening can usually be achieved using muscle relaxants.

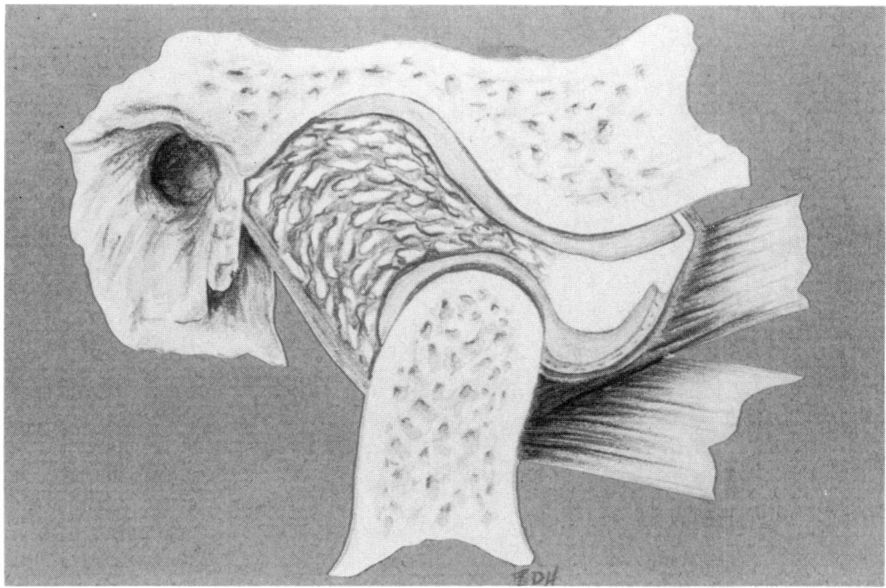

FIG 13–9.
Completely forward, displaced articular disk seen in severe type of internal derangement of the TMJ.

Conditions that may not respond to muscle relaxants include myofibrositis, scleroderma, and myofibrositis ossificans.

Difficulty passing a nasotracheal tube may be encountered in a variety of circumstances. Midface trauma can distort anatomy to the point where this approach would not be the best alternative. In addition, midface trauma with fracture through the cribriform plate and associated cerebrospinal fluid leak may make another route for establishment of an airway necessary (Fig 13–10). Deformities of the region, whether they are congenital (choanal atresia), traumatic (deviated nasal septum), or surgically acquired (pharyngeal flap) (Fig 13–11), may represent challenges to nasal intubation.[11]

In patients with a pharyngeal flap the use of a rubber catheter to guide the endotracheal tube through the nasopharynx may be considered, as well as the use of a fiberoptic nasal endoscope. In instances where the patient may be in intermaxillary fixation following an osteotomy, an alternative may lie in passing an oral endotracheal tube with the tube lying behind the last molars with the teeth wired together (Fig 13–12).

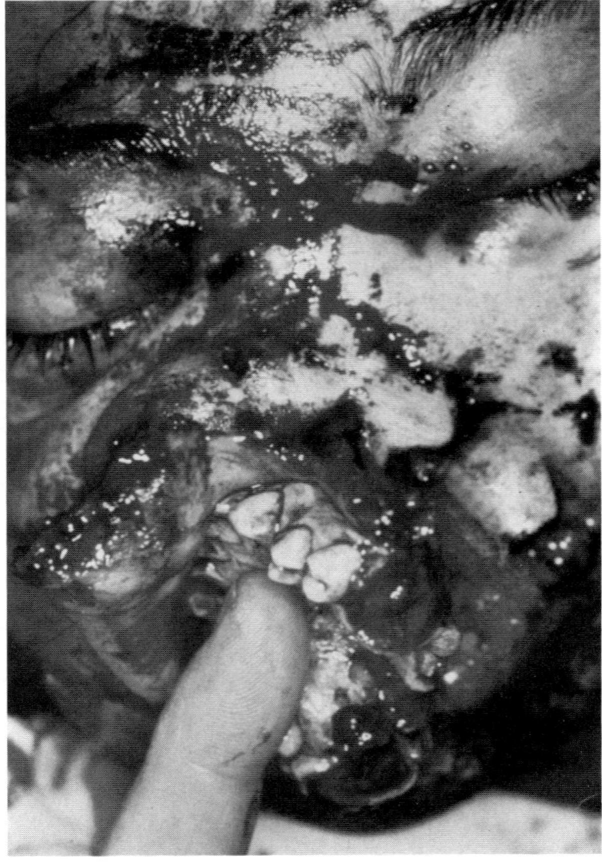

FIG 13–10.
Severe distortion of anatomy of upper airway–associated trauma. Such cases represent significant problem in airway establishment and ultimately suggest tracheostomy as soon as it can be appropriately established.

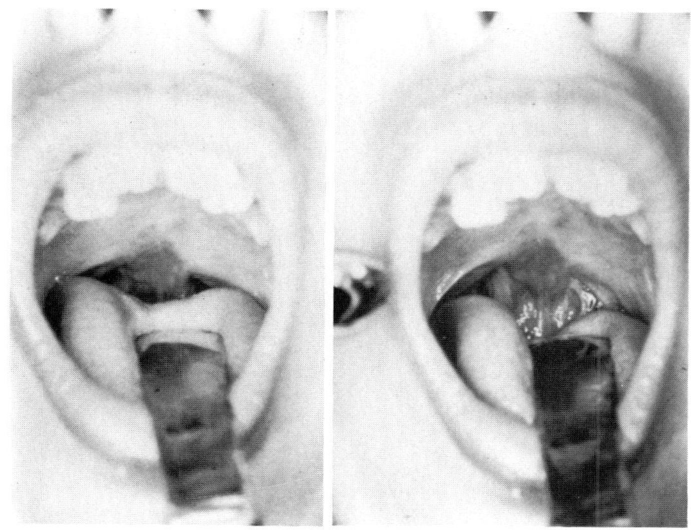

FIG 13–11.
Compromised space associated with pharyngeal flap. Note narrow lateral ports that compromise opportunity for passage of nasal endotracheal tube.

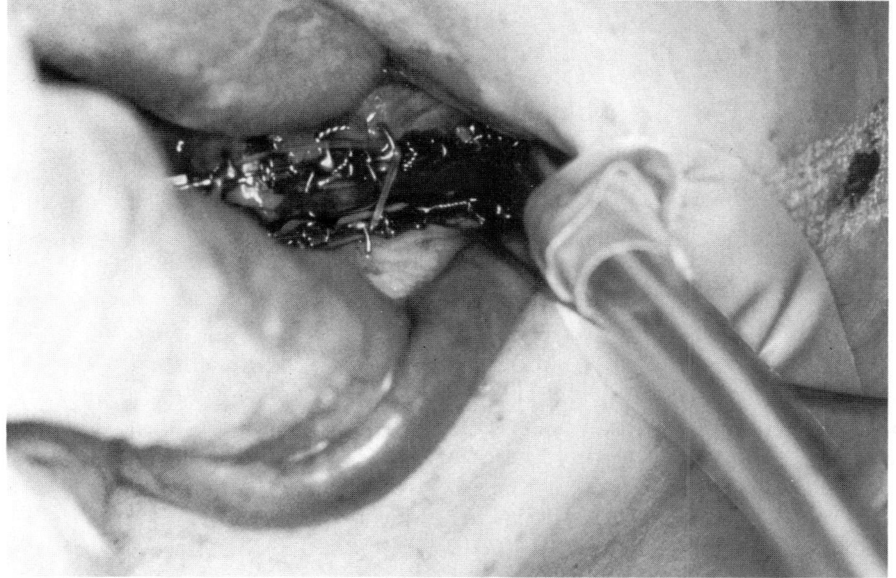

FIG 13–12.
Use of oral endotracheal tube in an instance of surgery involving intermaxillary fixation of the jaws.

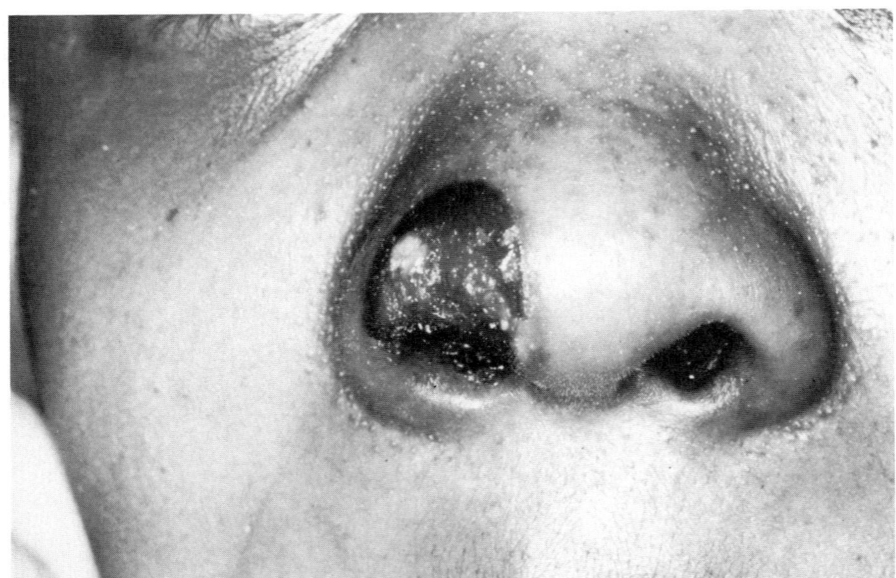

FIG 13–13.
Pressure necrosis of nares caused by excessive pressure from the nasoendotracheal tube during a surgical procedure.

NASOTRACHEAL INTUBATION CONSIDERATIONS

The use of a decongestant to facilitate endotracheal tube insertion into the nasal passages without excessive bleeding is recommended. There is some question, however, as to whether attempts to dilate the nares in preparation for endotracheal tube placement is of benefit.[12] Care should be taken when the nasal endotracheal tube is secured to avoid excessive pressure against the nares, which may produce ischemia and possible necrosis (Fig 13–13).

Occasionally the nasotracheal tube will be placed inadvertently in the esophagus instead of the trachea.[13] When this is noted by failure of lung ventilation, the tube may be withdrawn out of the esophagus into the hypopharynx. The mouth and the opposite nares are then occluded and respirations maintained until the patient has adequately oxygenation for the next attempt at intubation. Withdrawing the endotracheal tube up into the nasopharynx and disconnecting the oxygen source with reconnection to the face mask for face mask ventilation produces excessive trauma to the nasal cavity and wastes additional time before reventilation.

FIBEROPTIC NASAL LARYNGOSCOPIC CONSIDERATIONS

The use of a fiberoptic nasal endoscope to place an endotracheal tube may be indicated in patients with limited mouth opening and when the larynx cannot be visualized with a laryngoscope. A variety of techniques involve an approach with the patient awake, and other techniques involve sedation of the patient. In some instances the patient is asleep with a light, general anesthetic, allowing the patient to maintain ventilation with an inhalation agent. The ad-

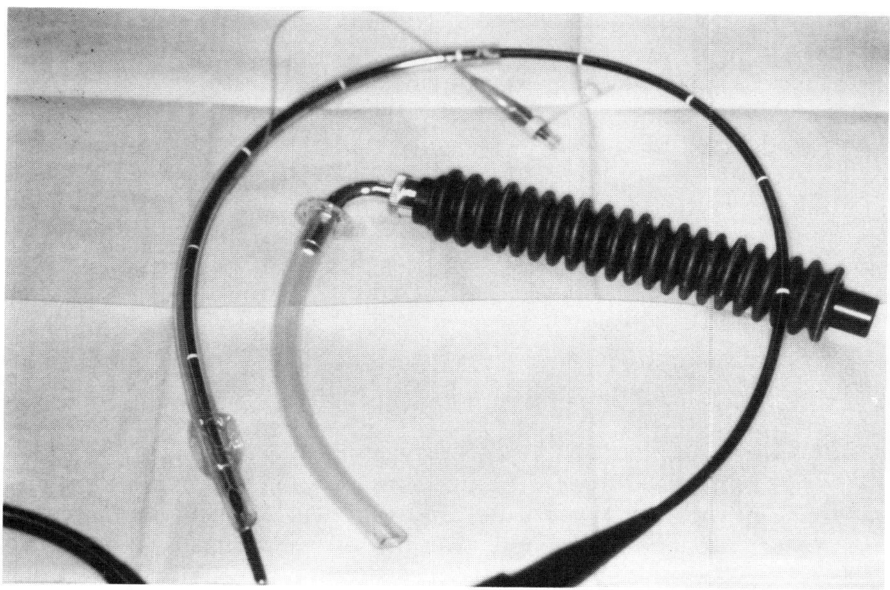

FIG 13–14.
Equipment used to simultaneously provide insufflation of patient who is asleep maintaining spontaneous respirations under general inhalation anesthesia while fiberoptic endoscope is being placed through opposite nares in preparation for passage of a nasal endotracheal tube.

vantage to the former approach is that the patient maintains spontaneous respirations and all protective reflexes. The disadvantage to this technique is the psychic trauma that often accompanies it.

Maintaining spontaneous respiration under general anesthesia circumvents emotional stress to the patient but carries the risk of inadvertent deepening of the anesthesia with loss of spontaneous respirations and possible loss of airway. Relative to the latter approach, the technique involving simultaneous oxygen–inhalation agent insufflation through one nostril with simultaneous use of the fiberoptic endoscope through the opposite nostril allows for control of the patient while tracheal identification and entrance are attempted (Fig 13–14).[14]

INJURIES ASSOCIATED WITH INTUBATION

Dental injuries may occur with inadvertent traumatic forces against the maxillary incisors by the laryngoscope. It is most frequently seen in the hands of inexperienced personnel and less frequently seen in association with a patient who has a difficult airway. Fractures at the crown of the incisor may be managed through referral to the local dentist after the patient is discharged from the hospital. Teeth that are partially or completely avulsed from the socket, however, should have immediate attention. If the tooth is partially avulsed, it should be pressed back into its normal position. The tooth that has been avulsed should be placed in saline and a consultation from the oral surgery service obtained.

Ideally, an avulsed tooth should be replaced into its socket immediately. However, the practical concerns of aspiration of the nonsecured tooth during the remainder of general anesthesia or the recovery period makes this approach somewhat risky. As a result, the reimplantation of the tooth should probably be delayed until after the operation, when the tooth can be secured in place by a dentist using direct bonding or wiring techniques. Such avulsed teeth normally require root canal therapy within the next 1 to 2 weeks.[15]

Within the last 10 years much has been published about TMJ abnormalities. Of 561 patients that I saw for TMJ derangements, 15 patients stated that their problem began following general anesthesia. This finding has also been noted by other authors.[16] Because of an increase in the incidence of litigation related to dental and medical procedures allegedly causing TMJ problems, it would be prudent for the anesthesiologist to inquire about previous TMJ complaints.

If a history of clicking, popping, catching, locking, or joint pain is identified,[17] the patient's preexisting condition should be discussed with him or her, with emphasis placed on the fact that any maneuver of such a joint may cause a flare-up. These patients should be informed that flare-ups are also known to be caused by such routine jaw movements as yawning, yelling, and biting into food.

Should a patient develop postanesthetic TMJ complaints, the initial management would be soft diet, avoidance of wide opening, anti-inflammatory medications, and moist heat to the symptomatic joint and muscle regions for approximately 2 weeks. If the complaint is not resolved within this time period, the patient should be referred for more definitive management of the complaint.

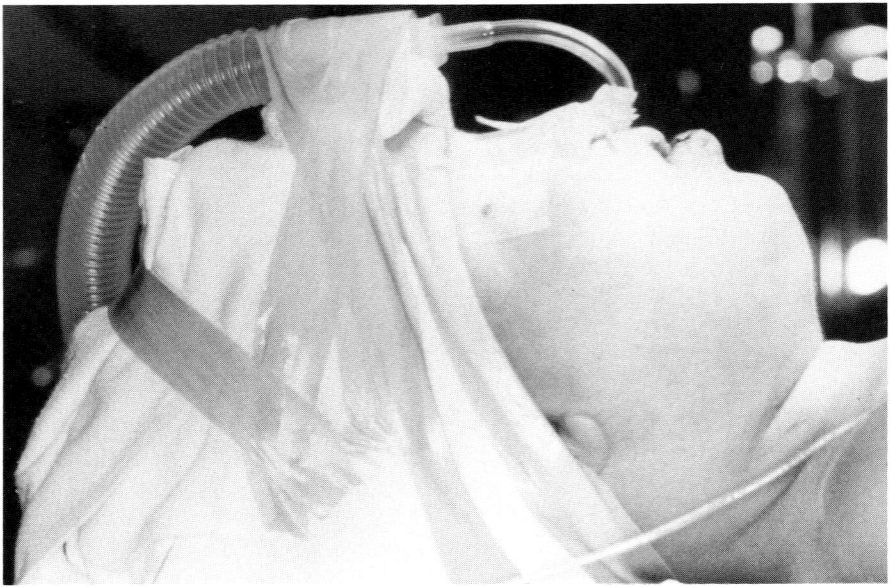

FIG 13–15.
Example of securing the endotracheal tube as a means of avoiding unexpected uncoupling during surgery.

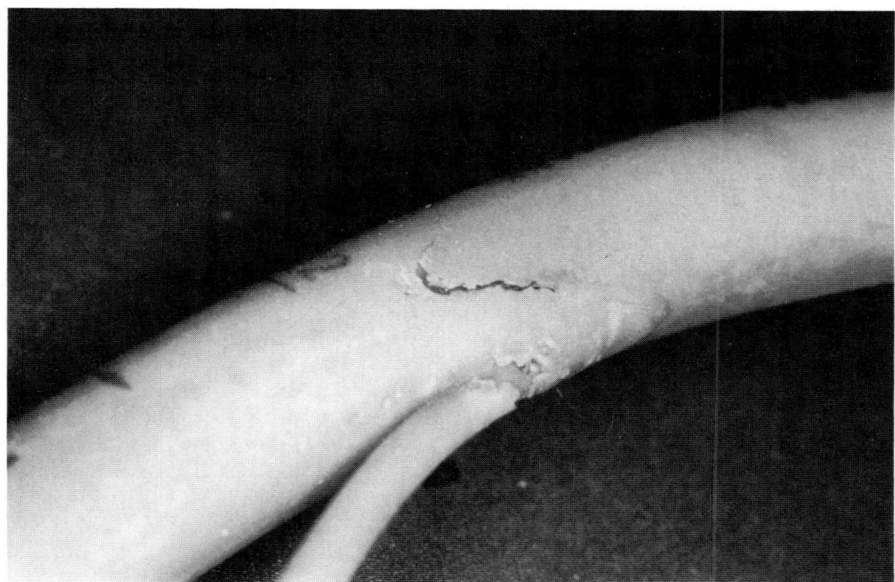

FIG 13–16.
Endotracheal tube with laceration caused by surgical instrument during maxillary osteotomy.

INTRAOPERATIVE AIRWAY PROBLEMS

Intraoperative airway difficulties may be related to uncoupling of connectors or tube displacement. Before the surgical phase is initiated, it is important to secure the endotracheal tube in a manner that will prevent the uncoupling of the connector and at the same time prevent the tube from being extracted out of the larynx (Fig 13–15).[18] The latter concern would be most apt to occur in the posterior of the mouth and during pharyngoplasties. The use of a suturing technique around the endotracheal tube to the anterior vestibule of the mandible helps provide additional security to this end.

Trauma to the endotracheal tube or cuff can also be a concern. Pretesting of the inflatable cuff is standard procedure. The use of McGill's forceps has the potential to rupture soft cuffs. Certain maxillary osteotomies may produce direct injury to the cuff by surgical saws and drills (Fig 13–16).[19, 20] Finally, obstruction of tubes may occur with intraluminal clots or herniated cuffs.[21, 22]

POSTANESTHESIA AIRWAY CONSIDERATIONS

The management of the patient's airway in the recovery room has special problems related to the emergence from the general anesthetic with the patient's sensorium and reflexes still depressed. Many of these patients have had surgery in the maxillofacial region with resultant postsurgical oozing and surgical edema.[23] In instances of palatal or pharyngeal surgery, the posterior airway is diminished relative to the presurgical period. Following osteotomies or fractures of the maxilla or mandible, the patient may be placed in intermaxillary fixation.

In the recovery room the airway in doubt should remain intubated. For surgical procedures involving the oral and nasal cavities, a semiprone position with the patient's head dependent, relative to the larynx, is indicated. The patient should be lying on his or her side such that the endotracheal tube is in the upper naries, allowing drainage to occur from the most dependent nostril and out of the oral cavity. In children with closure of soft palate or pharyngoplasties, the use of a deep tongue suture taped passively to the cheek will allow forward positioning of the tongue should acute airway obstruction occur (Fig 13–17). The use of a Briggs adapter with humidified air facilitates good gas exchange and upper airway physiology.

Regarding patients in intermaxillary fixation, additional considerations include the use of the nasoendotracheal tube as a nasopharyngeal airway following extubation, allowing the tube to remain in the posterior pharynx for a period of time. Normally if the airway is extubated while the patient is awake, he or she must be spontaneously breathing and swallowing appropriately before

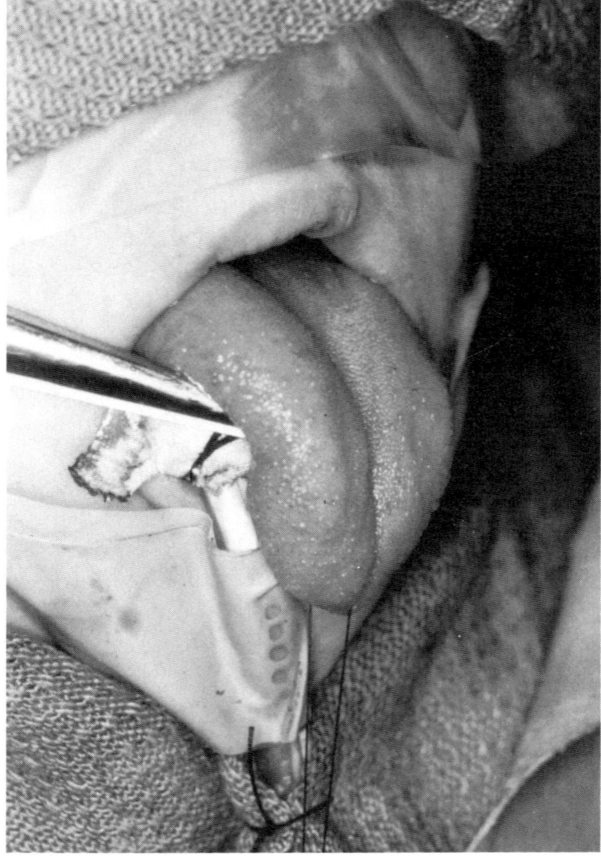

FIG 13–17.
Use of tongue suture in soft palate and pharyngeal surgery during immediate postoperative period to provide for emergent airway.

extubation. Additional measures to facilitate airway protection include using intrasurgical corticosteroids, using nasal decongestants, having wire cutters at the bedside, removing gastric contents before the patients leave the operating room, and using nasal airways if necessary.

Management of the airway in oral and maxillofacial surgery is expressed in a variety of settings and circumstances. Optimum success toward these goals requires knowledge of the anatomy and physiology of this region, as well as a careful preparation and approach to these problems.

REFERENCES

1. Hutton JB, Hoggins GS: Severe facial trauma resulting in airway obstruction. *Oral Surg* 1986; 62:476.
2. Steinhauser P: Ludwig's angina: Report of a case in a 12 year old boy. *J Oral Surg* 1967; 25:251.
3. Strauss H, Tilghmann DM: Ludwig's angina, emphysema, pulmonary infiltration and pericarditis secondary to extraction of a tooth. *J Oral Surg* 1980; 38:223.
4. Hill CM: Death following dental clearance in a patient suffering from ankylosing spondylitis: A case report with discussion on management of such problems. *Br J Oral Surg* 1980; 18:73.
5. Patterson H, Kelly JH, Strone M: Ludwig's angina: An update. *Laryngoscope* 1982; 92:370.
6. Hough RT, Fitzgerald BE, Latta JE, et al: Ludwig's angina: A report of two cases and review of the literature from 1945 till January 1979. *J Oral Surg* 1980; 38:849.
7. Topazian RG: Etiology of ankylosis of the temporomandibular joint: Analysis of 44 cases. *J Oral Surg* 1964; 22:153.
8. Carlsson GE, Popp S, Oberg T: Arthritis and allied diseases of the temporomandibular joint, in Zarb Z, Carlsson GE (eds): *Temporomandibular Joint Function and Dysfunction*. St Louis, CV Mosby Co, 1980.
9. Farrar WB: Characteristics of the condylar path and internal derangements of the TMJ. *J Prosthet Dent* 1978; 39:319.
10. Travell JG, Simmons DG (eds): Masseter muscle, in *Myofascial Pain and Dysfunction, the Trigger Point Manual*. Baltimore, Williams & Wilkins Co, 1983, p 225.
11. Kline SN: Anatomy related to intubation and general anesthesia. *Anesth Progr* 1969; 16:274.
12. Adamson DN, Theisen FC, Barrett KC: Effect of mechanical dilatation on nasotracheal intubation. *J Oral Maxillofac Surg* 1988; 46:372.
13. Birmingham PK, Cheney FW, Ward RJ: Esophogeal intubation: A review of detection techniques. *Anesth Analg* 1986; 65:886.
14. Stella JP, Kageler WV, Epker BN: Fiberoptic endotracheal intubation in oral and maxillofacial surgery. *J Oral Maxillofac Surg* 1986; 44:923.
15. Camp JH: Treatment of the avulsed tooth. Ad Hoc Committee on the Treatment of the Avulsed Tooth of the American Association of Endodontists: *J Am Dent Assoc* 1983; 107:706.
16. Taylor RC, Way WL, Hendrickson RA: Temporomandibular joint problems in relation to the administration of general anesthesia. *J Oral Surg* 1968; 26:327.
17. Kent JM (ed): Temporomandibular disorders: "Doctor, my jaw hurts." *Patient Care* 1983; 17:108.
18. Altemir FH: Pericranial fixation of the nasotracheal tube. *J Oral Maxillofac Surg* 1986; 44:585.
19. Schwartz LB, Sordill WC, et al: Difficulty in removal of accidently cut endotracheal tube. *J Oral Maxillofac Surg* 1982; 40:518.

20. Fagraius L, Angelillo JC, Dolan EA: A serious anesthesia hazard during orthognathic surgery. *Anesth Analg* 1980; 59:150.
21. Feingerb SE, Klein SL: Airway obstruction with the Rae endotracheal tube. *J Oral Maxillofac Surg* 1983; 41:262.
22. Glinsman D, Paulin EG: Airway obstruction after nasal-tracheal intubation. *Anesthesiology* 1982; 56:229.
23. Handler SD, et al: Airway management in the repair of craniofacial defects. *Cleft Palate J* 1979; 16:16.

Chapter 14

Pediatric Difficult Airways

Niall Wilton

Management of the difficult pediatric airway requires knowledge of developmental anatomy and the differences between the adult and pediatric airway (Figs 14–1 to 14–4). Many of the skills and techniques used in the management of difficult airways in children are the same as those used for difficult airways in adults but with adaptations for pediatric practice.

BASIC EQUIPMENT

Oral Airways

Oral airways are designed to bypass possible sites of obstruction between the mouth and larynx. To perform this function, they must be the appropriate length. An airway that is too short may push the base of the tongue posteriorly, thus causing airway obstruction, whereas one that is too long may push the epiglottis over the laryngeal aperture to produce airway obstruction. The appropriate-size airway is one that extends from the corner of the mouth and ends just cephalad to the angle of the mandible.

Nasal Airways

Nasopharyngeal airways are useful in pediatric airway management. Soft red rubber tubes (Rusch, Inc., Germany) are available, or an airway may be fashioned from an endotracheal tube. It is wise to place a safety pin through the end of such an airway to prevent it from being inhaled if it becomes unfastened. The appropriate length can again be estimated by measuring the distance from the nares to just cephalad to the angle of the mandible, allowing for an appropriate curve. The airway should be long enough to overcome obstruction at the level of the base of the tongue. A nasopharyngeal airway that is too

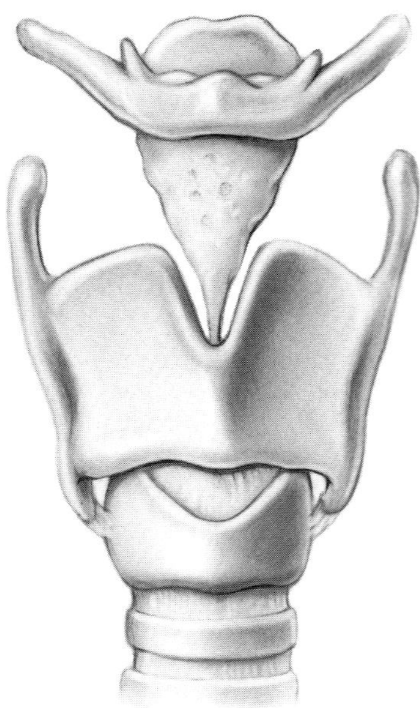
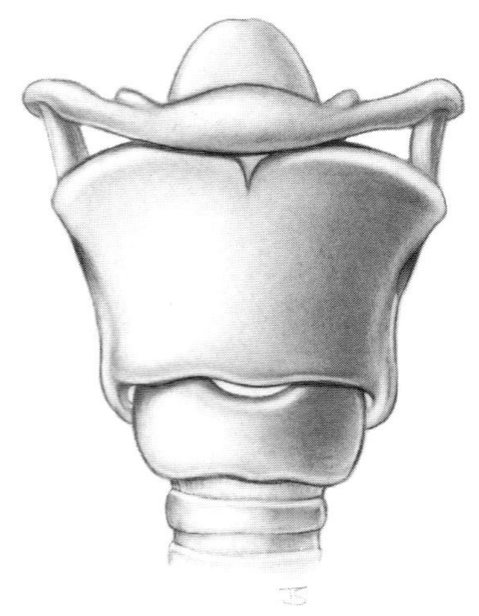

FIG 14–1.
Front view of the larynx. Note overlapping of hyoid, thyroid, and cricoid on infant. (Courtesy of M. L. Norton, M.D.)

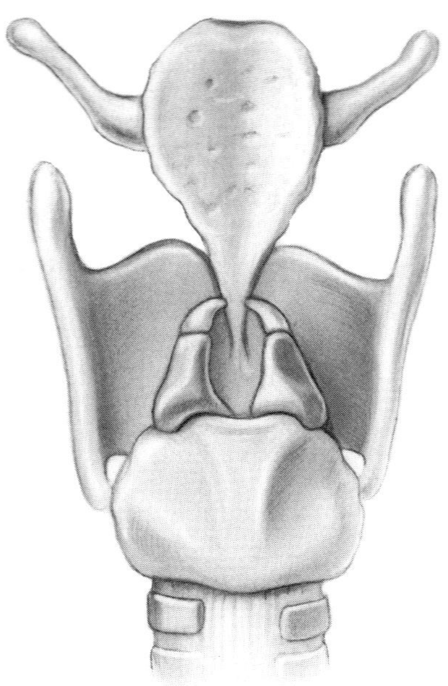
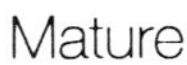
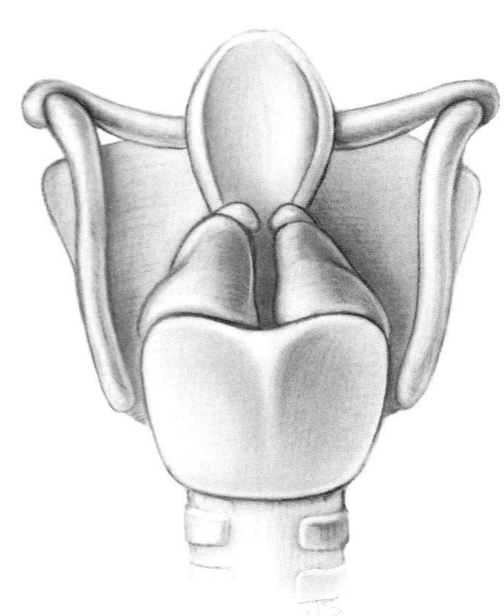

FIG 14–2.
Back view of the larynx. Note shape of the intrinsic laryngeal cartilages (arytenoids, especially) and positioning of the aryepiglottic folds. (Courtesy of M. L. Norton, M.D.)

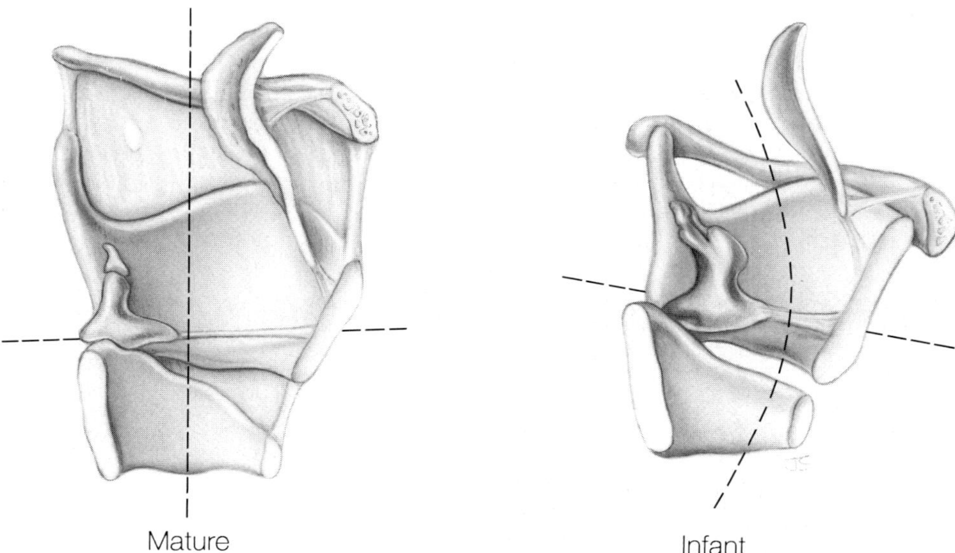

FIG 14–3.
Lateral view of the larynx. Note axes and arytenoids, vocal folds, and epiglottic ligaments. (Courtesy of M. L. Norton, M.D.)

long may pass via the hypopharynx into the esophagus so that even though the site of obstruction is bypassed, ventilation will still not be possible.

In an anesthetized patient it may be appropriate to purposefully advance the airway into the esophagus and then withdraw the airway until breath sounds are heard. The airway should be inserted dorsally, perpendicular to the patient's face. This is important to ensure that the airway passes through the inferior meatus of the nares under the inferior concha, which is the largest of the three meati. If resistance to insertion occurs, one should check to see that the tube is directed toward the inferior meatus, then try the opposite nostril. If resistance still occurs, a smaller size airway should be selected.

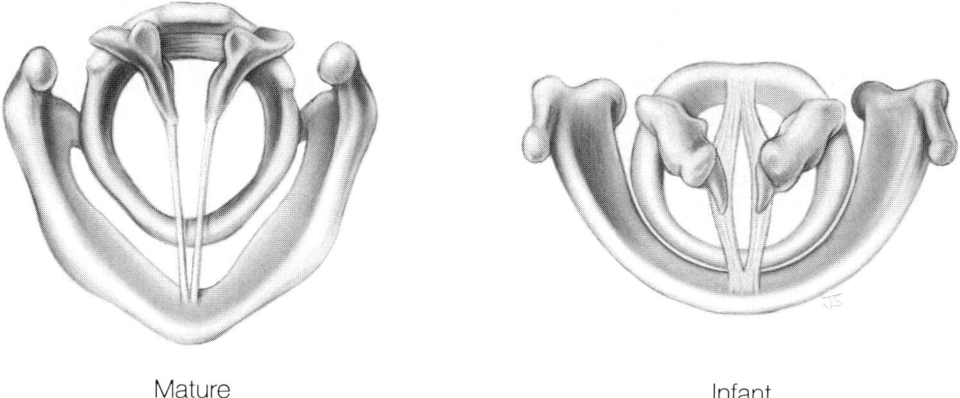

FIG 14–4.
Superior view. Note shape and positioning of the intrinsic laryngeal cartilages (arytenoids, etc.) and vocal folds. (Courtesy of M. L. Norton, M.D.)

Masks

Both cushion masks and noncushioned masks (Rendell-Baker) are available for airway management. The mask should achieve an airtight fit. With a cushion mask this requires a mask that fits over the bridge of the nose and seats over the mentum. Some anesthesiologists prefer the noncushioned Rendell-Baker mask. This mask has a lower volume of displacement (i.e., dead space) and is designed to fit in the groove of the chin rather than over the mentum (Fig 14–5). It also forces the user to displace the mandible away from the mid-

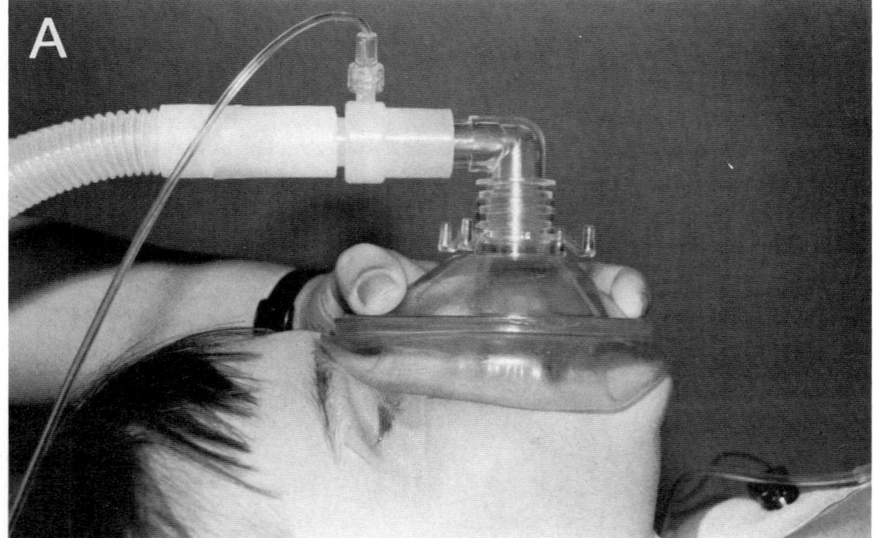

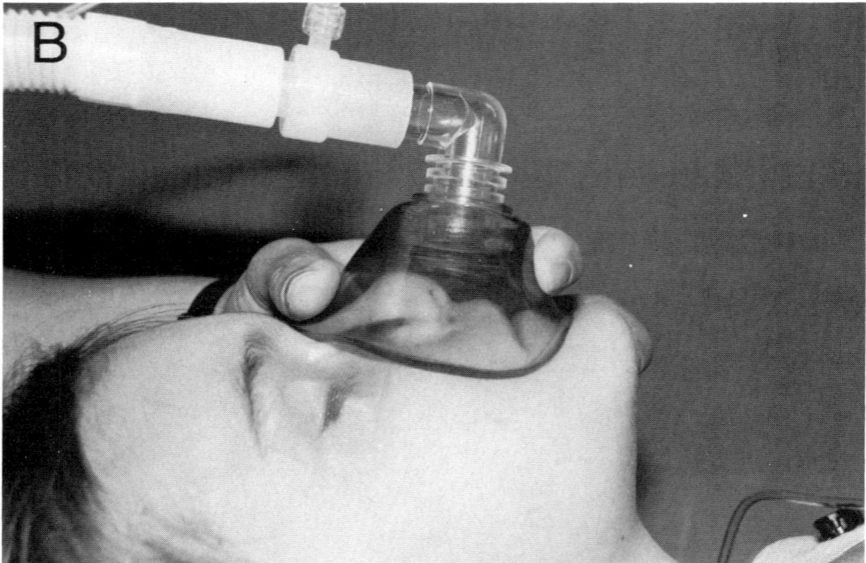

FIG 14–5.
Face masks. **A,** cushion mask. **B,** Rendell-Baker mask. Note position of the Rendell-Baker mask in the groove of the chin.

face, thus potentially displacing the tongue anteriorly and improving airway management.

INTUBATION EQUIPMENT

Laryngoscope Blades

A straight blade is usually used for laryngoscopy in neonates, infants, and young children. The relative macroglossia and cephalad positioning of the larynx (C-3 to C-4 vs. C-5 in the adult) produce a decrease in space between the base of the tongue and the epiglottis (vallecula) that causes inadequate visualization of the larynx when a curved blade is used. The straight blade is usually passed posterior to the epiglottis, unlike the curved blade laryngoscopes in adults. This is necessary because the epiglottis tends to be angled more posteriorly and lies over the laryngeal aperture, which may not be visible when the epiglottis is elevated by placing the tip of the blade in the vallecula. The most commonly used blades are the straight Miller blades (Fig 14–6). Also, in chil-

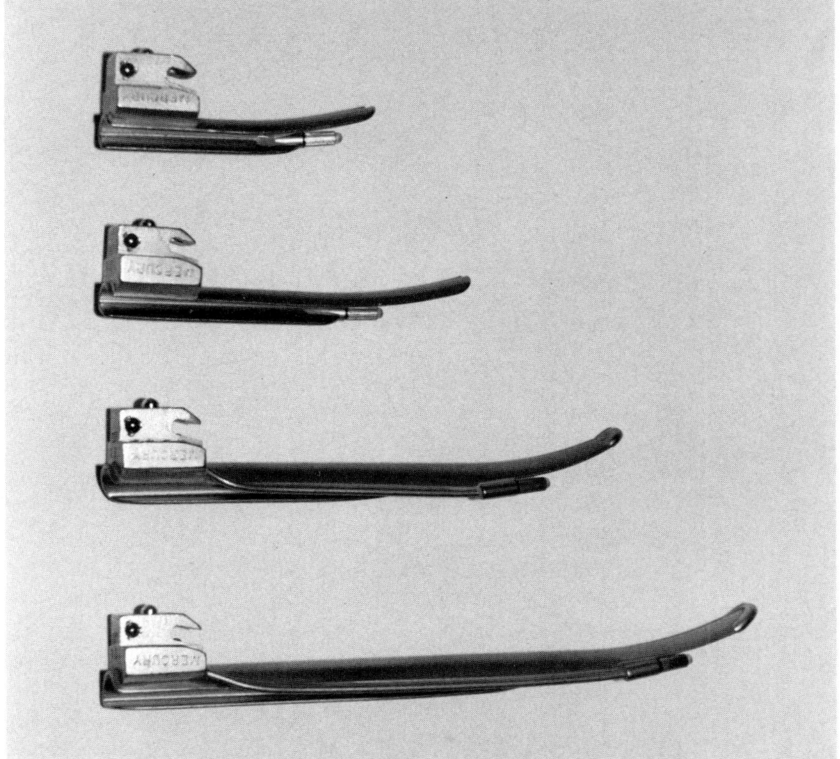

FIG 14–6.
Miller blades viewed from the right. *Top* to *bottom:* Miller 0 for neonates and Miller 1, 2, and 3 for adolescents. Note braiding on Miller 2 and 3, allowing use similar to that of curved blades by placement of the tip in the vallecula. Also note that the light source may be placed on the left (Miller 0 and 1) or right (Miller 2 and 3), depending on the manufacturer.

dren, a straight blade with a flat cross section designed to be placed in the vallecula, the Seward blade, is frequently used (Figs 14–7 and 14–8). A guide to the laryngoscope blades commonly used for children may be found in Table 14–1.

Endotracheal Tubes

With the changing diameter and length of the larynx and trachea with age, several different endotracheal tubes of varying diameter and length are required. The narrowest part of the upper airway in neonates, infants, and young children is the cricoid cartilage. It is not until 8 to 10 years of age, with the growth of the cricoid cartilage, that the narrowest part of the airway is at

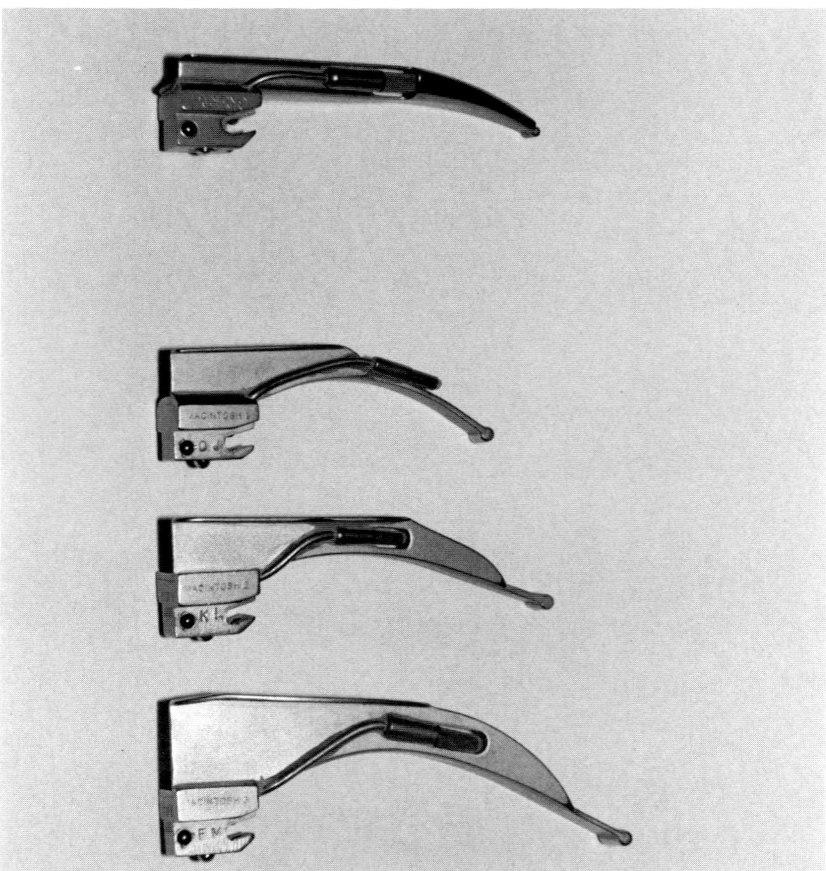

FIG 14–7.
Seward and Macintosh blades viewed from the left. *Top* to *bottom:* Seward 1; Macintosh 1, 2, and 3. All of these are designed to be placed in the vallecula. The extreme curve of the Macintosh 1 limits visibility and has little use in routine pediatric practice. Note increasing posterior depth of Macintosh blades, designed to sweep the tongue away and keep line of vision clear. The light source is always positioned on the left side.

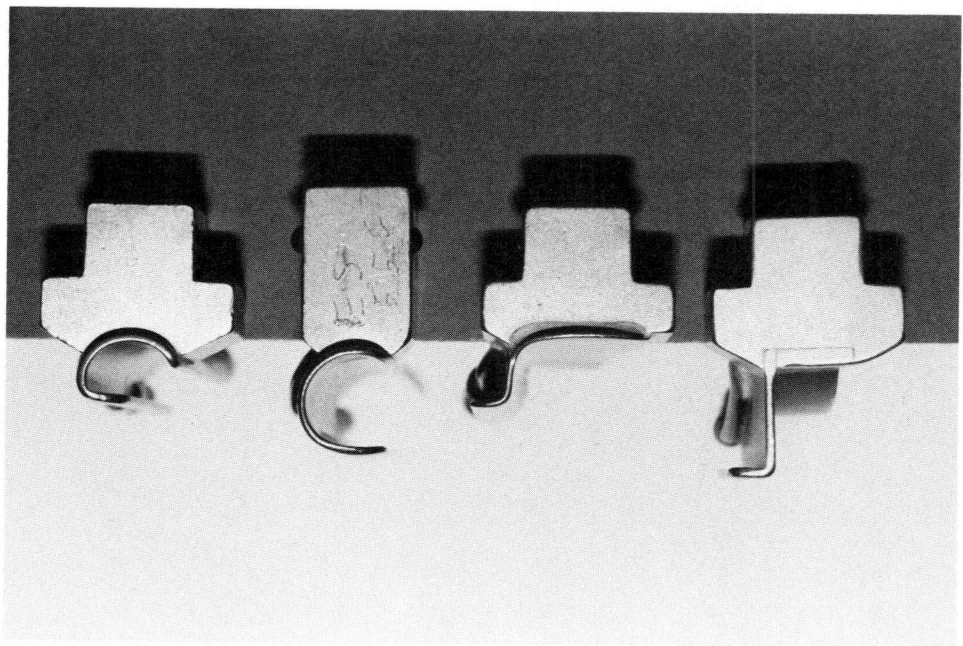

FIG 14–8.
Laryngoscope blades seen end on (*left* to *right*): size 1 Miller, Wisconsin, Seward, and Macintosh blades. The deeper **C** in the Wisconsin blade makes it easier to pass the endotracheal tube down the bore of the laryngoscope blade, but in comparison with the Miller, makes it more difficult to pass the endotracheal tube from the right side. Flange on Seward blade is noticeably less deep than on the Macintosh blade and is usually deep enough to prevent the tongue from sliding across the line of vision. The flange may be easier to insert than the Macintosh blade because of the decrease in depth posteriorly.

the level of the vocal folds, as in adults. For most children less than this age, an uncuffed tube should be used. In these patients it is desirable to select an endotracheal tube that produces an audible air leak at 20 to 25 cm H_2O to prevent postintubation edema. The ideal length of an endotracheal tube should leave its distal end lying in the midtrachea. Although visual inspection and auscultation are the surest methods of confirming the appropriate length of in-

TABLE 14–1.

Guide to Sizes of Laryngoscope Blades
Commonly Used for Children

Age	Miller	Wis-Hipple	Seward	Macintosh
Premature	0	—	—	—
Neonate	0	—	—	—
1 mo–2 yr	1	—	—	—
2–6 yr	—	1.5	1	—
6–12 yr	2	—	2	2
≥12 yr	3	—	3	3

TABLE 14–2.
Guide to Internal Diameter and Length of Pediatric Endotracheal Tubes

Weight or Age	Internal Diameter (mm)	Oral Length (cm)	Nasal Length (cm)
<1,000 g	2.5	8–9	10–11
1,000–2,500 g	3.0	9–10	11–12
Neonate–6 mo	3.5	10	13
6–18 mo	4.0	11	14
18–24 mo	4.0–4.5	12	15
≥2 yr	$4.0 + \dfrac{\text{Age (yr)}}{4}$	$12 + \dfrac{\text{Age (yr)}}{2}$	$15 + \dfrac{\text{Age (yr)}}{2}$

sertion of an endotracheal tube, an approximate guide is outlined in Table 14–2.

TECHNIQUE

Positioning

Compared with an adult, the neonate has a large head in relation to the rest of his or her body. This means that the patient's cervical spine is slightly flexed at rest. The optimal position for intubation, cervical flexion with head extension, is produced by simply extending the patient's head. As the child ages and head size decreases relative to body size, the head will need to be elevated to produce cervical spine flexion.

Holding the Mask

It is important that the face mask be applied firmly without compressing the patient's airway, that is, there should be no pressure applied to soft tissues of the patient's face or neck. This is achieved by careful placement of the hand so that the thumb and first finger are applied to the mask, the middle finger is applied to the mentum, and the ring or little finger is applied to the bony angle of the mandible (Fig 14–9).

Laryngoscopy

Visualization of the larynx is achieved using techniques similar to those described for adults. Visualization is frequently improved by posterior displacement of the larynx using cricoid pressure. In neonates this posterior displacement can be achieved with pressure from the little finger (Fig 14–10). The standard insertion technique of displacing the tongue to the left sometimes causes problems in neonates and infants because of difficulty in controlling the tongue. If this occurs, better visualization may be achieved by inserting the straight blade laryngoscope in the midline and fixing the tongue between the mandible and the laryngoscope blade. If visualization of the larynx is inadequate using the standard insertion technique, insertion of the laryngoscope from the extreme right-hand corner of the mouth may improve it.

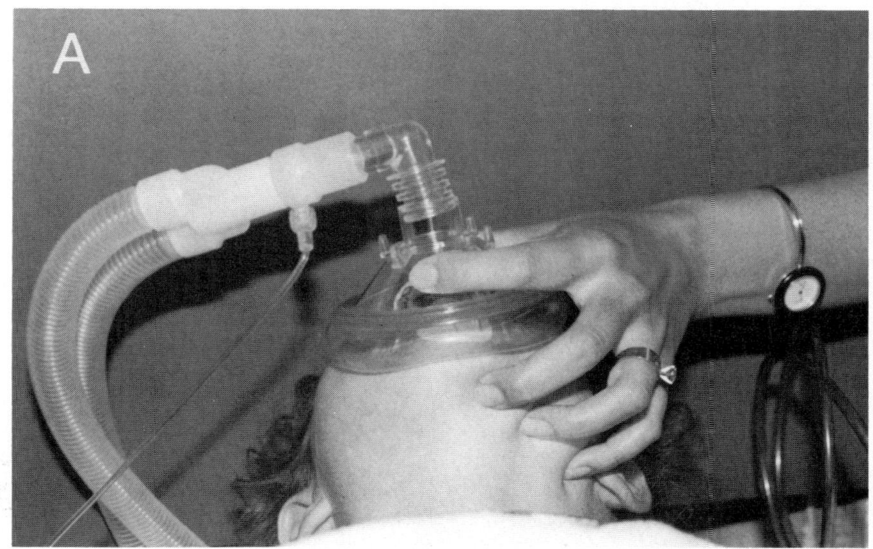

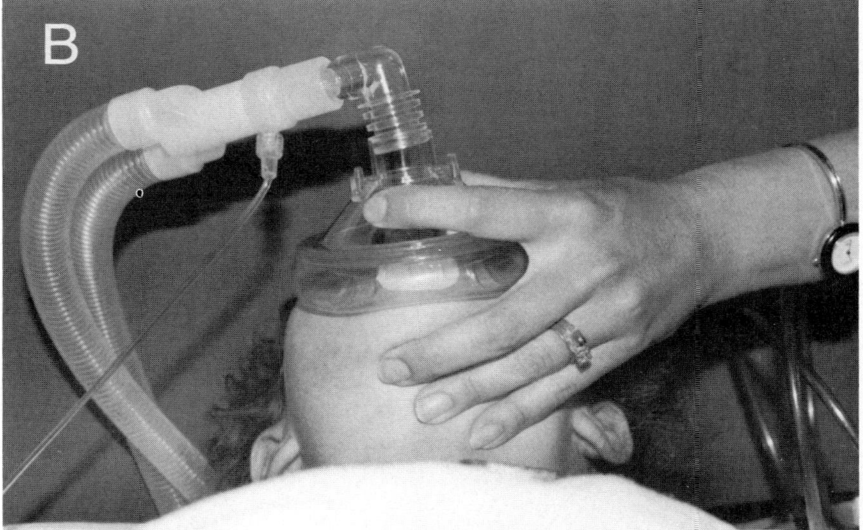

FIG 14–9.
A, correct hand position for holding the mask with fingers gently but firmly placed laterally over the ramus and angle of the mandible. **B,** incorrect hand placement, with fingers in midline compressing soft tissue structures in the floor of the mouth, thereby decreasing patency of the oral airway.

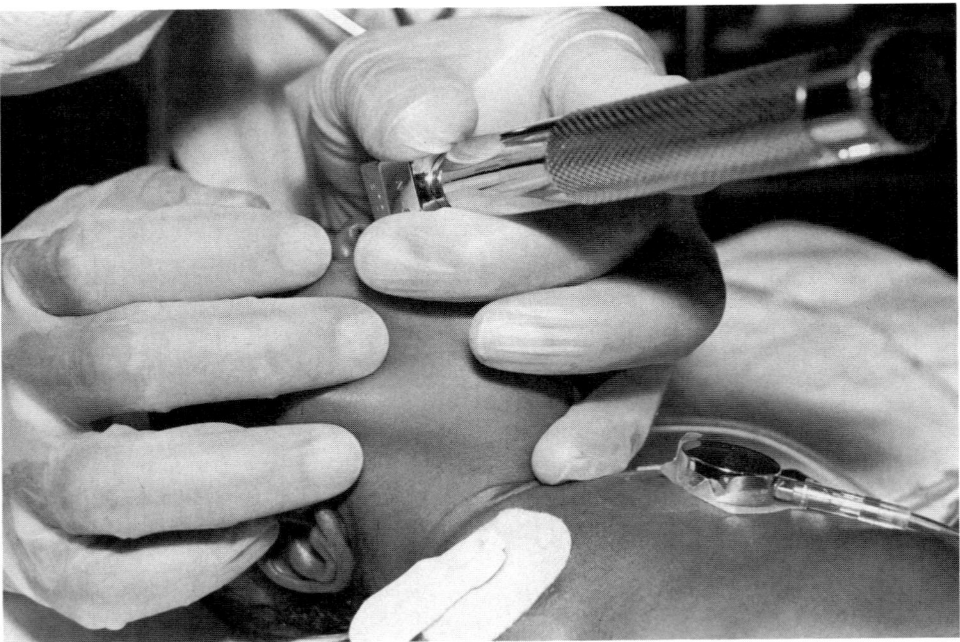

FIG 14–10.
Laryngoscopy in a neonate. Anterior displacement of the contents of the floor of the mouth by lifting the laryngoscope in the direction of the handle. Simultaneous pressure on the trachea just distal to the thyroid cartilage applied with the little finger moves the larynx posteriorly and improves visualization of the glottis.

OTHER TECHNIQUES OF INTUBATION

Light Wand Intubation

An endotracheal tube placed over the light wand may be used to facilitate intubation. The stylet should be bent at a distance from the top that corresponds to the distance from the angle of the mandible to the hyoid. In a low-light environment, the stylet is advanced over the tongue until a glow is visible. The stylet is manipulated, keeping it in the midline. When the glow is visible distal to the hyoid, the endotracheal tube is advanced into the trachea. Unfortunately only one size of light wand is currently available, which limits the smallest endotracheal tube to 5.5 mm.

Anterior Commissure Laryngoscope With Optical Stylet

In children with mandibular hypoplasia or macroglossia, the use of an anterior commissure laryngoscope inserted from the extreme right side may improve visualization of the larynx. An endotracheal tube (without a connector) applied over an appropriately sized telescope can then be advanced through the anterior commissure laryngoscope and into the trachea (Fig 14–11). For a neonate, a 9 mm laryngoscope used with a small telescope will allow intubation with a 3.0 or 3.5 mm endotracheal tube.

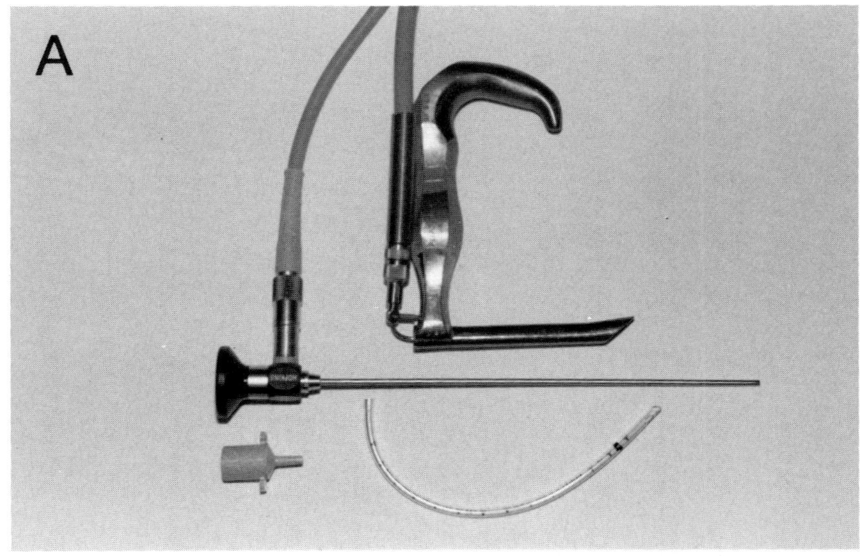

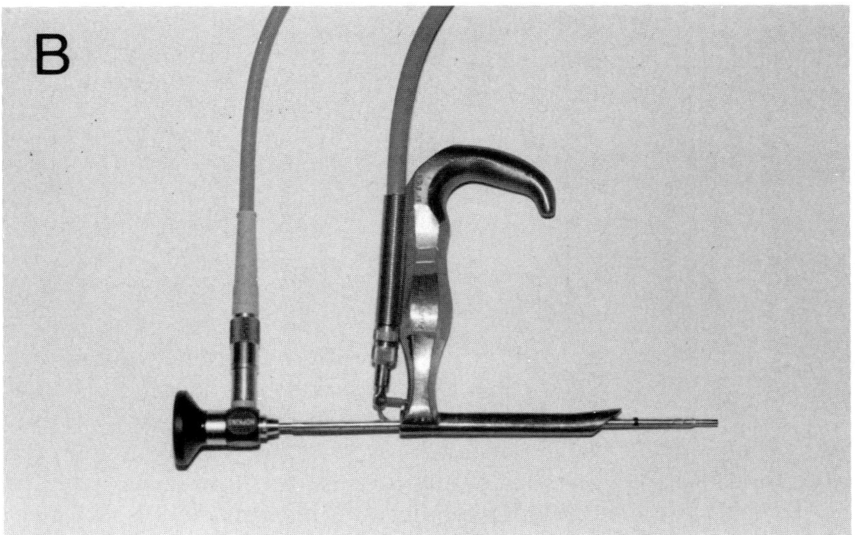

FIG 14–11.
Anterior commissure laryngoscope and telescope. **A,** individual components necessary for intubation. Visualization of larynx is achieved by the use of anterior commissure laryngoscope. **B,** optical telescope with the endotracheal tube placed over it is advanced through the laryngoscope maintaining visualization of larynx and trachea. Intubation is completed by advancing the endotracheal tube over the telescope.

Bullard Laryngoscope

The pediatric version of the Bullard laryngoscope (Fig 14–12) is a laryngoscope with a fixed preformed curve of approximately 90 degrees and an applied fiberoptic light source and image bundle to allow visualization at the tip. The advantage of this laryngoscope is that it can be introduced into the

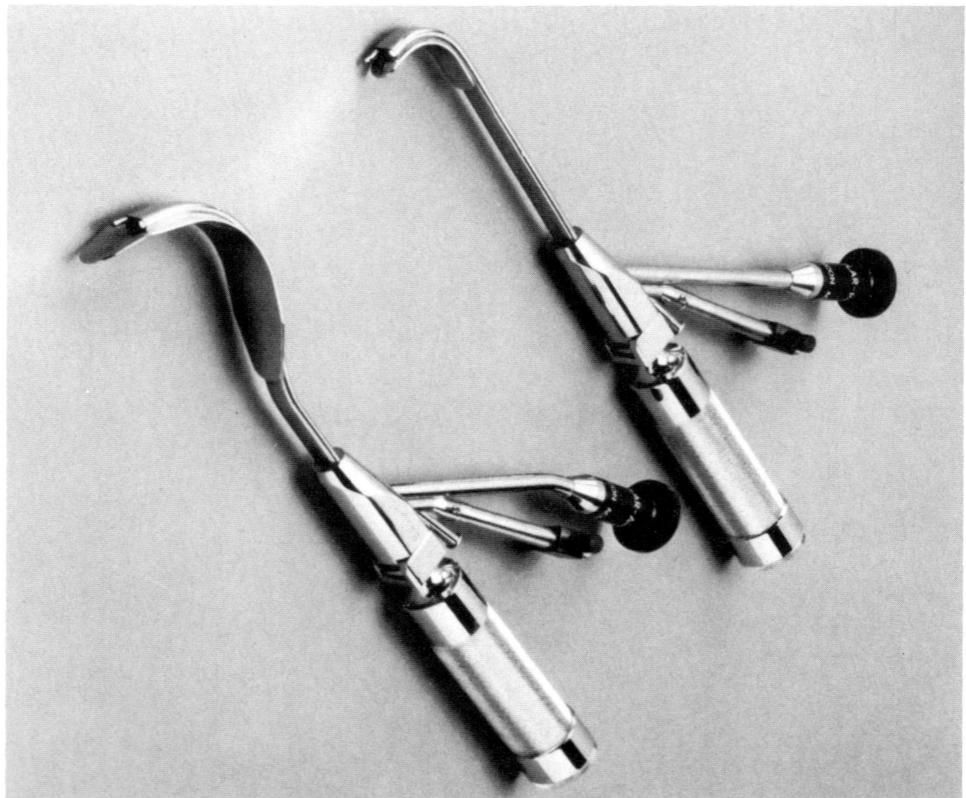

FIG 14–12.
Bullard laryngoscopes.

oropharynx with minimal mouth opening. With the patient lying supine, the laryngoscope is placed in the patient's mouth with the handle horizontal and then rotated vertically as the blade is advanced over the patient's tongue to allow visualization of the larynx. In small infants, however, one may experience difficulty in displacing the epiglottis sufficiently to allow visualization of the larynx, particularly when temporomandibular joint movement is impaired. The laryngoscope is supplied with an intubating stylet attached to the right side of the laryngoscope. Although useful in older children, in neonates and smaller infants the lateral offset of this device limits its use as an aid to intubation.

Fiberoptic Endoscopy as an Aid to Intubation

The fiberscope may be used to aid intubation in both the awake and anesthetized pediatric patient. Intubation using the fiberscope in the awake child is used less frequently than in adults who are awake because of the lack of patient cooperation. In children, fiberoptic endoscopy is often performed following an inhalational induction of anesthesia. If this is not appropriate, intubation of the "awake" patient is performed with the patient sedated. A combination of midazolam and ketamine following an antisialagogue such as atropine or glycopyrolate is most effective.

Where indicated, we use an Olympus LF-1 fiberscope for pediatric patients. Instead of using the suction channel to aspirate secretions, we prefer to pass oxygen at a flow of 2 to 3 L/min through the channel, which serves the dual purpose of maintaining the distal lens clear from secretions and increasing the inspired oxygen concentration.

The technique for nasal intubation in the awake child is essentially the same as for adults. If the oral route is chosen, the most difficult problem is maintaining the fiberscope in the midline. Unlike for adult patients, no specialized oral airways are available for pediatric patients. If an oral Guedel airway is selected and the convex surface cut away, the fiberscope can be kept in the midline (Fig 14–13). If this technique is used in the awake patient, it is important to ensure that the upper palate as well as the remainder of the oropharynx is anesthetized and be aware that although the airway offers some protection from damage to the fiberscope by teeth, it is not as effective as a bite block.

In anesthetized patients, anesthesia may be maintained with either nasopharyngeal insufflation or a specially adapted face mask (Fig 14–14). If airway management under inhalation anesthesia is trouble-free, endoscopy can be performed on the paralyzed patient with adequate oxygenation monitored by continuous measurement of oxygen saturation.

The Olympus LF-1 fiberscope will not allow endotracheal tubes of less than 4.5 mm to pass over the insertion tube. Smaller fiberscopes that will allow the passage of 3.0 mm endotracheal tubes are presently available, but they lack a suction port. In children less than 2 years old (or when intubation with an en-

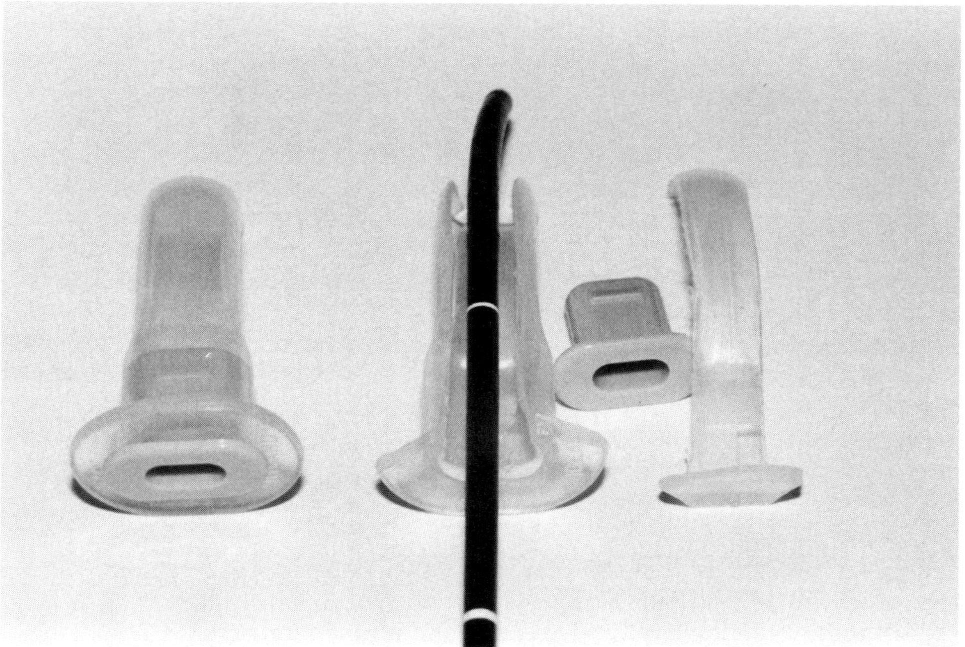

FIG 14–13.
Cutaway oral Guedel airway with fiberscope in place. This use of airway allows the fiberscope to be kept in midline and the endotracheal tube then to be advanced over the fiberscope.

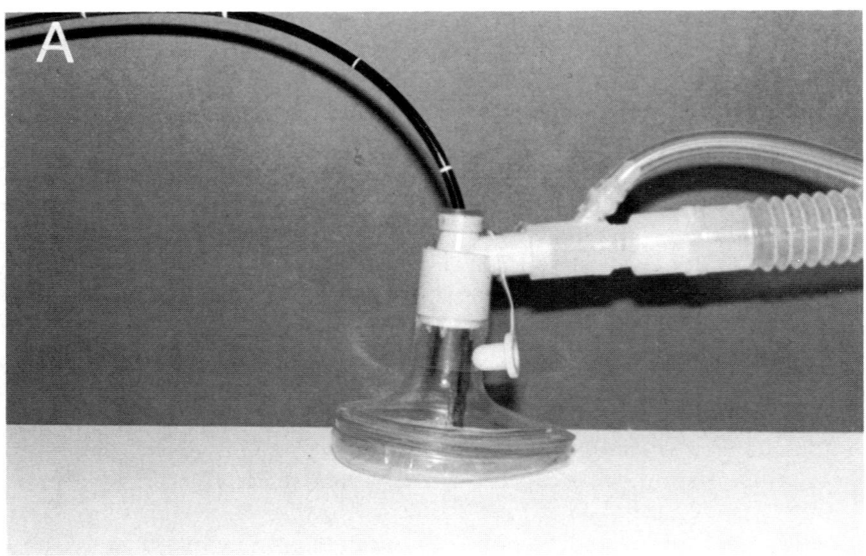

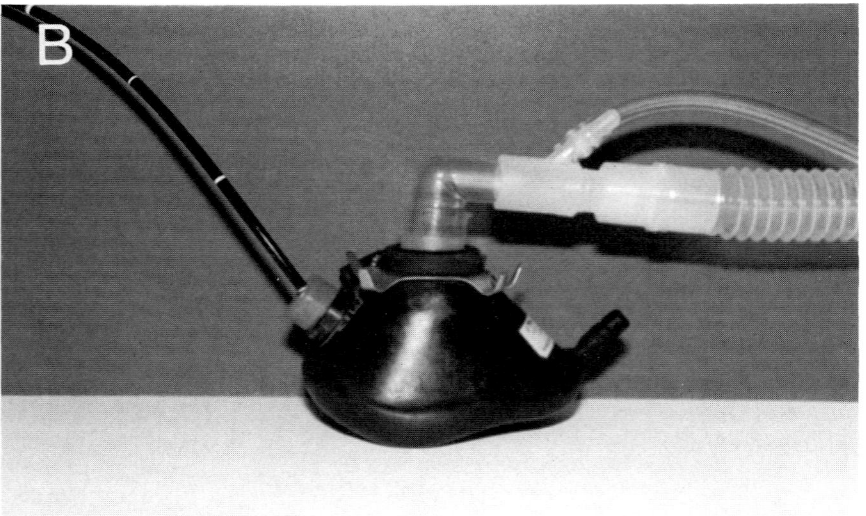

FIG 14–14.
Two techniques that allow mask ventilation and fiberoptic laryngoscopy simultaneously in small infants. **A,** use of Portex connector and clear cushion mask. **B,** use of smallest size Patil-Syracuse mask with separate hole and diaphragm for insertion of fiberscope.

dotracheal tube of less than 4.5 mm internal diameter is required), the LF-1 fiberscope may still be used. Using the suction port, one can pass a guide wire (0.35 mm) through the laryngeal aperture and into the trachea (Fig 14–15). The wire can be left in place, the fiberscope removed, and an endotracheal tube advanced over the wire. It may be advisable to reinsert the fiberscope through the opposite nostril as a visual aid because in neonates and infants the endotracheal tube may get held up at the laryngeal inlet.

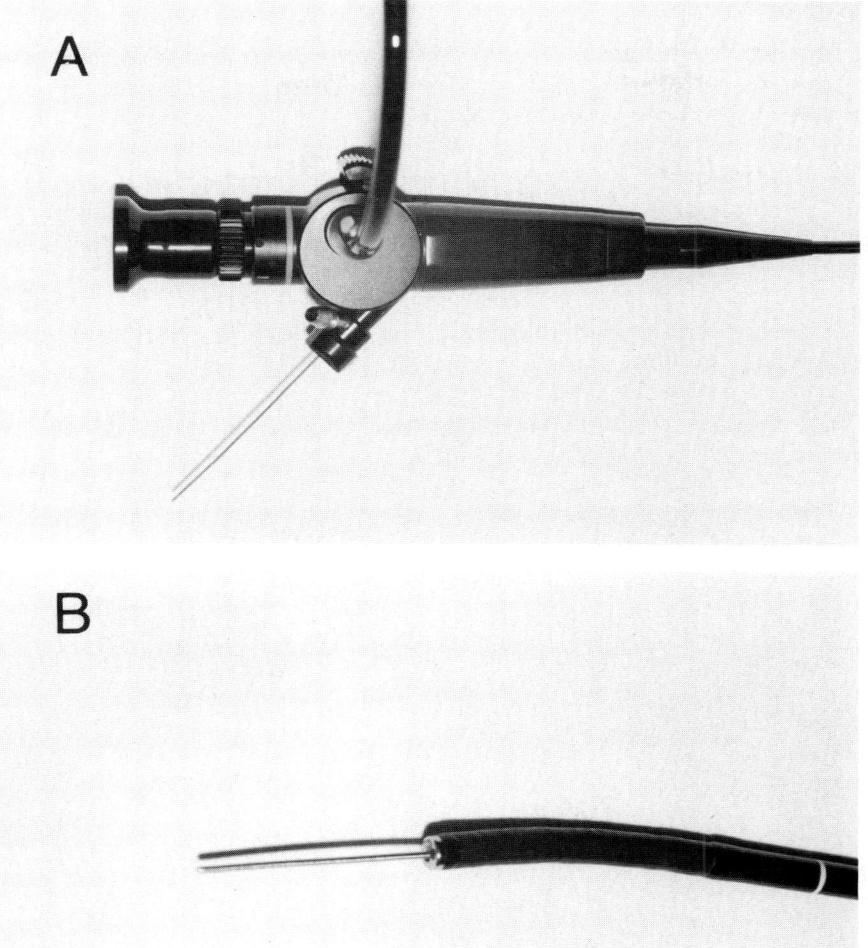

FIG 14–15.
Proximal **(A)** and distal **(B)** ends of fiberscope showing guide wire in place in suction port.

ACTUAL OR POTENTIAL COMPROMISED AIRWAYS

Patients without congenital anomalies may have a compromised airway as a result of many differing etiologies. Each condition usually has its own etiology and presenting symptom complex that determine the management sequence. The following conditions are discussed in order of the anatomic site that they affect rather than based on their etiology.

1. *Supraglottic* area: (1) tonsillar obstruction (kissing tonsils and abscess), (2) retropharyngeal abscess, and (3) epiglottitis.
2. *Glottic* area: (1) laryngeal papillomatosis and (2) laryngospasm.
3. *Subglottic* area: (1) croup (laryngotracheobronchitis) and (2) postintubation edema.
4. *Foreign bodies* aspirated to any site.

Supraglottic Area

Tonsillar Obstruction: Kissing Tonsils and Sleep Apnea Syndrome

Etiology.—Hypertrophied lymphoid tissue leads to partial or intermittent complete airway obstruction (Fig 14–16).

Natural History.—Episodes of partial and complete airway obstruction lead to periods of severe hypoxia, particularly during sleep. This can lead to right-sided heart failure and altered sleep-wake cycles, plus mental impairment.

Symptoms and Signs.—Typically, the patient snores nocturnally, leading to progressive daytime somnolence and lack of concentration.

Investigation.—Flow-volume loops may show abnormalities. Sleep studies show periods of hypoxia (see Chapter 12).

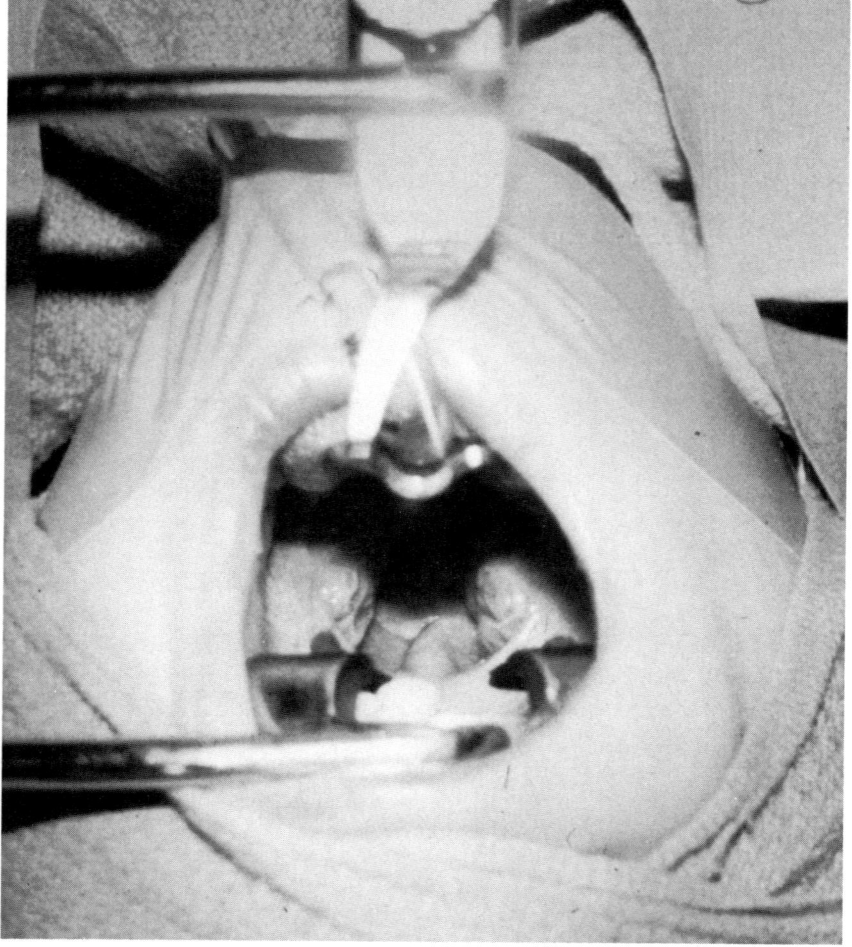

FIG 14–16.

Tonsillar obstruction. These large tonsils met in midline to produce tonsillar obstruction before the mouth gag was inserted.

Management.—Tonsillectomy may improve the airway in some of these patients. Airway management may be difficult because of encroachment of the tonsils into the hypopharynx, which is exacerbated by a decrease in muscle tone during anesthesia. This is often exacerbated by the fact that many of these patients are morbidly obese.

Retropharyngeal Abscess

Etiology.—Bacterial inflammation of retropharyngeal space is often secondary to odontogenic or tonsillar infection.

Natural History.—If it is untreated, anterior displacement of the posterior pharyngeal wall into the oropharynx may cause airway obstruction. Rupture of the abscess may result in aspiration, pneumonia, or asphyxiation.

Symptoms and Signs.—Symptoms and signs include dypsnea and dysphagia, plus a large fluctuant mass in the posterior wall of the pharynx. Trismus may occur when ondontogenic infection is the initiating cause.

Investigation.—Lateral neck x-ray studies show thickening of the retropharyngeal tissues, sometimes with a defined abscess cavity (Fig 14–17).

Management.—The abscess is incised and drained. Airway management may be difficult in the presence of airway obstruction or trismus. WARNING: *Care should be taken to avoid contact with the posterior pharyngeal wall during laryngoscopy and intubation, because abscess rupture may be precipitated.*

Epiglottitis

Etiology.—Bacterial inflammation caused by *Hemophilus influenzae* involves the epiglottis and supraglottic tissues.

Natural History.—It usually occurs in children 6 months to 7 years, with rapid onset and progression of symptoms and signs of upper airway obstruction.

Symptoms and Signs.—Symptoms and signs include rapidly worsening dyspnea often with drooling and dysphagia in a pyrexial patient who has no cough. The patient frequently will be sitting up, tachypneic, in obvious respiratory distress, using the accessory muscles of respiration.

Investigation.—Lateral neck x-ray studies show (1) swelling of the epiglottis (thumb sign), (2) thickening of the aryepiglottic folds, (3) loss of vallecula, and (4) dilated hypopharynx (Plate 8,A).

Management.—Management of mild symptoms includes observation and use of antibiotics. For progressive dyspnea with respiratory distress, endotracheal intubation is achieved following inhalational induction of anesthesia, which tends to be prolonged because of suboptimal gas exchange. Airway management is greatly facilitated by keeping the patient sitting upright using jaw thrust and continuous positive airway pressure. Intubation may be

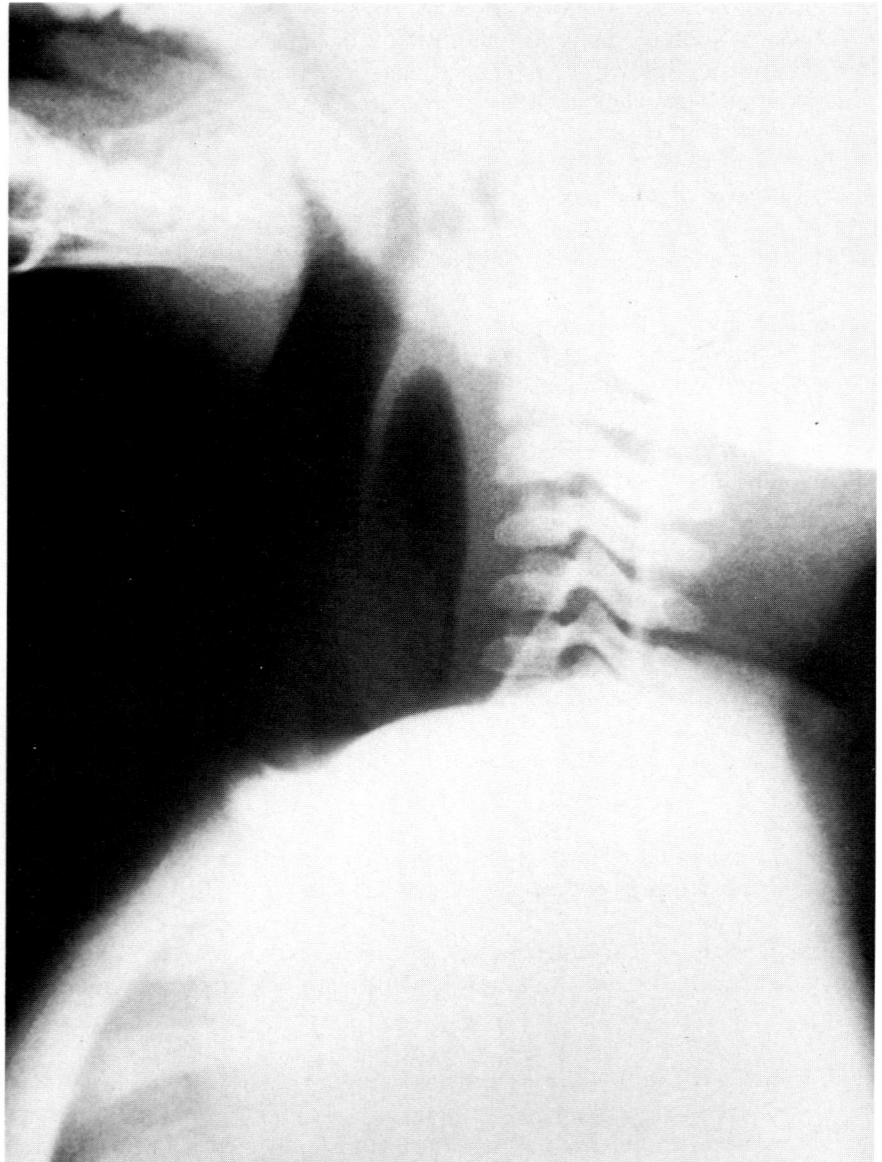

FIG 14–17.
Retropharyngeal abscess. Roentgenogram shows marked thickening of the cervical prevertebral fascia displacing upper pharynx and esophagus anteriorly. An unusual clear radiolucent abscess cavity is also seen.

extremely difficult because of inflammation altering the normal glottic architecture (Plate 8,B). If the laryngeal introitus cannot be identified, chest compression may produce bubbles at the site of the introitus. An endotracheal tube at least one size smaller than would be anticipated, with a stylet, should then be inserted. The endotracheal tube is left in place until the constitutional signs of the illness resolve and a leak is discernible around the endotracheal tube.

Glottic Area

Laryngeal Papillomatosis

Etiology.—The etiology is viral.

Natural History.—Hoarseness and dysphonia with increasing symptoms and signs of respiratory distress are present. It tends to recur because treatment is not curative.

Symptoms and Signs.—Symptoms and signs vary from the patient with hoarseness and no respiratory distress to a patient with marked stridor and severe respiratory distress.

Investigation.—Pharyngoscopy or indirect laryngoscopy is performed (Fig 14–18).

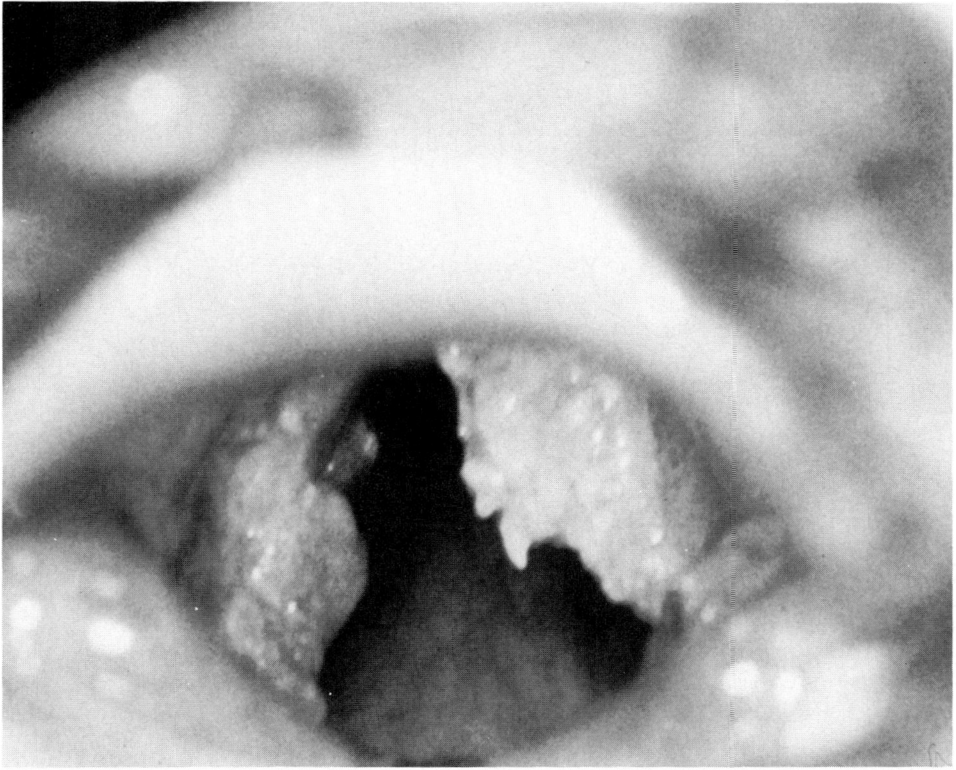

FIG 14–18.
Laryngeal papillomatosis. View at laryngoscopy with epiglottis superior. Note deranged architecture of the vocal cords covered with papilloma. Lack of smooth edge to the vocal cords provides a basis for changing character of voice, and gradual encroachment by papillomas across the laryngeal introitus provides the basis for airway obstruction.

Management.—Carbon dioxide laser is used to ablate the papillomas. Difficulty in airway management is proportional to the degree of respiratory distress. The airway is usually secured by endotracheal intubation, particularly if there are signs of respiratory distress, but this is not always necessary. During laser use it is essential that no combustible materials be presented to the laser beam, in particular, endotracheal tubes. Airway management can be achieved by a variety of techniques, including:

1. Nasopharyngeal insufflation with spontaneous respiration. Care must be taken to ensure that whatever is used to insufflate (either a nasopharyngeal airway or a suction catheter) remains hidden from the laser behind the soft palate.
2. Endotracheal intubation with a red rubber tube, wrapped with nonflammable metal tape. Ventilation may be either spontaneous or controlled. Care must be taken to ensure that none of the tube shows through the tape, particularly when it is curved to lie in the airway.
3. Jet ventilation using an 18- or 16-gauge metal cannula applied to a suspension laryngoscope. The cannula is connected to a high-pressure oxygen source with a pressure regulator to allow intermittent ventilation.

Tracheostomy should be avoided because of the risk of seeding papillomas along the respiratory tract.

Laryngospasm

Etiology.—Stimulation of the larynx or epiglottis (usually on induction of or emergency from the anesthetized state) produces reflex airway obstruction involving vocal cords, false cords, and paraglottic structures.

Natural History.—Laryngeal closure leads to inadequate ventilation, which may progress to hypoxia and even death.

Symptoms and Signs.—Continuous respiratory effort with no or minimal signs of gas exchange in an anesthetized patient. High-pitched inspiratory stridor will be present only with partial obstruction. With continued respiratory effort, cyanosis will appear.

Management.—If possible, the source of stimulation is removed, and firm traction is applied to the angle of the mandibles. Continuous positive airway pressure and an increase in the inspired oxygen concentration to 100% is helpful with partial obstruction, but forced positive pressure ventilation is detrimental. If cyanosis persists despite the previous treatment plan, the administration of succinylcholine (to relieve spasm of the intrinsic and extrinsic laryngeal muscles) and positive pressure ventilation may be required.

Subglottic Area

Croup: Laryngotracheobronchitis

Etiology.—Subacute viral inflammation usually caused by parainfluenza virus or respiratory syncitial virus involves airways distal to the glottis.

Natural History.—This viral-like illness has an insidious onset with a low-grade fever and barking cough. It usually occurs in children less than 3 years of age.

Symptoms and Signs.—Dyspnea with inspiratory stridor, often with a barking cough, usually progresses over several days. The patient may go on to develop intercostal and sternal retractions with cyanosis.

Investigation.—Anteroposterior neck x-ray studies show edematous subglottic tissues producing so-called steeple, or sharpened pencil, sign (Fig 14–19).

Management.—Management consists of humidified oxygen therapy with racemic epinephrine, if indicated (Table 14–3). Racemic epinephrine should be diluted with 2 mL of normal saline and administered via a nebulizer. It may be repeated every 1 to 2 hours. Severe respiratory distress may require intubation for relief. Because of the prolonged course of the disease, combined with the production of inspissated and tenacious sputum, cricoid split or tracheostomy may be performed.

Postintubation Edema

Etiology.—Contact edema following endotracheal intubation.

Natural History.—The history is variable. The edema usually occurs within 1 to 2 hours following extubation. It may resolve spontaneously or may require racemic epinephrine or occasionally reintubation.

Symptoms and Signs.—Stridor and signs of airway obstruction following intubation.

Management.—Management consists of humidified oxygen and racemic epinephrine or reintubation, depending on the severity of respiratory distress.

TABLE 14–3.

Dosage of Racemic Epinephrine

Age (yr)	2.25% Solution (mL)
<1	0.2
1–3	0.3
3–6	0.4
>6	0.5

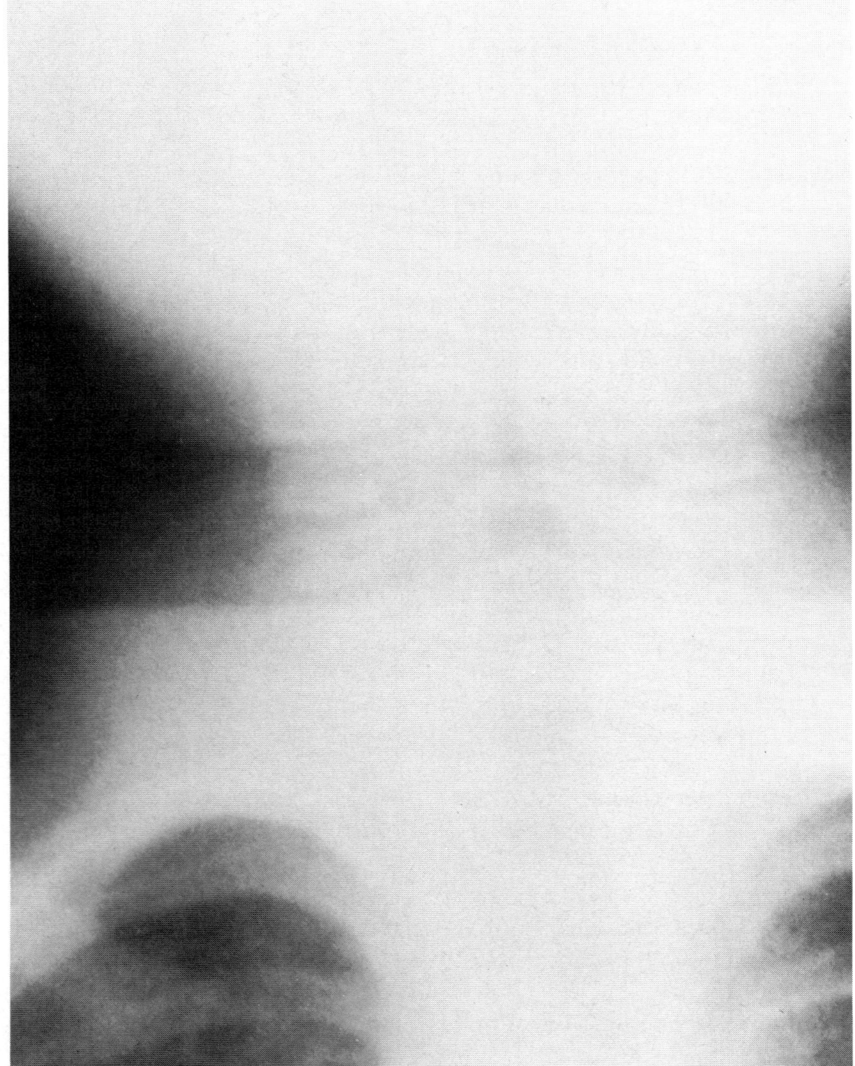

FIG 14–19.
Laryngotracheobronchitis. Anteroposterior neck roentgenogram showing gradual tapering of subglottic area because of edematous subglottic tissues.

The patient should be observed for 4 to 6 hours following either resolution of symptoms and signs or the last dose of racemic epinephrine.

Foreign Body Aspiration

Etiology.— An inhaled foreign body becomes lodged along the path of the upper airways, especially in the pyriform sinuses and the laryngeal vestibule.

Natural History.— The history depends on the site and nature of the inhaled object. Large objects lodged proximally may produce signs as a result of nearly complete airway obstruction or choking, whereas objects lodged distally may produce signs as a result of regional obstruction, atelectasis, or infection. Most foreign bodies lodge distally and are not radiopaque.

Symptoms and Signs.—The patient may have a history of choking while eating (especially peanuts and popcorn). Signs of proximal foreign body aspiration include dysphagia, severe respiratory distress, and cyanosis. Signs of distal foreign body aspiration include localized expiratory wheezing, persistent cough, and cyanosis.

Investigation.—Neck and chest x-ray studies will show foreign bodies directly only if they are radiopaque. Otherwise findings are the consequences of

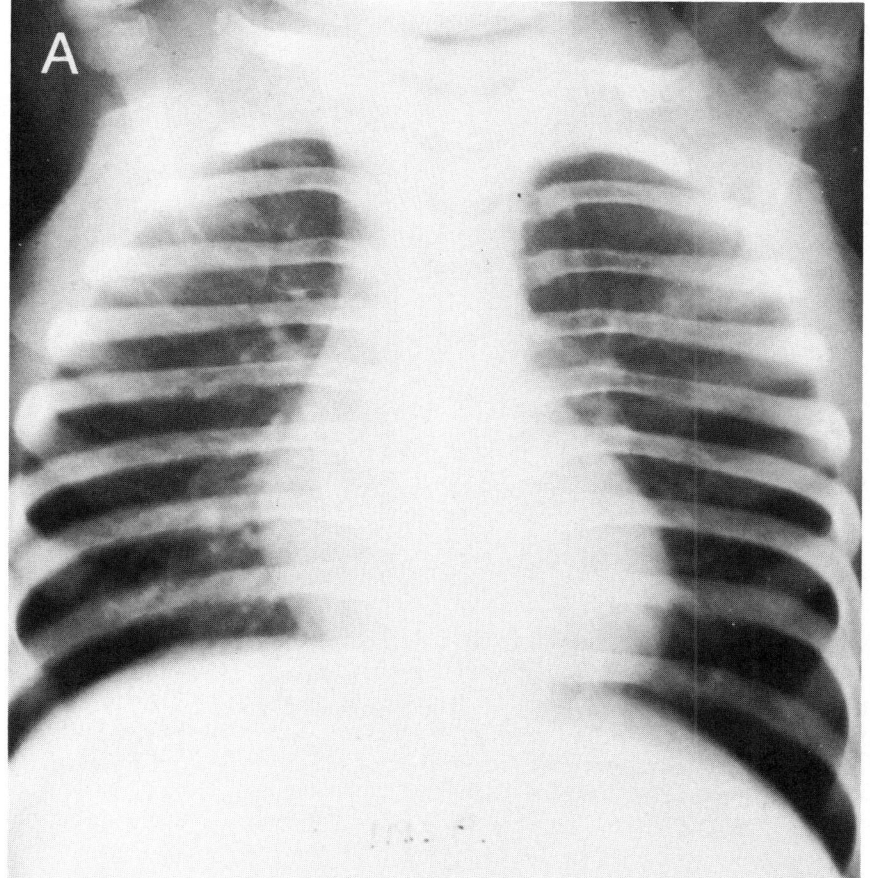

FIG 14–20.
Distal foreign body, showing both **(A)** inspiratory and **(B)** expiratory chest films. Inspiratory film appears normal, but on expiration, air distal to the site of obstruction is not exhaled, producing decrease in lung volume on the opposite side and a shift in mediastinum away from the side in which obstruction occurs. In this sequence the site of obstruction is on the patient's left side.

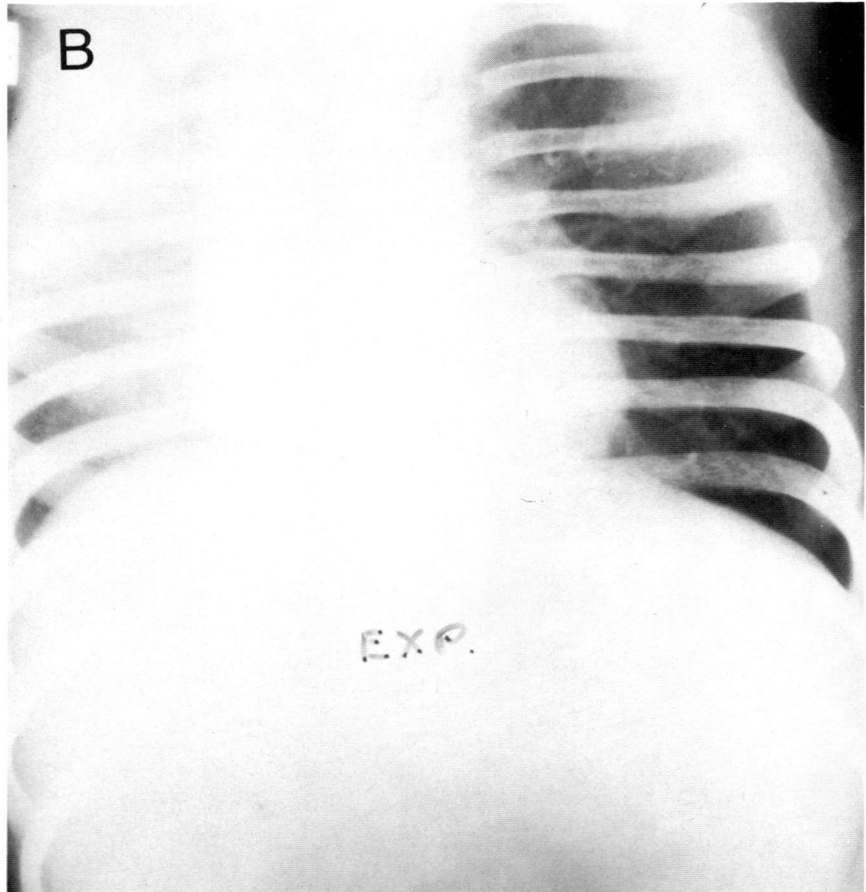

FIG 14–20   (cont.).

obstruction caused by the foreign body, that is, air trapping or regional atelectasis (Fig 14–20).

Management.—The foreign body is removed by bronchoscopy under general anesthesia. The aim of anesthetic management is to maintain spontaneous
ventilation to prevent displacing the foreign body distally. This is not always
possible, particularly in small infants; in this case gentle assisted ventilation often improves oxygenation, prevents hypercarbia, and does not affect the position of the foreign body.

Chapter 15

Anesthetic Management

Allan C. D. Brown

To an anesthesiologist a difficult airway is one that poses management challenges either by endotracheal intubation or by mask. One of the most frightening experiences for the practicing anesthesiologist is to find unexpectedly that, having induced anesthesia, he or she is unable to maintain the patient's oxygenation. The truly difficult airway that requires heroic methods to control is infrequent, although unanticipated difficulties with intubation have been variously reported in 3% to 5% of all patients requiring general anesthesia.[1] As other elements of anesthesia practice become more sophisticated, from the precision of anesthetic pharmacology to the refinement of anesthetic gas machines and monitors, the relative importance of airway management is increasing as a major contributor to anesthetic morbidity and mortality. Because death or serious morbidity can and does result from these technical misfortunes, the anesthesiologist is obliged to become familiar with the several management techniques that may be applied to avert disaster.

MANIFESTATION OF COMPROMISED AIRWAY

It is useful to divide patients with airway problems into three general groups according to the manner in which they are seen by the anesthesiologist: (1) patients in extremis (near death), (2) patients in distress, and (3) patients with occult impending obstruction.

Patients in extremis have severe airway obstruction associated with hypoxia, hypercarbia, delirium, or unconsciousness. This is an emergency in which cardiac arrest will supervene unless the airway is reestablished quickly. This is the sort of problem that manifests itself at the site of an accident, on arrival in the emergency room, or on the hospital ward in association with fulminating infection in or around the airway or with postoperative edema or hemorrhage in or adjacent to the airway. The overwhelming consideration is time, and the prime objective is to reestablish patient oxygenation immediately.

The treatment for hypoxia is to reestablish or maximize oxygenation. Since a patient in extremis may already be unconscious with total airway obstruction or in extreme distress with some residual airway, rapid assessment is required to determine initial management.

If the airway is totally obstructed, rapid laryngoscopy is required as a first step to ascertain whether an oral endotracheal tube may be passed. If laryngoscopy or intubation should prove in any way difficult (i.e., cannot be achieved with one attempt), all further efforts should be abandoned and an airway secured from below the larynx. This may be effected with an emergency tracheotomy, cricothyrotomy, or transcricothyroid or transtracheal jet ventilation. These maneuvers should be undertaken where the patient is first seen. Only when adequate oxygenation has been reestablished should the patient be moved to the operating room for formal tracheotomy. If the airway is not totally obstructed when first encountered, the patient is usually very agitated and may be sufficiently hypoxic to be confused and uncooperative. In this circumstance the prime consideration is to maximize effective oxygen intake with minimum airway interference, with the intent of avoiding turning partial obstruction into total obstruction. Thus 100% oxygen is administered by mask, and if hypoxia is relieved the patient is transferred to the operating room for formal tracheotomy.

The reader is cautioned not to take these two separate scenarios in a dogmatic context. A partial obstruction may turn total with minor stimulus and little warning. The purpose of the description is to concentrate attention on the fact that the prime consideration is to reestablish patient oxygenation. If a patient is moving any air into the lungs past an incomplete obstruction, he or she may respond well to 100% inspired oxygen by mask, but the airway still can become totally obstructed during transport. Thus the means for laryngoscopy and intubation and sublaryngeal airway control must accompany the patient to the operating room. However, the patient who does not respond well to raising the inspired oxygen concentration may be improved only by placing an oral airway. Note that this action can also precipitate total obstruction in an irritable airway, requiring the more invasive immediate intervention described earlier. Many such patients require nothing more than laryngoscopy to raise a relaxed tongue bulk or a swollen epiglottis to remove the obstruction and permit oxygenation. Intubation of the airway itself may pose no difficulty, where the prime problem is an incidental pathologic condition superimposed on an essentially normal airway. However, this fact cannot be known in advance of laryngoscopy, and because time is short, alternative means of gaining control must be available. The one pitfall that should be avoided in those patients who are confused and uncooperative is the use of sedative and anesthetic drugs, which can abolish any airway remaining to the patient.

Patients in distress represent the largest group of patients who require anesthesia but have a compromised airway. Such patients may exhibit stridor, labored breathing, tracheal tug, intercostal retraction, and agitation, but they are alert and cooperative. The distressed patient is usually becoming fatigued by the time the anesthesiologist arrives, but is still able to compensate for airway difficulties sufficiently to maintain adequate oxygenation. With such patients the anesthesiologist and the surgeon are permitted the luxury of time to plan for careful airway management.

Patients with respiratory distress through established or progressive partial obstruction of the airway are usually agitated and very conscious of dyspnea. They tend to adopt a sitting or erect posture and endeavor to "straighten" their airway to reduce resistance to breathing. The neck is flexed and the head extended, sometimes with protrusion of the tongue. The fists are clenched and arms rigid and forced into the bed, thereby fixing the pectoral girdle, which enables the full force of the accessory muscles of inspiration and expiration to be brought into action. Such an appearance of struggling for air must be recognized as characteristic and calls for prompt but not immediate action to relieve the situation.

Patients with occult impending obstruction on cursory physical examination give few clues to suggest the management problems that will follow the induction of anesthesia. They volunteer little information in their history to suggest airway difficulties, and the first intimation that the unwary anesthesiologist may have of an occult airway problem is when the patient is medicated or manipulated. This situation occurs in patients with some supraglottic tumors and base of tongue neoplasms or with congenital deformities, usually arising from the second branchial arch, for which the patient normally compensates with muscular effort.

The major challenge in this group of patients is to detect that a problem exists before anesthesia induction. This enables a full evaluation to be undertaken in such a facility as a difficult airway clinic and the formulation of an anesthesia plan that has some assurance of success. The detection of the initial problem frequently relies on eliciting a careful detailed history, with specific leading questions as required. Of particular interest are previous anesthetic intubation difficulties, a history of heavy snoring, or obstructive sleep apnea. Sleep apnea may be represented only as a story of unexplained early wakening, but when the patient's spouse or bedmate is questioned, a true history of "choking" followed by the patient's awakening is obtained. A history of congenital abnormalities of hearing and the heart should also alert the anesthesiologist to the possibility of involvement of structures arising from the second branchial arch.

For convenience we discuss the problems posed as falling into these three distinct groups for the following reasons: (1) the short time available for successful management of the patient in extremis, (2) the urgent but carefully considered management of the patient in distress, and (3) the diagnostic acumen and experience required to detect a patient with occult problems that require careful anesthetic management.

However, this division is artificial, and in reality the groups tend to merge into a continuum, where management depends on the degree of hypoxia, hypercarbia, and distress, which in turn dictates the rapidity of intervention. Within this continuum two distinct problems may exist, separately or together: (1) the truly difficult airway, where abnormal anatomy and superimposed pathology render the maintenance of a mask airway or the technical feat of intubation difficult, and (2) the relatively more normal airway with only pathologic changes leading to obstruction, which, once bypassed, do not pose intubation or mask problems. In the absence of hypoxia there is sufficient time to unravel these problems in the individual patient and develop a cogent anesthetic plan in conjunction with the operating surgeon.

MANAGEMENT OF COMPROMISED AIRWAY

General Principles

Where the absence of hypoxia permits the time required for patient evaluation, an anesthetic plan offering some reasonable hope for success in every patient with a compromised airway may be made. The options for anesthetic management depend very much on the preferences and skills of the anesthesiologist. Whatever options are decided on, two precautions should be observed in every patient:

1. The patient's spontaneous respiration should not be abolished until the airway is secured.
2. The surgeon should be scrubbed and standing by *in the operating room,* ready to do an immediate tracheotomy if required.

The prime objective in management is to bypass the obstruction and to gain control of the airway, either from above the larynx with an endotracheal tube or from below with a tube passed through a tracheotomy or cricothyrotomy incision. Passing an endotracheal tube through the larynx from above is always more desirable, because the long-term morbidity associated with this approach is less than that associated with a tracheal incision.[2] However, the anesthesiologist must consider whether the patient's obstructive process can be expected to resolve within the time limit that an endotracheal tube may be left in place. The surgeon should be consulted. If the technical difficulties posed by the patient's condition are great and a tracheotomy would be needed later in any case, the patient's interest may be best served with a tracheotomy under local infiltration anesthesia in the first instance.

Whenever possible the airway should be controlled with a cuffed endotracheal tube when a tracheotomy is performed to protect the airway against operative bleeding or technical difficulties in placing the tracheostomy tube. If the airway cannot be controlled from above a tracheotomy must be performed under local infiltration without the benefit of a cuffed endotracheal tube, which gives no protection against aspiration of blood and secretions and precludes sedation until the airway is controlled.

Premedication

The patient should be brought to the operating room without any narcotic or sedative premedication. Even small doses of sedatives can turn a partial obstruction into a complete obstruction with alarming rapidity. Should this occur on the ward, unseen and remote from those with the means to intervene effectively, the result can be fatal. The use of an antisialagogue such as atropine, glycopyrrolate, or scopolamine is optional. On the one hand, in patients with pathologic conditions that lead to difficulty in handling secretions, a preoperative antisialagogue may improve their agitation and general condition; on the other hand, the drying effect of antisialagogues can increase airway irritability and make the gentle positioning of instruments more difficult. The patient's usual medication for chronic medical conditions should not be forgotten. In patients with distress, swallowing may have been difficult for some time and routine oral medications may have been ignored, thus requiring appropriate parenteral administration before operation.

Transport to Operating Room

The patient in severe distress should be transported to the operating room on a stretcher accompanied by a source of oxygen with a mask and also a means of giving positive pressure assistance for ventilation, such as an Ambu-bag. In addition, a means of controlling the airway from below the larynx must accompany the patient, for example, an emergency tracheostomy tray, a crico-thyrotomy kit, or a jet ventilation cart. The purpose of the trolley is to permit the switch from spontaneous to controlled ventilation in the supine position. However, the patient should not be forced to lie down if the dyspnea is better tolerated in the sitting position. In a patient in less distress, it is appropriate to permit transport in a hospital wheelchair. In either situation it is important that the anesthesiologist and the surgeon fetch the patient in person, accompanied by at least one assistant, thereby providing two pairs of trained hands and a "runner" in the event of emergency.

Preparation and Monitoring

Once the patient has arrived in the operating room, three options for positioning for anesthetic induction are available, depending on the clinical circumstances:

1. The *sitting position* with the operating table appropriately conformed for the patient's comfort is the most common position for the patient in distress. It facilitates respiratory excursion and permits the patient to maintain the fixity of the pectoral girdle. It is an ideal position for the application of a topical anesthetic and for most intubation maneuvers in the awake patient. However, should direct rigid laryngoscopy be required, the anesthesiologist will still need to work from behind the patient's head and will usually require something stable on which to stand, such as an operating room lift, to achieve the correct working height relative to the patient's head.

2. The *right tonsil position* is used much less commonly for those patients who have active bleeding or free pus in the airway. The tonsil position, with or without a minimum of head-down tilt on the operating table, facilitates the passive drainage of liquids away from the larynx out of the mouth and dependent nostril. The position is used in conjunction with inhalation induction of general anesthesia. The type of problems managed in this way include post-tonsillectomy secondary hemorrhage, bleeding from biopsy sites in or around the larynx, and ruptured retropharyngeal abscess. The position is particularly useful in managing induction in the patient with active hematemesis.

3. The *supine position* is suitable only for patients with airway difficulties in the absence of significant respiratory distress. Thus it tends to be limited to those patients with occult problems where a viable anesthestic plan has already been formulated, with alternative approaches should obstruction occur during induction of anesthesia. Should vomiting or loss of the airway occur before intubation is achieved in this position, disaster may be averted by turning the

patient into the tonsil position, which will aid drainage and resuscitation maneuvers and tend to throw the patient's tongue forward, thus making a mask airway easier to maintain. In an emergency, turning a patient from one position to another requires the help of several trained assistants.

Two particular groups of patients are worth noting in passing: the morbidly obese patient and the woman in labor. The morbidly obese patient may derive airway difficulties from obesity itself or from several more usual causes of abnormal basic anatomy or disease. However, the sheer bulk of the patient makes it difficult to manage the induction of general anesthesia in anything other than the supine position, a moderate reverse Trendelenburg position on the table may facilitate respiratory excursion, although at some risk of hypotension and aspiration should vomiting occur.

The parturient requires that particular precautions be taken against hypotension, which makes the sitting position for induction of general anesthesia less desirable. The tonsil position is usually too uncomfortable for most of these patients, and the usual left lateral wedge tilt in the supine position must be remembered to guard against supine hypotension at term.

Once the patient has been placed in the appropriate position for the procedure intended, monitors are applied. The extent of invasive monitoring is dictated by the patient's overall medical condition. However, the minimum standards of noninvasive monitoring recently promulgated by the American Society of Anesthesiologists[3] should be adhered to with all patients, including end-tidal CO_2, pulse oximetry, indirect blood pressure, temperature, and electrocardiogram. A well-secured intravenous line is started as a conduit for resuscitation drugs, should they be required. The patient's limbs should not be strapped to armboards or to the table but should be restrained by assistants in the event of excitement during induction. This ensures that the patient's position can be changed quickly as needed and that the intravenous line and monitor attachments remain functional during induction.

ANESTHESTIC OPTIONS

Once the patient with known or potential airway difficulty has been evaluated, an anesthesia plan can be formulated. Because a difficult airway to the anesthesiologist usually translates into a difficult intubation, the first question to be asked is whether intubation may be avoided, thereby nullifying the difficulty. As a matter of convenience, it is too often forgotten that endotracheal intubation, like all other invasive medical procedures, has formal indications (Table 15–1). The indication for intubation in the particular patient should be established. Many patients who have airways difficult to intubate may be managed perfectly well with a mask for general anesthesia, provided the operative procedure is suitable. Even better, can general anesthesia be avoided altogether with local infiltration or conduction blockade?

However, the reverse of this argument must also be considered. Just because an operation can be managed with a local anesthetic technique does not relieve the anesthesiologist of the responsibility of planning for general anesthesia with endotracheal intubation. Intubation may be required in a hurry

TABLE 15–1.

Indications for Intubation

Ventilatory support
Airway protection
Airway patency
Access for surgery
Tracheal toilet
Special techniques
Reduction of dead space

during a local anesthetic procedure for several reasons. Even light sedation may lead to obstruction of a marginal airway in an awake patient. A spinal anesthetic may migrate too high. A technical complication (e.g., pneumothorax in association with a supraclavicular block) might demand emergency intubation. The patient's airway problem may worsen acutely during the operation, or he or she may not be able to tolerate the positioning for the time required to complete the operation.

Therefore, as a basic rule, no anesthetic drugs of any sort should be given to the patient until a formal plan to secure the airway has been formulated and the necessary equipment and personnel assembled. If the anesthesiologist decides that intubation is a reasonable course, a decision must be made between awake intubation and passing the tube under general anesthesia. Some physicians maintain that awake intubation is safer because the patient's protective reflexes are maintained, but experience suggests that this argument has been exaggerated. The technique of awake intubation is not pleasant for the patient, and even with the utmost care and concern, the patient's cooperation cannot be guaranteed. If one takes the time to meticulously prepare the patient with topical anesthesia to the oral structures, the base of the tongue, and the larynx, there certainly is a better chance for an atraumatic intubation, but this obviates the original argument for maintaining protective reflexes. The addition of sedative drugs may compound the problem further. Spraying the larynx with local anesthetic can itself produce laryngospasm in an irritable airway. It is true that with some patients, usually in the older age groups, complete faith in the physician may permit a trouble-free intubation, but this is not so in many cases. It is suggested that awake intubation be reserved for those patients in whom there is no firm indication for tracheotomy under local anesthetic but about whom the anesthesiologist has doubts in regard to safe airway management under general anesthesia.

Intubation Under General Anesthesia

If one accepts the premise that the careful passage of an endotracheal tube through the glottis under direct vision in a fully relaxed and asleep patient is least likely to cause any lasting damage to the patient's psyche or anatomy, then general anesthesia must be considered the method of choice for gaining control of the airway. The purpose of the preoperative assessment is to determine whether there are sufficiently weighty reasons involving patient safety or whether the experience of the anesthesiologist might dictate the less desirable approaches of either performing a tracheotomy under local infiltration or passing an endotracheal tube in the airway of a conscious patient who may not cooperate.

Factors likely to influence the anesthesiologist to recommend a tracheotomy under local anesthesia include a friable tumor above the larynx likely to bleed and thus to obscure vision or a large retropharyngeal or peritonsillar abscess, particularly if "pointing," which could rupture on contact with either the laryngoscope or the tube and contaminate the airway with pus. Any history of previous unsuccessful intubation attempts requires that serious consideration be given to a tracheotomy under local infiltration.

Induction of Anesthesia by Inhalation

If the induction of general anesthesia by inhalation is decided on, the patient is brought to the operating room with no premedication other than antacids or an H_2 blocking drug, and is made comfortable on the operating table, in the sitting position if necessary. The patient's neck is prepared for tracheotomy. The patient is then preoxygenated by mask for at least 5 minutes. Preoxygenation does not improve the moment-to-moment oxygen supply to the tissues to any great extent, but it does create an oxygen reserve in the patient's functional residual capacity (FRC) that may be of importance if induction is subsequently troublesome. Denitrogenation also facilitates the speed of inhalation induction. When all is prepared, the anesthesiologist should check that the surgeon is scrubbed and ready before beginning induction.

Intravenous induction agents are avoided, and relaxants should not be used; either can result in loss of muscle tone that can lead to complete obstruction before it is known whether the patient can be ventilated artificially. A reliable estimate of dose-response cannot be made with even small doses of thiobarbiturates, particularly in the patient who is already fatigued. The patient should be instructed quietly, in simple language, as to what to expect. He or she should be told about the characteristic smell of inhalation agents and be reassured that the experience is not unpleasant. The patient should not be requested to breathe deeply, because in the presence of anxiety it can lead to hypocapnia and periods of apnea that interfere with the induction process. Deep breathing also leads to increased peak inspiratory flow rates, perceived by the patient as an increase in the obstruction to breathing, leading to further agitation. The patient should be talked down quietly and with confidence and should not be asked any questions after induction has begun. Particularly stormy inductions have been observed in patients struggling against the depressant effects of anesthesia in an attempt to answer a question from the anesthesiologist, which, as far as the patient knows, may be critical to his or her care and safety. However, the anesthesiologist should be talking to the patient constantly until the patient has lost consciousness, remembering that hearing is the last special sense to be obtunded.

During induction the anesthesiologist must ensure that nothing is done to stimulate the patient during the first or second stage of anesthesia. This includes the nurse making any last-minute adjustments or the surgeon palpating or trying to prepare the neck for tracheotomy. Similarly, the anesthesiologist must be gentle in his manipulations, to minimize stimulation. The support given to the patient's jaw must be gentle, and the pressure used to maintain a good seal with the mask must be the least possible. Along with these precautions, I prefer not to make any cuff blood pressure measurements during the early stages of induction, but rely on an impression of blood pressure from the continuous gentle palpation of the temporal or facial pulse. Silence should be maintained by other personnel in the operating room until induction is complete.

Patients will usually tolerate an initial inhaled concentration of 1% of any of the three commonly used halogenated agents (fluothane, enflurane, or isoflurane) in oxygen while conscious. The vaporizer with the chosen agent is turned on after preoxygenation. The patient is allowed to breathe this mixture for 10 to 15 breaths, then nitrous oxide is introduced to the extent that permits the maintenance of a satisfactory inspired oxygen concentration in that patient. The patient will move more rapidly through the second stage of anesthesia because of the second-gas effect. The percentage of inspired vapor is increased 1% at a time, allowing 5 to 10 breaths between each increment so that the anesthesiologist may detect any developing irritable response to the new concentration. The total carrier gas flow is maintained at a high level (8–10 L/minute), particularly if a circle absorber is being used, so that the set concentration is presented to the patient as soon as possible. The factors limiting the rapidity with which the inspired concentration may be increased are airway irritability and the maintenance of adequate blood pressure.

During this whole process the anesthesiologist should be watching for developing difficulty in maintaining the patient's airway. He or she must develop that nicety of judgment required to decide at which point signs of increasing obstruction or a tiring patient dictate the abandonment of induction, while still permitting the agents to be vented spontaneously. Should total obstruction occur without warning, an oral airway should be inserted. If the airway is inserted too early, this manipulation may itself result in laryngeal spasm. If an oral airway is already in place or does not lead to immediate improvement, rapid but gentle laryngoscopy should be attempted. Frequently, lifting a swollen epiglottis is all that is required to reestablish the airway, and intubation may be possible even if the patient is not fully relaxed. One should insert a nasal airway only as a last resort, because nasal bleeding adds more difficulties to be overcome. If the obstruction is not caused by the epiglottis or the base of the tongue, the problem may be at the glottis itself. Even if the anatomy is grossly abnormal or distorted, one can usually detect some residual entrance to the trachea. This may amount to nothing more than a dimple in the edematous folds of the false cords. In such circumstances, if an antisialagogue has not been used the anesthesiologist can "follow the bubbles" in the spontaneously breathing patient. Once the entrance has been found, with the laryngoscope still in place, a soft flexible stylet may be inserted as an endotracheal tube guide, or a small rigid pediatric bronchoscope may be passed to control the airway. If anesthesia is too light or if, even with gentle probing, the entrance to the trachea cannot be found, the surgeon should be called on to perform an immediate tracheotomy before severe hypoxia develops.

Should the induction process prove stormy, the anesthesia assistants should be instructed to restrain the patient's movements rather than prevent them. If the patient tries to sit up, the anesthesiologist should not resist.

Rather, he or she should maintain a gas seal and try to continue induction without disturbing the patient's pattern of respiration any further. The anesthesiologist should follow the patient's movements, restraining only those that are likely to cause injury to the patient. A high-volume suction capability must be available, together with a hard suction tip (e.g., Yankauer) to deal with any vomiting during the excitement stage.

The objective of the whole exercise is to achieve a smooth transition from consciousness to stage 3 anesthesia, at which time laryngoscopy and intubation may be undertaken safely. Spontaneous respiration must be maintained so that the process can be reversed in the face of insurmountable difficulty. This is why intravenous drugs are not given. Obsessive attention to the details of technique is required. As the stages of anesthesia are traversed, the patient can be lowered to the supine position, if sitting. Any interference with the airway is delayed as long as possible. The initial rate of induction should be sufficiently rapid to minimize the chance of excitement, but as induction proceeds and the relaxation of muscle tone becomes apparent, the rate should be slowed to assess any loss of airway in time to retreat. Once the anesthesiologist is satisfied that the patient is in the third stage of anesthesia, vital signs should be checked and the carrier gas mixture adjusted to increase the oxygen reserve in the FRC before intubation maneuvers. Any loss of the nitrous oxide anesthetic effect because of the increase in oxygen percentage must be compensated for by increasing the inspired vapor concentration if a stable level of anesthesia is to be maintained.

A variation of this procedure is required if a patient is bleeding in the oropharynx or the airway (e.g., post-tonsillectomy hemorrhage). If the patient is a child, the problem is complicated further by the small airway. Children with secondary hemorrhage usually swallow the blood and may develop signs of shock before the situation is recognized. If irritability is observed in a postoperative patient, after hypoxia has been excluded as a cause, secondary hemorrhage should always be considered before pain medication is prescribed.

The anesthesiologist is presented with several concurrent problems: a patient who has just had an anesthetic with persisting drug effects and who has hypovolemia with a stomach full of blood and active bleeding above the airway. A large-bore needle for intravenous infusion should be inserted immediately. If shock is evident, transfusion is indicated, even though a rise in blood pressure may make the pharyngeal bleeding worse. The situation will not improve until the bleeding points are secured; therefore the patient should be returned to the operating room without delay in the tonsil position (i.e., semiprone; Fig 15–1).

Once in the operating room, the patient should be placed on the operating table in the same tonsil position, on the right side (if the anesthesiologist holds the laryngoscope in the left hand) with no support under the head, to facilitate gravity drainage of blood away from the larynx. Assistants are instructed to stand on either side of the table to hold the patient in position. The same preparations for induction are made. An endotracheal tube of appropriate size is selected, together with one a full size smaller to deal with any narrowing of the glottis following the previous intubation. When possible, a transparent plastic mask is selected. The same induction procedure is followed, but the oxygen concentration in the carrier gas mixture is maintained at 50% or higher. Blood

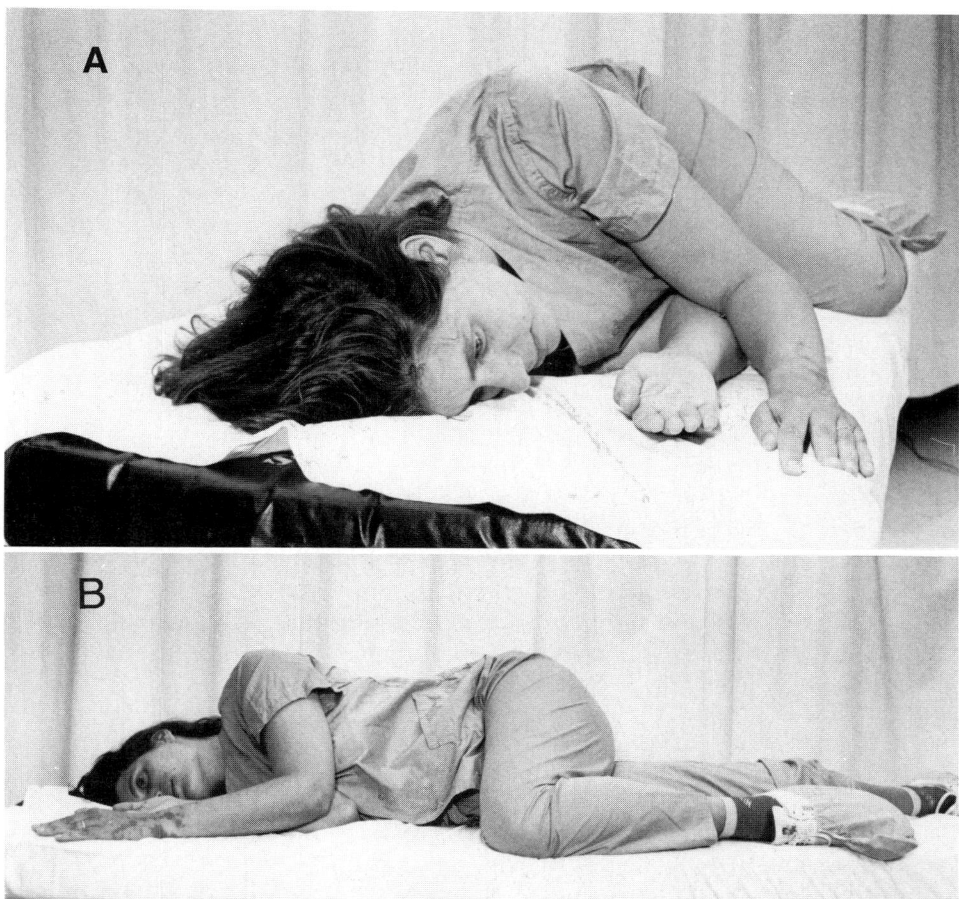

FIG 15–1.
Right tonsil position permits anesthetist, holding laryngoscope in left hand, to visualize larynx in normal way. **A,** patient lies on right side with body leaning forward at 45 degrees. **B,** position of left leg and arms stabilize pelvic and pectoral girdles. No pillow under head permits width of shoulder to incline pharynx downward to facilitate drainage away from larynx.

accumulating under the mask is allowed to drain intermittently by raising the lower edge. When adequate anesthesia is achieved for laryngoscopy, the table is raised to the appropriate height for the individual anesthesiologist, and the assistants are asked to roll the patient gently into the full right-lateral position and hold him or her there. With no supports under the head, the bleeding points are below the larynx, and a few degrees of head-down tilt will prevent the passive draining of any blood down the trachea. The laryngoscope is introduced, but instead of lifting in the usual sagittal plane the direction of lift is now 45 degrees upward and outward from the sagittal plane, exposing the larynx for intubation over any blood pooling inside the right cheek. When intubation is complete, the table is lowered and the patient turned into the supine position, secured, and presented to the surgeon.

Intubation Under Local Anesthesia

If the anesthesiologist elects to intubate the airway of the awake patient, some measures usually have to be taken to modify or obtund upper airway protective reflexes and to allay the patient's anxiety. In the very young and the old and frail, intubation of the awake patient may be achieved without any drugs at all, but this is neither usual nor, perhaps, kind.

The introduction of instruments into the upper airway is a potent stimulus to gagging in most patients and vomiting in some. Therefore, if the case is elective, it is a wise precaution to ensure that the patient has had nothing by mouth and has been premedicated with H_2 blocking drugs and antacids as considered appropriate. In addition, the use of an antisialogogue is a useful precaution to facilitate the use of topical local anesthetics and to ensure that they come into direct contact with mucous membranes and are not washed away or diluted by the secretions stimulated by airway manipulation.

If the problems presented by the airway are complex and both oral and nasal access are available, it is prudent to prepare both routes for intubation rather than having to repaint the pharynx and the glottis latter if the initial access choice is unsuccessful. The concern here is to avoid exceeding the total safe drug dosage for the topical anesthetic chosen.

The major problems associated with preparing the awake patient for airway intubation with local anesthetic topical paint-up include, in order of frequency:

1. Patient agitation and intolerance for the procedure
2. Toxic dose of the drug chosen
3. Induction of vomiting
4. Profound vagal response to manipulations in the pharynx
5. Induction of laryngeal spasm during paint-up
6. Allergic response to the local anesthetic

Most of these adverse events can be avoided or minimized by gentle, unhurried technique. However, a few points are worth noting. If a patient becomes increasingly agitated during preparation for intubation, it must be remembered that this could be caused by further deterioration in the airway problem itself rather than intolerance for the paint-up procedure. If the anesthesiologist elects to use a sedative or an anxiolytic such as one of the benzodiazepines to counteract the patient's agitation, the same caveats apply as for premedication, and the risk of airway loss because of loss of muscle tone must be remembered. Similarly, the patient, usually prepared in the sitting position, is much more vulnerable to drug-induced hypotension and loss of consciousness.

The toxic dose for the commonly used local anesthetics is relatively well defined (Table 15–2). However, where mixtures are used these numbers are less reliable. It is of particular importance to note that the anesthesiologist may not be the first person to attempt intubation over a short time. It is not uncommon for intubation of the airway with the patient under topical anesthesia to be attempted in the emergency room before the anesthesiologist is consulted. Therefore it is important to establish which drugs have already been used, in what dosage, and in what time frame.

TABLE 15–2.

Local Anesthetic Drugs for Airway Management

	Topical		Injection	
Drugs	Respiratory Tract	Total Dose Without Epinephrine (mg)	Nerve Block	Total Dose Without Epinephrine (mg)
Ester group				
Cocaine HCL	4%–5% (5–4 mL)	200	Not used	—
Procaine	Ineffective	—	1%–2% (100–50 mL)	1,000
Benzocaine	Lozenges	100	Not used	—
Amide group				
Lidocaine	2%–4% (10–5 mL)	200	1%–2% (50–25 mL)	500
Bupivacaine	Not used	—	0.25%–0.75% (200–65 mL)	500

Because most sensory innervation to the upper airway is derived from the vagus nerves, adequate vagolytic premedication will usually avoid the problem of a profound vagal response. However, laryngeal spasm and induced vomiting cannot be completely prevented, but may be minimized by working gently and taking sufficient time to ensure that each stage of the topical paint-up is effective before commencing the next stage deeper in the upper airway. Allergic responses to local anesthetics are extremely rare, and it is not usual practice to test every patient for sensitivity. However, if a history of adverse responses to previous local anesthetics is obtained, the drug group concerned should be avoided if it is identified, or a conjunctival sensitivity test should be undertaken before proceeding.

Technique of Topical Paint-up

The purpose of the topical application of anesthetic drugs to the upper airway is to render the patient as comfortable as possible during what is a very unpleasant experience for most. It is also used to obtund protective airway reflexes sufficiently to enable inspection of the airway to the level of the glottis and the subsequent passage of an endotracheal tube, while not completely abolishing protective reflexes to give some protection against the aspiration of blood, pus, or vomitus in the awake patient. These two objectives are probably mutually incompatible, despite repeated claims to the contrary, particularly when patient sedation is added to the equation! Any patient with an airway that has had anesthesia topically applied must be considered at risk from aspiration.

The technique may be used in two distinct ways with minor variations, depending on the objective to be achieved. If the patient has not already been fully evaluated, the anesthesiologist will need to know the details of the problems he or she faces and may wish to view the airway directly before deciding on the final techniques to be used for intubation. For this purpose the topical block of sensory input to the level of the vocal folds is all that is required. If the object is intubation, the addition of laryngeal muscle relaxation is helpful to facilitate the passage of the tube through the glottis.

The patient is brought to the operating room and placed on the table in the sitting position with the back supported by a suitably conformed table. Monitoring devices are applied and anesthesia machine checks are completed. If the patient is in respiratory distress, the surgeon stands ready in the operating room to perform emergency tracheotomy. (It is assumed that the patient's anatomy has already been examined in the preoperative period and that the state of dentition and patency of both nostrils are known.)

First, the oral cavity is prepared. The patient's lips and gingivae are sprayed with topical anesthetic, followed by spraying of the anterior two thirds of the tongue, including the edges. The patient is asked to swallow any residual fluid left in the mouth after each application. Then the patient is allowed to rest. Next the upper surface of the posterior tongue is sprayed, together with the fauces, soft palate, and uvula. Again the patient is asked to swallow, then allowed to rest. Finally the visible posterior wall of the oropharynx is sprayed.

Second, the nasal cavity is prepared. The nostril is first sprayed, with the patient inspiring through the nose. Then a long cotton-tipped swab soaked in 4% cocaine solution is passed back along the base of the nostril over the hard palate to ensure that the route that will be followed by the nasal tube is unobstructed. The patient's grimace will denote that the tip has reached the posterior nasopharyngeal wall. The single long swab is then withdrawn, and pledgets soaked in 4% cocaine solution are passed slowly and gently to the nasopharynx with nasal forceps, which are then withdrawn, leaving the pledgets in place. The patient is then allowed to rest. It is unnecessary to prepare the nose with multiple swabs and pledgets in the manner of a surgeon undertaking an intranasal operation. Only the lower part of the nasal cavity in the region of the inferior turbinate will come into contact with a nasal endotracheal tube, and it is this area that requires anesthesia and vasoconstriction. Finally, the patient is asked to open his or her mouth and protrude the tongue while the nasopharynx behind the soft palate is sprayed from below. The patient is again allowed to rest.

Third, the hypopharynx is prepared. It is my preference to ask the patient to gargle 5 mL 4% viscous lidocaine solution. The patient is then asked to concentrate on breathing, slowly and deeply through the mouth, with eyes shut if preferred. Leaving the nasal packing in place facilitates this exercise.

The patient is asked to protrude the tongue, which is firmly grasped with a gauze swab between the finger and thumb of the anesthesiologist's left hand while the right hand manipulates the spray. The lateral and posterior hypopharyngeal walls are sprayed blind from behind the tongue. The patient is then allowed to rest.

The tongue is pulled forward again, and using an angled spray tip (e.g., a deVilbiss varidirectional spray; Fig 15–2), the base of tongue and vallecula are sprayed blind from behind the tongue. The patient is allowed to rest. Finally, again with the tongue pulled forward and the spray tip directed inferior and anterior, the glottis is sprayed blind while the patient takes a deep breath. In many patients these steps are sufficient to allow visualization of the glottis with both fiberoptic and rigid instruments. However, in a large minority of patients sufficient discomfort and reflex activity are still present to hamper proceedings. Usually the most sensitive areas are the vallecula (innervated by the glossopharyngeal nerve), the epiglottis, and the larynx itself. Should further

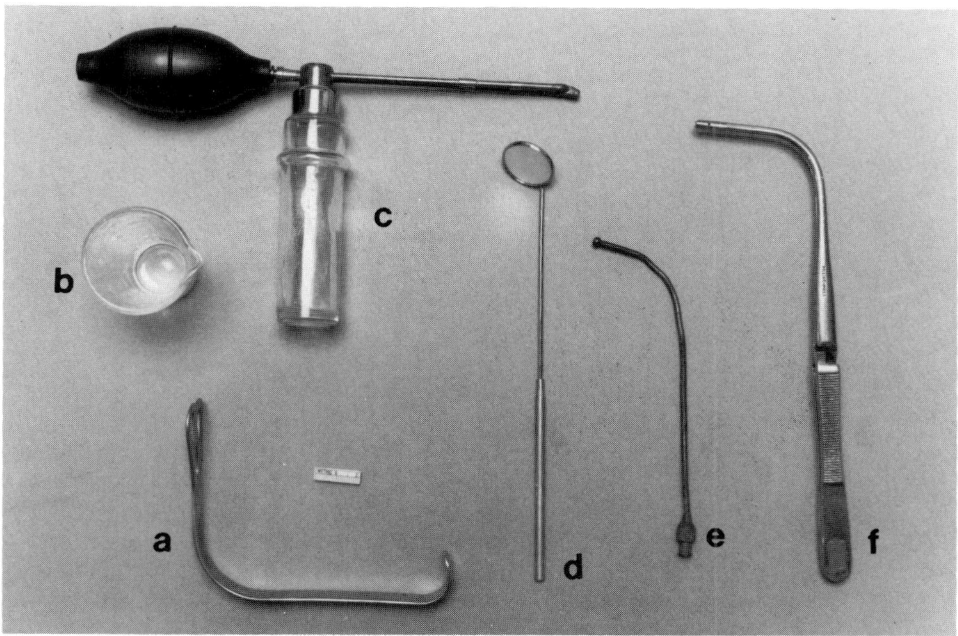

FIG 15–2.
Contents of a standard topical paint-up tray. Tongue blade *(a)*, graduated medicine glass *(b)*, DeVilbis atomizer with adjustable tip *(c)*, indirect laryngoscopy mirror *(d)*, Malleable cannula *(e)*, and Jackson (Krause) forceps *(f)*.

blind spraying not resolve the problem, several additional techniques are available.

More topical anesthetic drugs may be introduced under direct vision through the suction channel of a fiberoptic laryngscope or bronchoscope. This is usually best achieved via the nasal route. If the anesthesiologist is practiced in indirect mirror laryngoscopy, a malleable cannula may be used to drip local anesthetic vertically into the vallecula, onto the larynx, and indeed down the trachea. Blocking the posterior surface of the epiglottis, however, requires a sure block of the internal branch of the superior laryngeal nerve, which may be achieved in two ways.

Jackson (Krause) forceps (see Fig 15–2,F) are made to conform to the curve of the tongue. Self-retaining jaws are used to hold pledgets of gauze soaked in anesthetic solution. The patient is asked to open the mouth, and the tongue is pulled forward and held. The forceps are introduced over the side of the tongue, avoiding pressure on the ipsilateral pillar of the fauces. The tips are slid over the tongue base and down into the ipsilateral pyriform fossa, where they may be palpated in the neck next to the thyroid cartilage (Fig 15–3). With the handle held horizontally, the patient is asked to hold the forceps in place for 30 seconds with the teeth. This also acts as an effective distraction for the patient. The procedure is then repeated on the opposite side.

Percutaneous block of the superior laryngeal nerve (Fig 15–4) may be achieved by identifying the posterior horn of the hyoid bone on each side in the neck. A skin wheel is raised over this landmark, and a small needle is directed down-

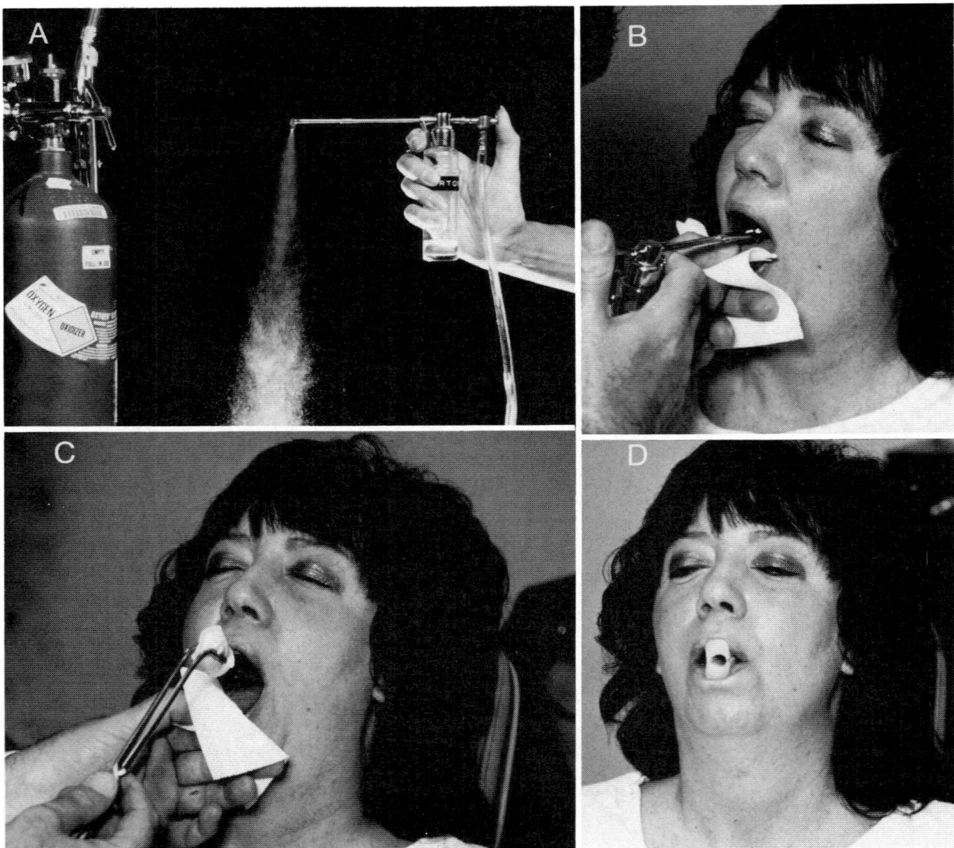

FIG 15–3.
A, DeVilbis varidirectional anesthetic spray powered by oxygen cylinder rather than hand bulb for convenience. **B,** patient's tongue is held forward as paint-up proceeds. **C,** Jackson forceps with anesthetic-soaked gauze pad in self-retaining jaws are advanced over tongue into each pyriform fossa. **D,** sufficiently good block obtained to tolerate Berman airway.

ward and anteriorly at a 30-degree angle to the skin. Two milliliters of 2% lidocaine are injected as the needle is slowly withdrawn. The procedure is repeated on the opposite side. If only the internal branch of the superior laryngeal nerve is blocked, mucosal sensation down to the level of the vocal folds will be obtunded. However, if the superior laryngeal nerve trunk itself is blocked before it divides just posterior and inferior to the posterior horn of the hyoid, the cricothyroid muscle will also relax, making any local reflex closure of the false vocal folds less of a problem.

Percutaneous cricothyroid block (see Fig 15–4) of the lower larynx and trachea is usually required in addition to internal laryngeal block if intubation in an awake patient is to be attempted. Both sensory and motor innervation of the intrinsic muscles of the larynx is conducted through branches of the recurrent laryngeal nerves, which, because they come to lie submucosally in the trachea, are amenable to topical blockade.

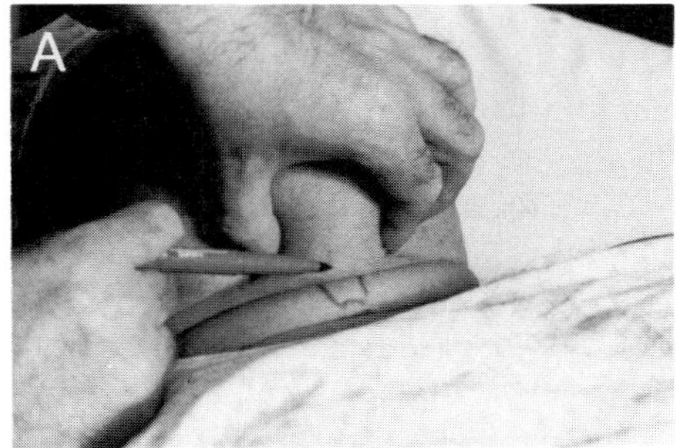

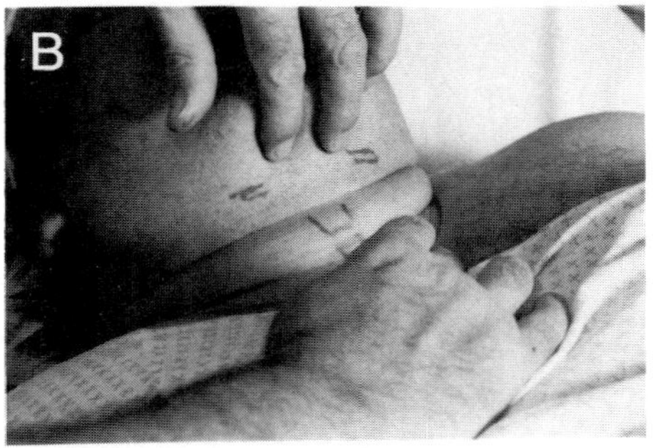

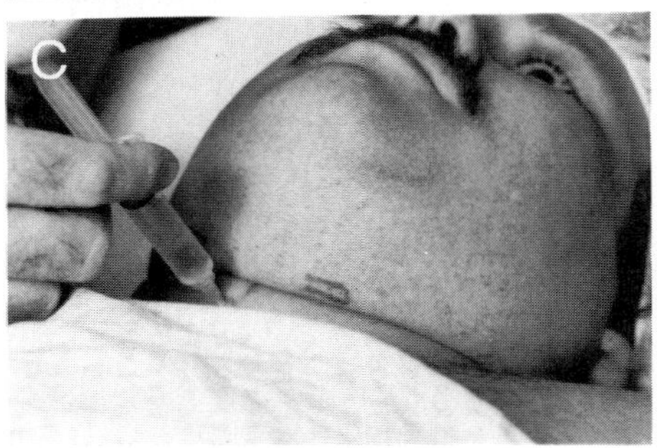

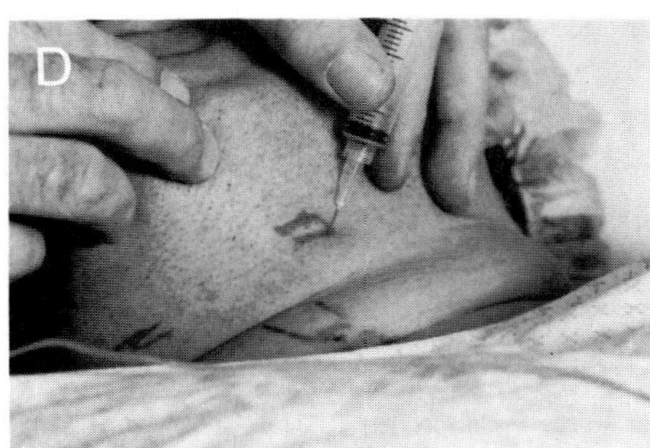

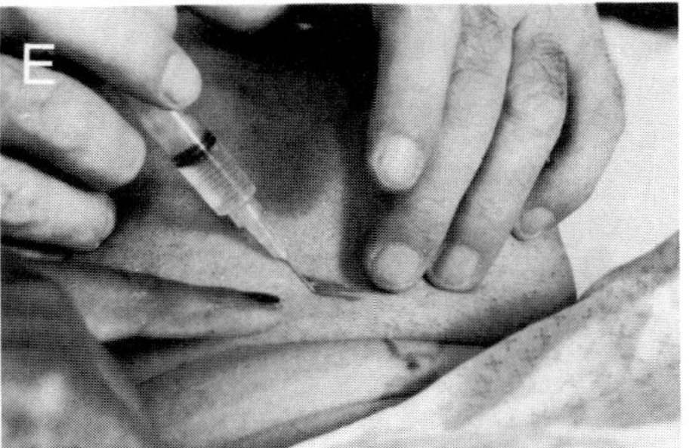

FIG 15–4.
A and **B,** cricoid and thyroid cartilages are identified and marked and cornua of hyoid identified. **C,** skin is prepared with antiseptic solution, and skin wheel is raised; 4 mL 2% lidocaine solution is injected through cricothyroid membrane into trachea. Position of needle is first checked by aspirating air from trachea through anesthetic solution. **D** and **E,** left and right superior laryngeal nerves are blocked, in turn, with 2 to 3 mL 2% lidocaine solution. Short, fine needle is advanced 1.0 cm downward and forward from lower edge of hyoid cornua at 30 degrees to skin with patient's head turned to opposite side. Before injection, syringe is aspirated to ensure that tip is not in pharynx (air) or in a blood vessel. Anesthetic is then injected as needle is continuously withdrawn.

A skin wheel is raised in the midline over the cricothyroid membrane, which connects the inferior edge of thyroid cartilage above to the superior edge of the cricoid cartilage below. The membrane, measuring 3 by 4 mm in the adult, fills the cricothyroid visor angle. A short needle on a syringe containing 4 mL 2% lidocaine is introduced vertically through the skin wheel into the trachea. The patient usually coughs as the tracheal lining is pierced, and correct positioning is confirmed by aspiration of air through the anesthetic solution injected. The needle and syringe are then withdrawn.

INTUBATION TECHNIQUES

The following section illustrates how techniques may be assigned utility and priority within an anesthetic plan for difficult intubation based largely on experience with the patients and problems presented in this atlas.

Difficult airways are either anticipated or unanticipated. If anticipated, this atlas describes a systematic method of evaluation of the airway problems involved and the management options available to maintain the patient's spontaneous respiration and oxygenation while a methodical sequence of techniques is applied to control the airway. If difficulty is unanticipated, the patient has usually received an intravenous induction agent followed by a depolarizing muscle relaxant before the problem is recognized, and now the overriding concern is the supply of oxygen left in the patient's FRC, which will dictate the time available to recoup the situation.

However, in both presentations the same four groups or combinations of problems are noted:

1. *Access.* Can an endotracheal tube be introduced into the pharynx?
2. *Visualization.* Can the larynx be visualized by normal anesthetic laryngoscopy?
3. *Target.* Can the glottis be seen within the laryngeal "funnel," and is it narrowed or obstructed?
4. *Escape.* If an endotracheal tube cannot be passed from above, does the anatomy of the neck permit rapid oxygenation from below the larynx?

In all patients in whom neck anatomy suggests a difficult escape route, even where airway difficulties are not anticipated, anesthesia management should be more circumspect.

In the following description, certain techniques have been selected as examples with particular utility in overcoming one of the groups of problems posed in either access, visualization, or intubating a difficult airway. The emphasis in the examples is on simplicity, and ease and rapidity of use. The use of fiberoptic instruments as intubation guides is not discussed, because other published sources already cover this aspect of management well.[5, 6] In addition, the time available and bleeding following early attempts at intubation frequently preclude the use of fiberoptic instruments in patients with unanticipated difficult airways. The need for every anesthesiologist to be able to perform a selection of simple intubating techniques is emphasized. Figure 15–5 demonstrates the success rate that may be achieved with simple techniques as

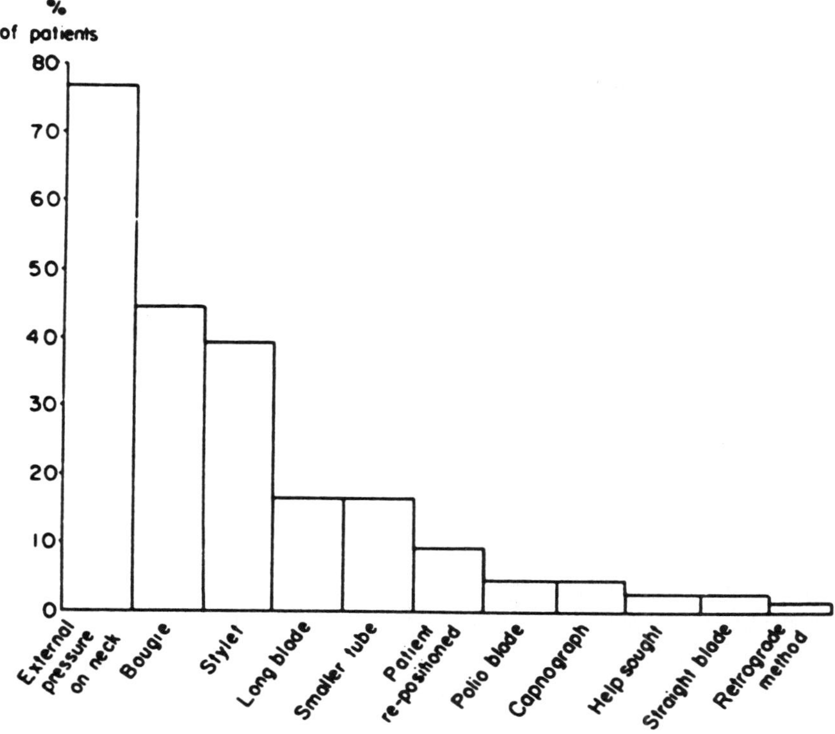

FIG 15–5.
Completed questionnaires with regard to initial choice of technique for management of difficult airway. Simple methods were chosen initially and are shown in order of preference. One third of respondents used these methods alone and had no experience with more complex methods. (From James Q, Latto IP: Unpublished data presented to the Welsh Society of Anaesthetists, 1982.)

described earlier. The careful repositioning of the patient's head into the true "sniffing" position and the selection of an endotracheal tube 1 mm smaller than the anticipated size is frequently all that is required to turn a failed intubation into a success on the second attempt. Figure 15–6 shows the order of choice of simple techniques that one group of experienced anesthesiologists has found particularly useful in difficult situations.

However, where simple maneuvers fail, other techniques must be used, and although each of the following may be used in more than one situation, each is described as being particularly suited to a given set of problems under the classification previously described.

Problems of Access

Access to the oropharynx may be sought through the mouth or through the nose. The nasal route may be obstructed by polyps, bony spurs, septal deflections, or tumors requiring oral intubation. The oral route itself may be restricted by limited mouth opening because of temporomandibular joint disease or trismus, enlarged tongue, or tumors in the oral cavity. Thus, although there

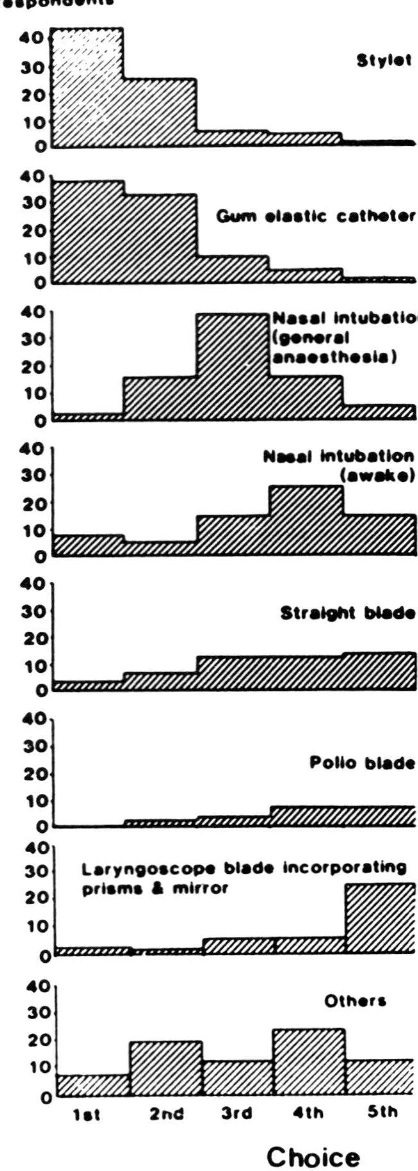

FIG 15–6.
Order of choices of simple techniques in prospective study of 43 cases of difficult intubation. (From Eastley R, Latto IP, Ng WS, et al: Unpublished data, 1984.)

may be room for a laryngoscope, it may not be possible to manipulate an endotracheal tube as well. If the nasal route is dictated because of the patient's condition, blind nasal intubation may be the technique of choice (Fig 15–7). The major risks associated with this technique are infection, bleeding, and trauma to the posterior pharyngeal wall. With base of skull fractures there is the remote possibility of the tube entering the cranium. The inherent risks are minimized by preparing the nose with vasoconstrictors and using a properly designed nasal tube that has a longer bevel than is usual with oral tubes but that does not have a Murphy's port, which can act as a curette during nasal passage. This nasal tube should be made of a material that is soft but does not

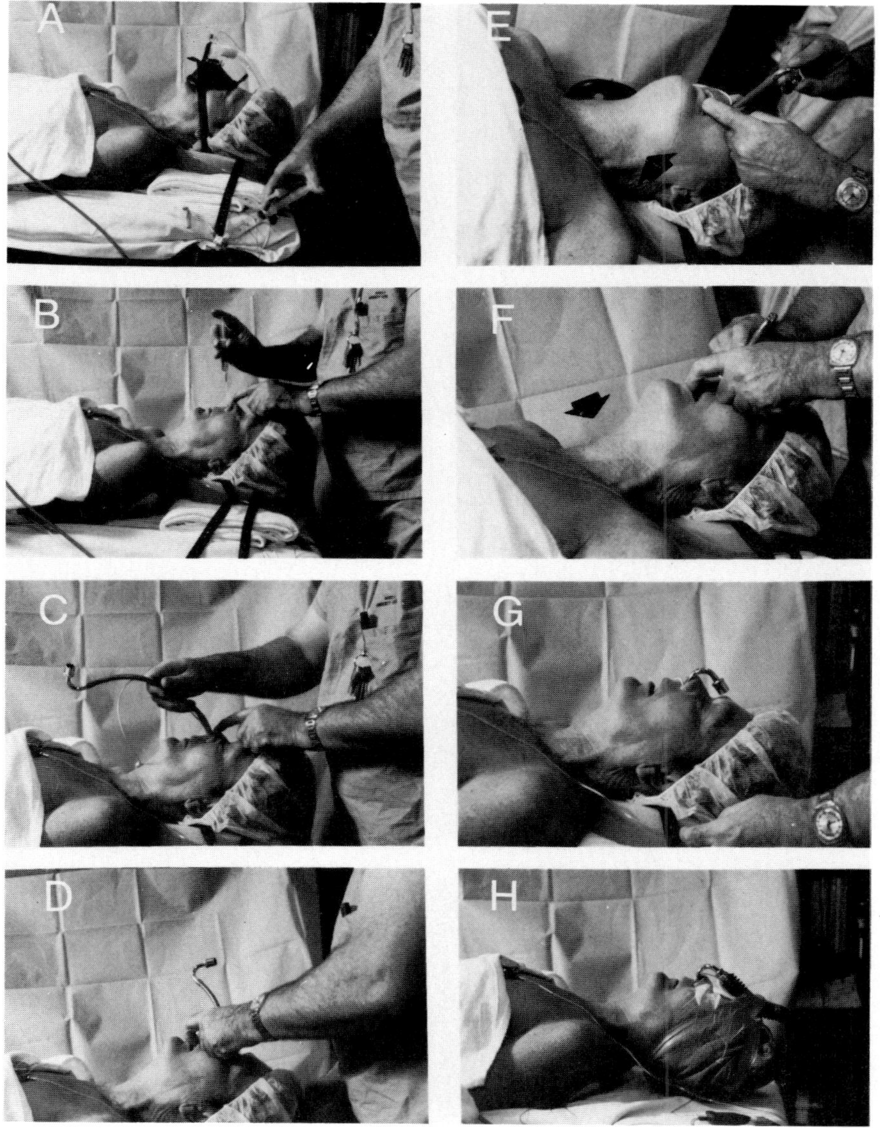

FIG 15–7.
Technique of blind nasal intubation. Here patient is relaxed with succinylcholine. **A,** 7.0 mm cuffed Magill red rubber tube has been cut to length while patient is fully preoxygenated. **B,** after induction, 2 mL 4% cocaine solution are instilled vertically into each nostril. **C,** tip of nose is elevated to allow tip of tube to pass over helix of chosen nostril. **D,** with patient's head in sniffing position, the tube is passed along floor of nasal passage against the junction of the nasal septum with floor of nostril to minimize trauma to inferior turbinate. Gentle click is felt as tip emerges into pharynx. **E,** with patient's head held in sniffing position, tube is advanced further until tip is seen to deform neck or cause thyroid cartilage to move. Here, tip of tube is off midline, deforming neck in left pyriform fossa. **F,** tube is withdrawn 3 to 4 cm to bring tip up above aryepiglottic fold, permitting rotation of tube and tip toward midline. Tube is readvanced, and another click is felt as tube enters trachea. "Mouse" is seen under skin as tip is advanced down trachea. **G,** tube is advanced so that tip of metal connector lies inside nostril. Upper section of tube is completely surrounded by bone and immune to kinking. Auscultation of lungs confirms that tube is not too long. **H,** black rubber corrugated connector ensures that metal connector is held away from nasal ala to prevent pressure ulceration.

lose its shape at body temperature, thereby allowing accurate manipulation. These properties are best embodied in the red rubber Magill nasal tubes. If access through the nose is not feasible and oral access is also restricted, the retrograde catheter technique (Fig 15–8) offers much. However, this technique takes time and requires the patient to be breathing spontaneously, either awake or asleep. If awake, the patient's hypopharynx is left unanesthetized, and the patient is encouraged to spit the slack catheter fed into the pharynx from below the larynx out through the mouth.

Problems of Visualization

Visualization of the larynx depends primarily on the ability of the laryngoscopist to reduce the angle between the planes of the oral and pharyngeal cavities in the sniffing position with the selected laryngoscope blade (Fig 15–9). This requires compression or deflection of the tongue mass within the arch of the mandible and the larynx being in its normal position.

If the arch of the mandible is small or the tongue is less than normally compressible because of infiltration or scarring, normal laryngoscopic techniques may not bring the glottis into view. Similarly, if the larynx is high and immobile, tucked under the base of the tongue, normal laryngoscopy will be ineffective.

In such a situation two approaches may achieve success. The tube changer, a long malleable stylet, which is also hollow, may be introduced under direct

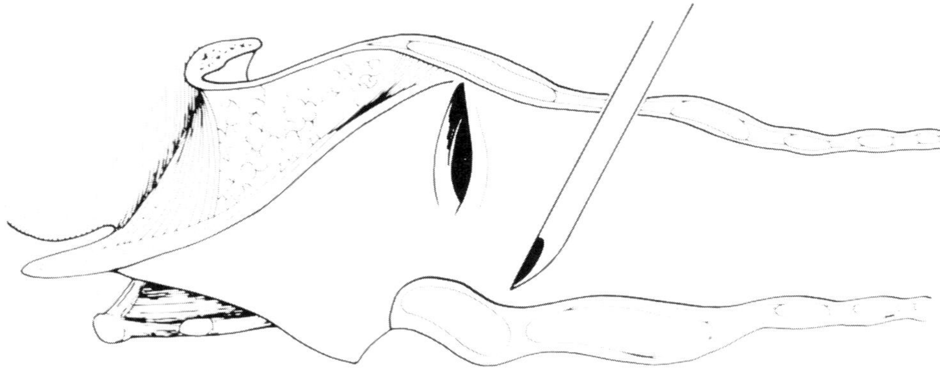

FIG 15–8.
Retrograde catheter technique using standard epidural set. Following percutaneous transcricothyroid topical block, Tuohy needle is introduced to trachea through cricothyroid membrane with bevel pointing cephalad. Epidural catheter with guide wire is fed through needle and put through glottis. Lateral control is achieved by rotating needle while anteroposterior control is achieved by rotating needle about its fulcrum at point of insertion. After passage of catheter, patient is asked to spit it out through mouth if awake, or catheter is picked up with forceps under direct vision in pharynx. Guide wire and Tuohy needle are then withdrawn and both ends of catheter secured with forceps with catheter used as guide for passage of endotracheal tube from above. If tube will not pass into trachea, one size smaller should be tried. Other maneuvers described to persuade tube tip over posterior laryngeal margin include feeding catheter through Murphy's port, then up inside tube, or passing suction catheter or gum elastic catheter down tube and into trachea to act as larger guide over and beside original catheter.

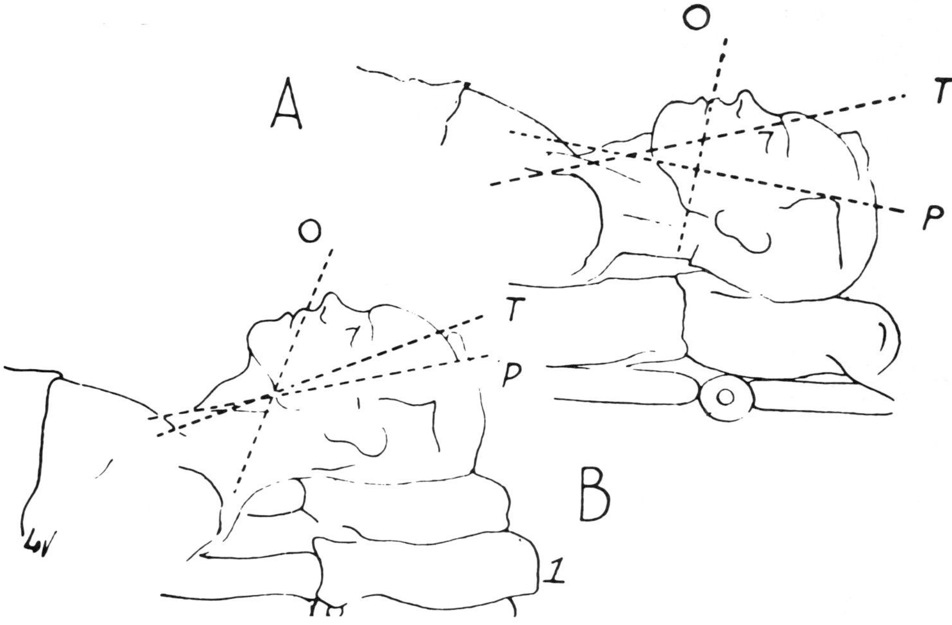

FIG 15–9.
Sniffing position. **A,** patient lies supine, and relative inclinations of oral cavity *(O)*, pharynx *(P)*, and trachea *(T)* in sagittal plane are indicated. **B,** sniffing position shows support of head giving flexion of lower cervical spine with extension of upper cervical spine and head, thereby reducing angle between planes *T* and *P*. This leaves angle *N* between *O* and *T* and *P* to be reduced by laryngoscopy for visualization of larynx. (Note the angle of *T* relative to the horizontal with respect to aspiration risk.)

vision (Fig 15–10), then passed blindly, anterior to whatever part of the posterior larynx can be seen. Once in place, the stylet is sufficiently stiff to pull at least part of the larynx back into view in most cases. The stylet then acts as a guide over which a range (lower limit 6.5 mm) of endotracheal tubes may be introduced.

Another technique that is useful in such a situation is the light wand (Fig 15–11), which may also prove successful when fiberoptic intubation attempts have failed. The disadvantage of the technique is that most larger diameter tubes must be trimmed to a suitable length for the light wand that may not be acceptable for some surgical procedures. With increasing neck obesity or skin pigmentation the chances of success diminish. Both techniques may also be used where oral intubation is a necessity but access through the mouth is restricted.

Problems with Target

The ability to pass an endotracheal tube through the glottis may be limited by the physical size of the glottic chink or the airway below. The position of the glottis may not be immediately evident because of swelling of supraglottic laryngeal structures or because of rotation and deformities of the larynx itself. A profuse crop of laryngeal papillomas may effectively camouflage the en-

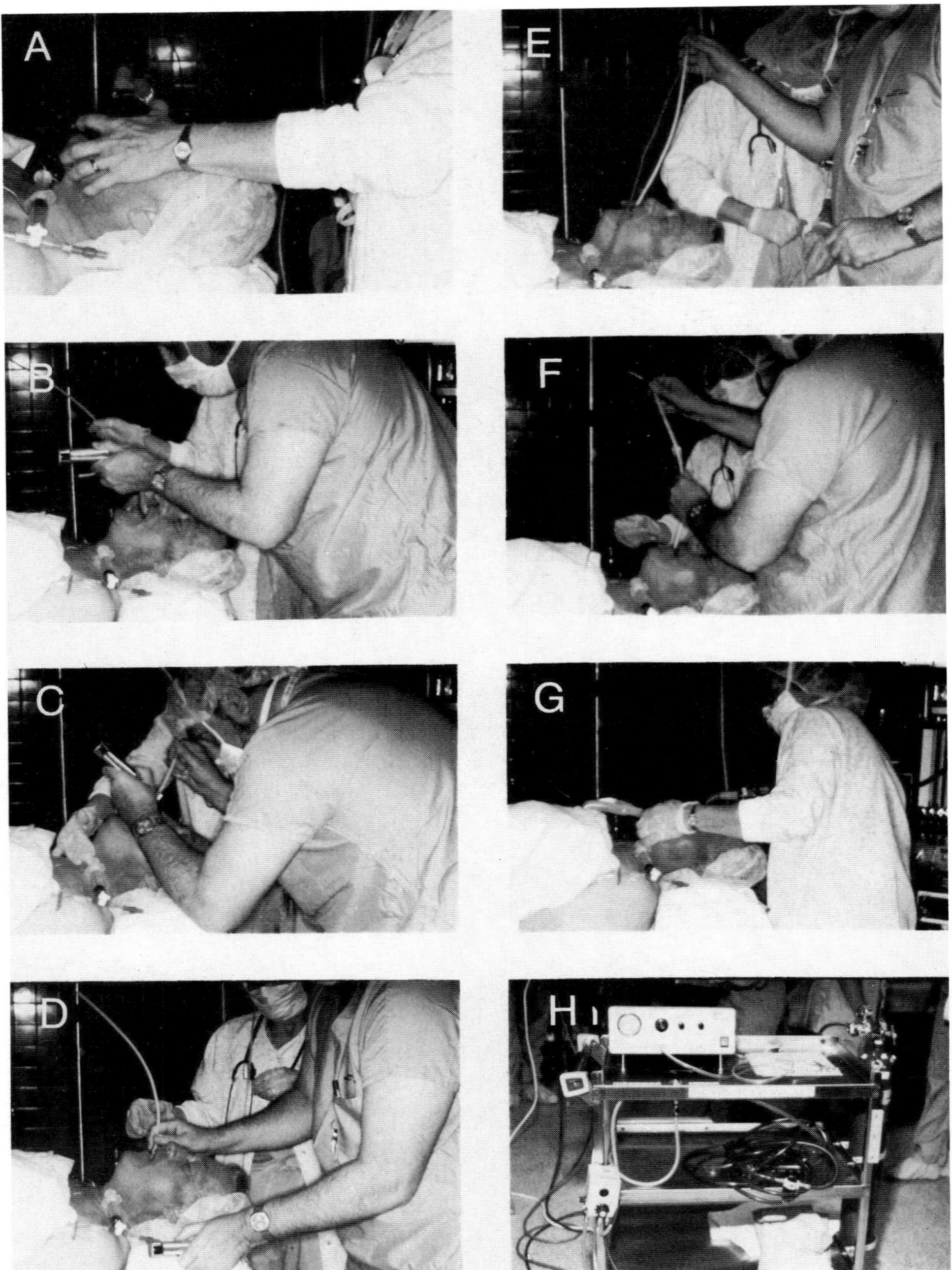

FIG 15–10.
Patient with known difficult airway secondary to postradiation scarring, giving incompressible base of tongue and difficulty in visualizing larynx. **A,** after preoxygenation, general anesthesia is induced by inhalation. **B** and **C,** after third stage, anesthesia tube changer is introduced under direct vision with Miller no. 4 straight blade. Posterior rim of larynx is seen with no view of glottis. **D** and **E,** once tube changer is placed, jet ventilator is attached. At low inflation pressures, two cycles confirm correct placement and chest deflation by auscultation. **F** and **G,** patient is paralyzed and trachea successfully intubated while patient is continuously jet ventilated. **H,** jet ventilation cart used incorporated Bird N_2O/O_2 blender and Wolf Injectomat automatic jet ventilator.

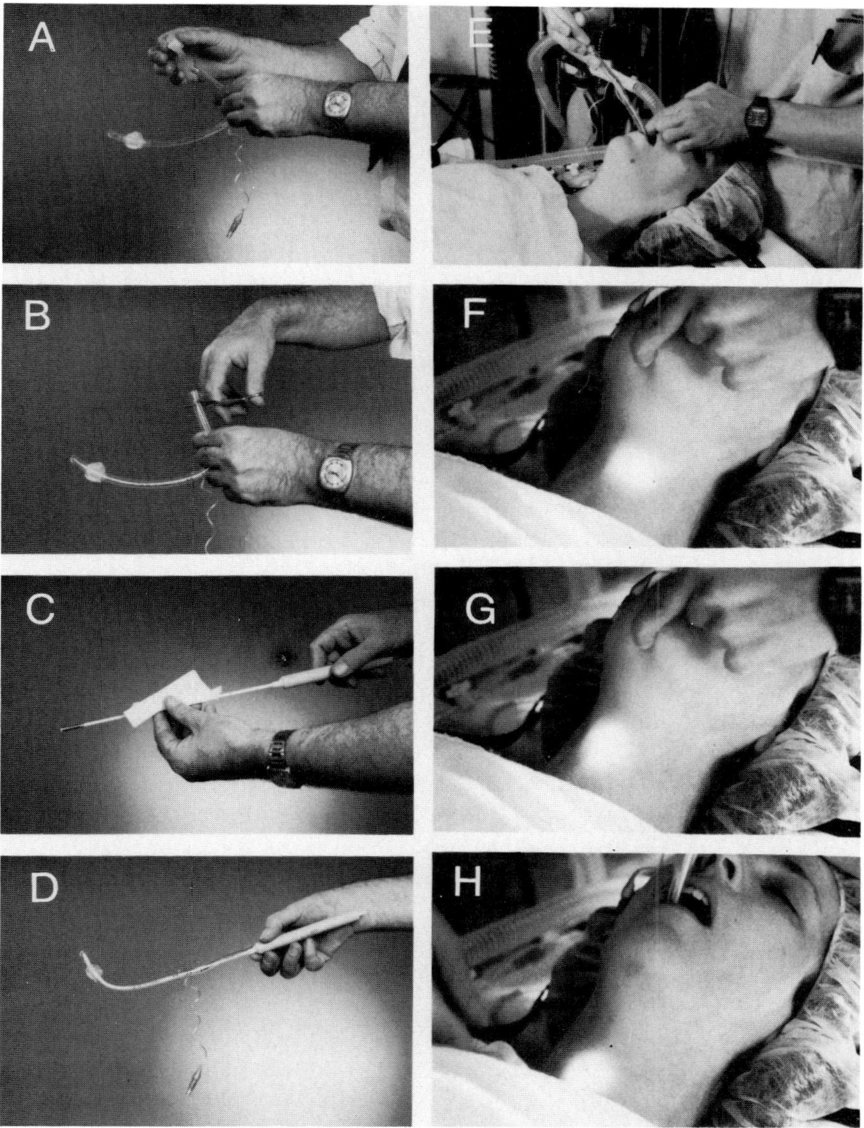

FIG 15–11.

A and **B,** light wand technique. Tube connector is removed (≥6.5 mm size) and tube cut so end abuts handle while bulb lies at tip without protrusion. **C,** wand is lubricated. **D,** tube is passed onto wand and tip bent just short of 90 degrees in hockey stick shape. **E,** table is lowered so that anesthesiologist is looking down on the patient's neck without bending forward. Patient's head is steadied in sniffing position while wand is passed over tongue in midline. **F,** patient's mandible is then lifted with left hand during further advance. If mass of tongue deflects wand to side or there is resistance to advance, wand is passed laterally into pyriform fossa (transillumination is seen on left side) with wand handle held back against upper teeth. **G,** once position of tip is identified, wand is withdrawn 3 to 4 cm slowly and rotated medially until it passes glottis. Flare of light down trachea will be seen. **H,** wand is advanced gently in this direction, and shadows of tracheal rings will confirm correct position. Wand is then withdrawn from tube and tube connector reattached. *(Do not lose it!)* Normal position checks are made.

trance to the airway. The problem in such situations is to first find the entrance to the airway, then determine the size of tube that will fit through the opening.

These problems require the ability to probe for the glottic opening without traumatizing the larynx. This is better done with a small diameter soft stylet rather than the endotracheal tube itself. The gum elastic stylet (modeled on the Tiemens urinary bougie) is ideal for this purpose (Fig 15–12). It is introduced with the endotracheal tube; but unlike an ordinary stylet, 2 to 3 inches of it are allowed to protrude beyond the tube tip, to be used as the probe and then the guide over which the tube is slid into place. It is of great help in this situation if the patient is breathing spontaneously, without antisialogogue, because the laryngoscopist can "follow the bubbles" with the stylet tip. Should the initial tube be too big for a fixed glottic or subglottic restriction, the original tube may be withdrawn from the larynx over the stylet and smaller tubes passed over or beside it.

If the problems are complex, involving mixtures of laryngeal rotation and other factors, continued oxygenation and ventilation of the patient under general anesthesia may be ensured by transcricothyroid jet ventilation (Fig 15–13) while supralaryngeal probing takes place. However, special care must be exercised to prevent barotrauma. The possibility of a fixed restriction in the expiratory pathway should be excluded, if possible. If any doubt exists, jet ventilation should be commenced at low inflation pressures (<14 psi), low rate, and at high inspiratory/expiratory ratio, while chest deflation and the escape of gas through the larynx are confirmed. Once the adequacy of gas escape is established, the patient should be relaxed to prevent him or her from raising the intrathoracic pressure by straining against ventilation. While still in the recovery room, all patients who have undergone jet ventilation should have a postoperative chest radiograph taken to check for barotrauma.

Escape Routes

Potential failure of anesthetic management must be considered in every patient with a difficult airway, and a clear plan of action to reverse the situation

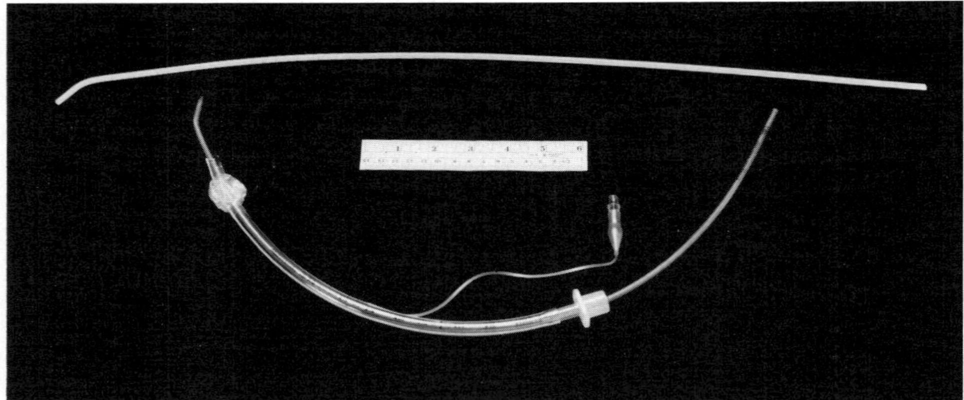

FIG 15–12.
Relative position of gum elastic bougie within endotracheal tube when used as probe. Above is similar device made of solid Teflon, which, although malleable, is not quite as soft as gum elastic variety.

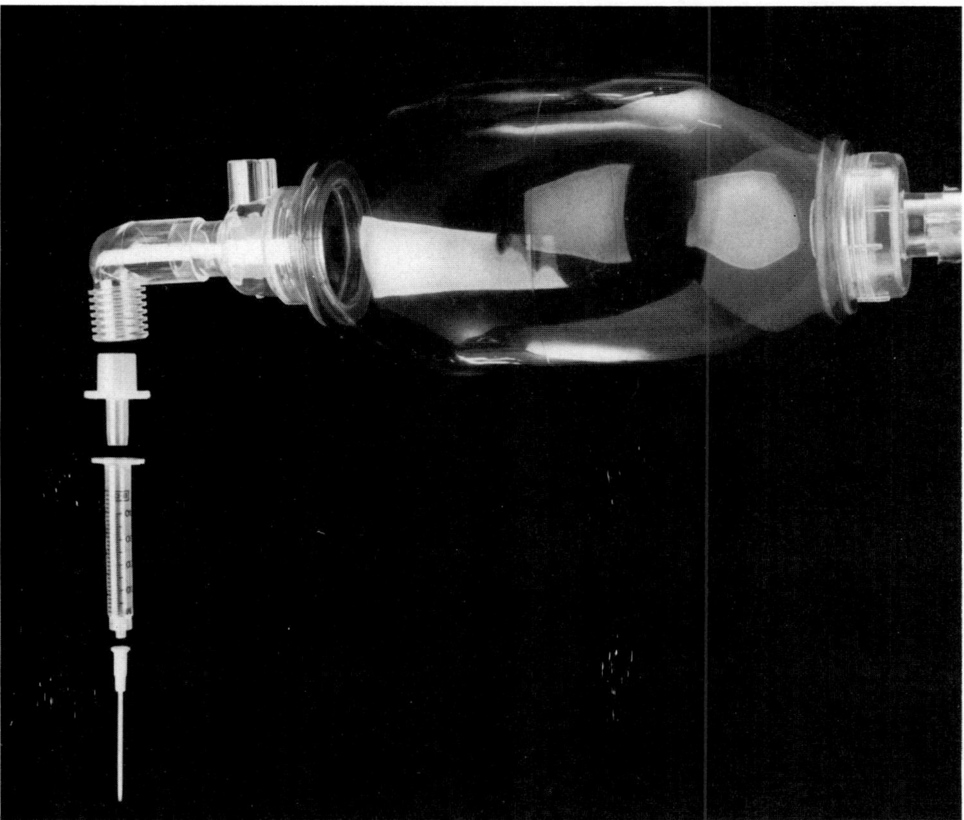

FIG 15–13.
Readily available equipment that permits low-pressure transcricothyroid ventilation. Standard 3 mL plastic syringe barrel connected to 7.0 mm endotracheal tube connector permits connection of standard self-inflating bag and nonrebreathing valve with IV cannula used as tracheal injector.

must be made in advance. This means not only a formulated plan but that all personnel involved in the operating room understand what is expected of them and the signal to implement it.

The most desirable escape plan is to maintain the patient's spontaneous respiration throughout anesthetic manipulations, but when the decision is made that the anesthetic intubation attempts have failed, a reasonable trial should be made to allow the patient to recover from whatever medications have been given, then proceed to a calm, elective tracheostomy under local anesthesia. However, should the ideal prove elusive, several methods of achieving oxygenation of the patient from below the larynx are available in an emergency. Jet ventilation can be effective as a lifesaving measure in an emergency, and the catheter-injector can be placed anywhere in the trachea if required. If the expiratory pathway is obstructed or barotrauma has occurred, a second catheter placed beside the first may improve the situation and allow enough time for an emergency tracheotomy to be completed. Jet ventilation depends on special equipment that may not always be available in an emergency, so some have described the use of various ad hoc combinations of widey available equipment to achieve low-pressure oxygenation through an injector (see Fig 15–13). This will buy time, but it is far less effective than jet ventilation.

Finally, several devices are now available in presterilized packaging for performing an emergency cricothyrotomy large enough to allow not only oxygenation but also sufficient reciprocal ventilation to control CO_2 levels and protect the airway either by suction or the introduction of a cuffed tube (Fig 15–14).

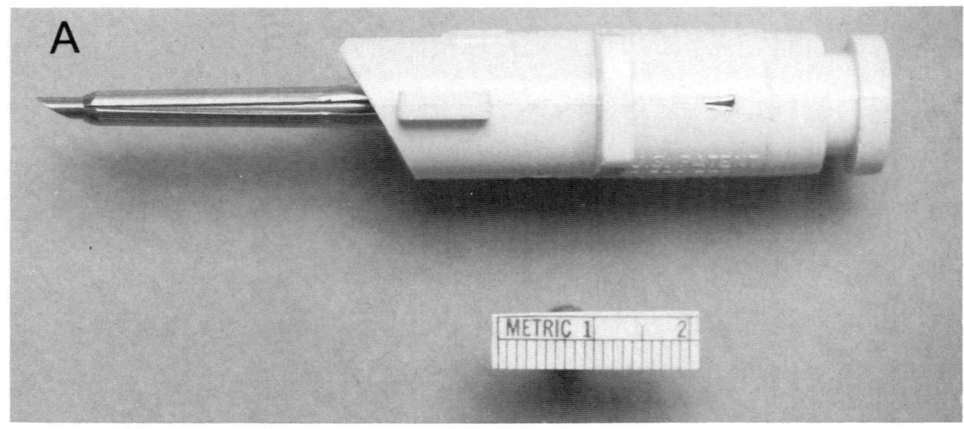

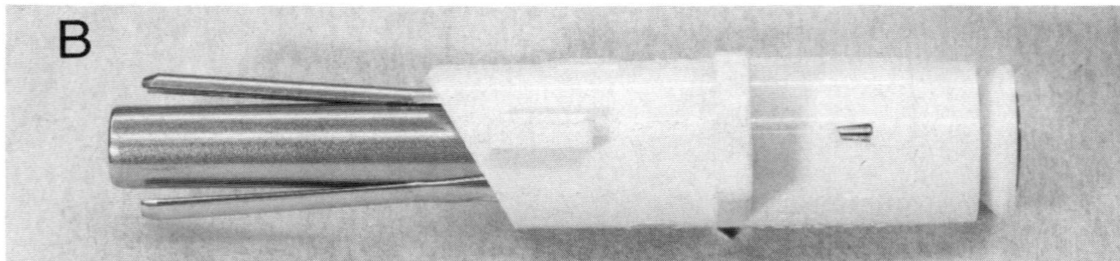

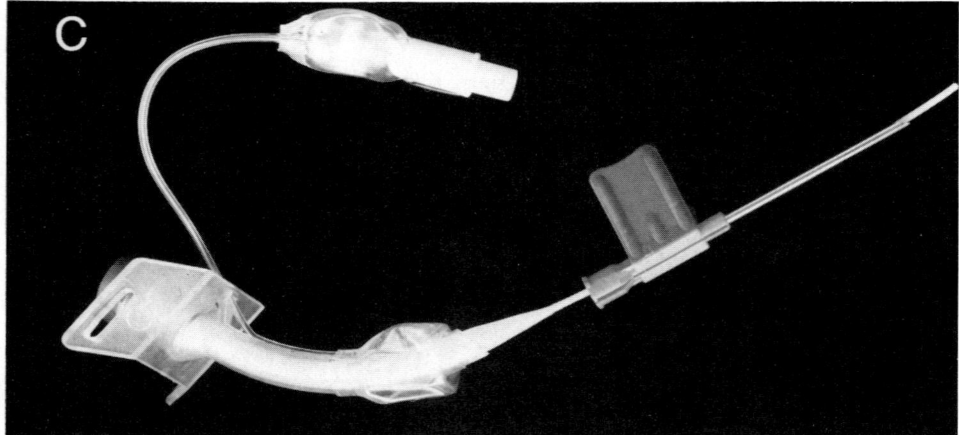

FIG 15–14.
Examples of emergency cricothyrotomy devices that permit reciprocal ventilation with 15 minute connectors. Nutrake configured for insertion **(A)** and ventilation **(B).** Pertrach device **(C).** The tube on dilator is shown with split needle to introduce filiform section into trachea. After insertion of filiform part of dilator through needle into trachea, needle is split apart and removed.

All such emergency maneuvers rely on the operator's ability to identify the exterior anatomic landmarks of the airway in the neck. Patients with gross fat deposits in the neck, fixed flexion deformities, or extreme swelling from any cause are not good candidates for such procedures. Therefore the original anesthetic management plan should take this lack of a reasonable escape route into account.

CONCLUSION

Several published reports suggest that difficulty with intubation is more common than generally supposed. The contribution of the difficult airway to anesthetic morbidity and mortality is significant and probably of increasing importance as other causes are overcome by improved monitoring and pharmacologic techniques. It has been estimated that at least 90% of difficult intubations should be anticipated,[8] but this can be achieved only by careful, routine examination of the airway in all patients requiring anesthesia. If a problem is detected, successful management can be expected only if a full preoperative evaluation is undertaken to establish the nature of the problem and the level in the airway involved. Most problems can be conveniently compartmentalized into problems of access, visualization, or target, or combinations thereof. Most intubation techniques are particularly suited to overcoming one of these problem types, but may be useful in more than one. Simple techniques are commonly successful in most patients with a difficult airway, and the equipment required for simple techniques is more generally available in an emergency. Therefore the anesthesiologist should make every effort to ensure facility with several simple techniques suited to overcoming the problems posed by each of the three groups described, as well as fiberoptic skills.

Thus an argument is made for mastering a group of techniques applicable in terms of access, visualization, or target, remembering that the problem highest in the airway is the usual determinant of the primary technique that can be used. This approach is recommended to formulate an elective anesthetic management plan and to simplify the management decisions under the pressure involved with the unanticipated difficult airway, rather than trying to memorize one of the more complex decision trees that have been published in the literature. In all patients requiring anesthesia, the anesthesiologist should cultivate the habit of examining the neck to identify the feasibility of a sublaryngeal emergency airway. Patient safety is best ensured by maintaining spontaneous respiration until the airway is secured or by exercising sufficient caution, combined with experience, to know when the management plan has failed, always remembering that falling oxygen saturation level on the pulse oximeter is a late manifestation of impending disaster.

REFERENCES

1. Aro L, Takki S, Aromaa V: Technique for difficult intubation. *Br J Anaesthiol* 1974; 43:1081.
2. Stauffer JL, Olson DE, Petty TL: Complications and consequences of endotracheal intubation and tracheostomy. A prospective study of 150 critically ill adult patients. *Am J Med* 1981; 70:65.

3. Caplan RA, Posner KL, Ward RS, et al: Adverse respiratory events in anesthesia: A closed claims analysis. *Anesthesiology* 1990; 72:828.
4. Standards for basic intraoperative monitoring, in *ASA Directory.* Chicago, American Society of Anesthesiologists, 1990, p 660.
5. Shaw JD, Lancer JM: *A Color Atlas of Fiberoptic Endoscopy of the Upper Respiratory Tract.* Chicago, Year Book Medical Publishers, 1987.
6. Patil V, Stehling L, Zander H: *Fiberoptic Endoscopy in Anesthesia.* Chicago, Year Book Medical Publishers, 1983.
7. Wies S: A new emergency cricothyroidotomy instrument. *J Trauma* 1983; 23:155.
8. Toye FJ, Weinstein JD: Clinical experience with percutaneous tracheostomy and cricothyroidotomy in 100 patients. *J Trauma* 1984; 26:1034.
9. Sia RL, Edens ET: How to avoid problems when using the fiberoptic bronchoscope for difficult intubations. *Anaesthesia* 1981; 36:74.

APPENDIXES

Further Depictions of Anatomic Features of the Airway

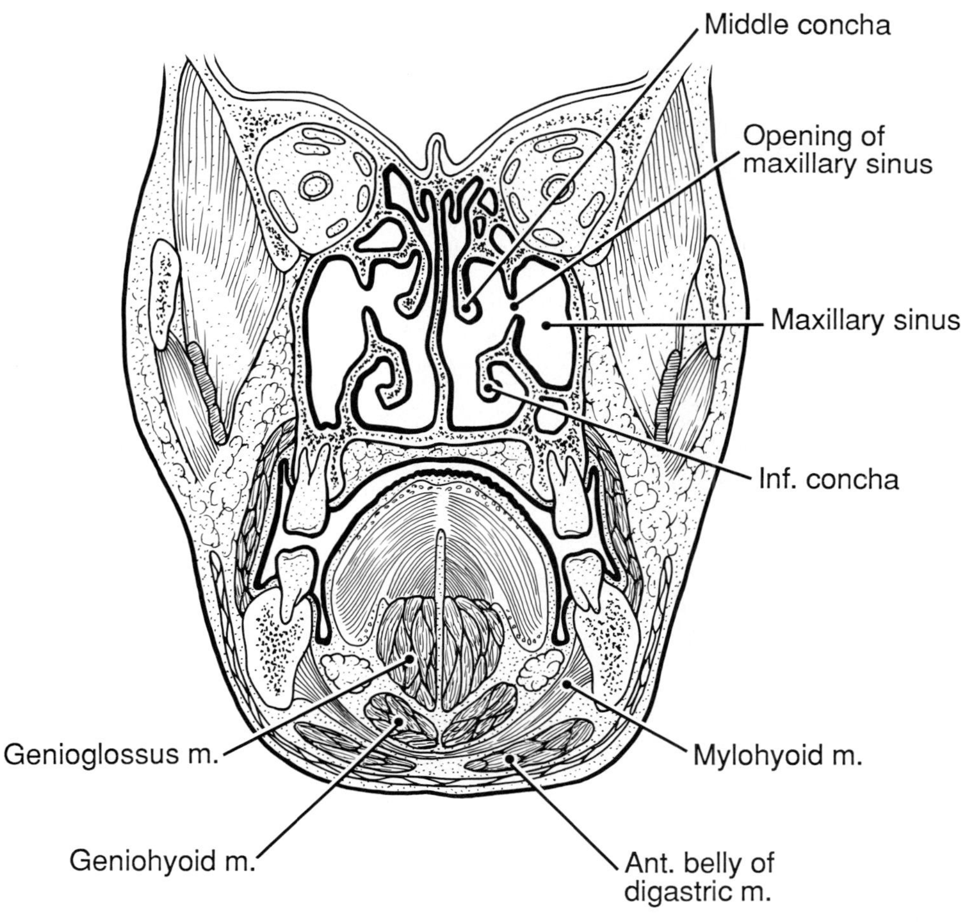

FIG A–1.
Relationship of nasal passages to oropharyngeal structures.

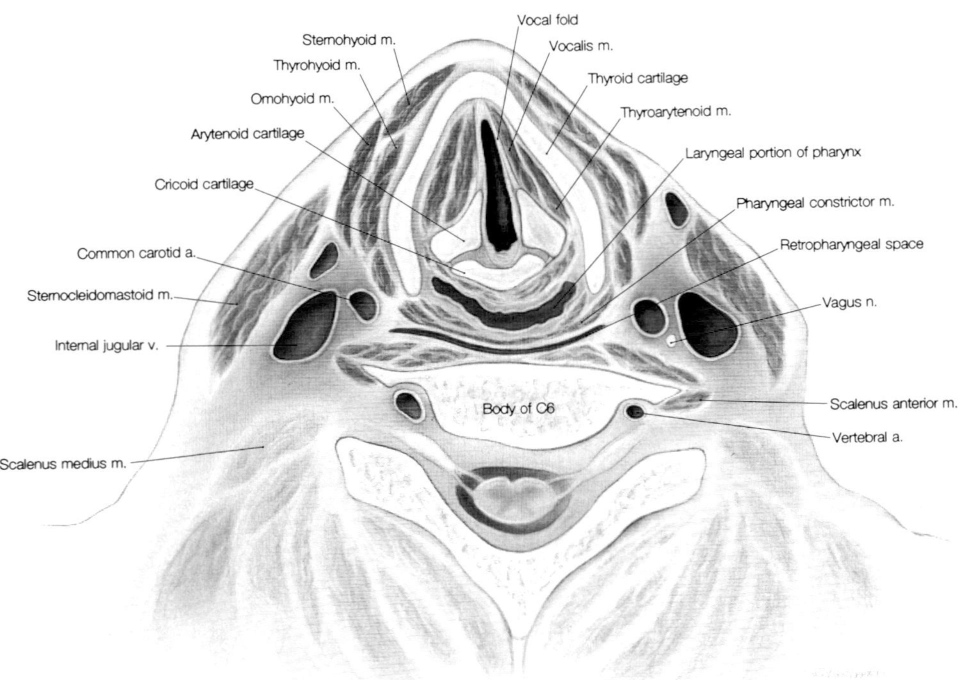

FIG A–2.
Transection of the neck at level of C-6.

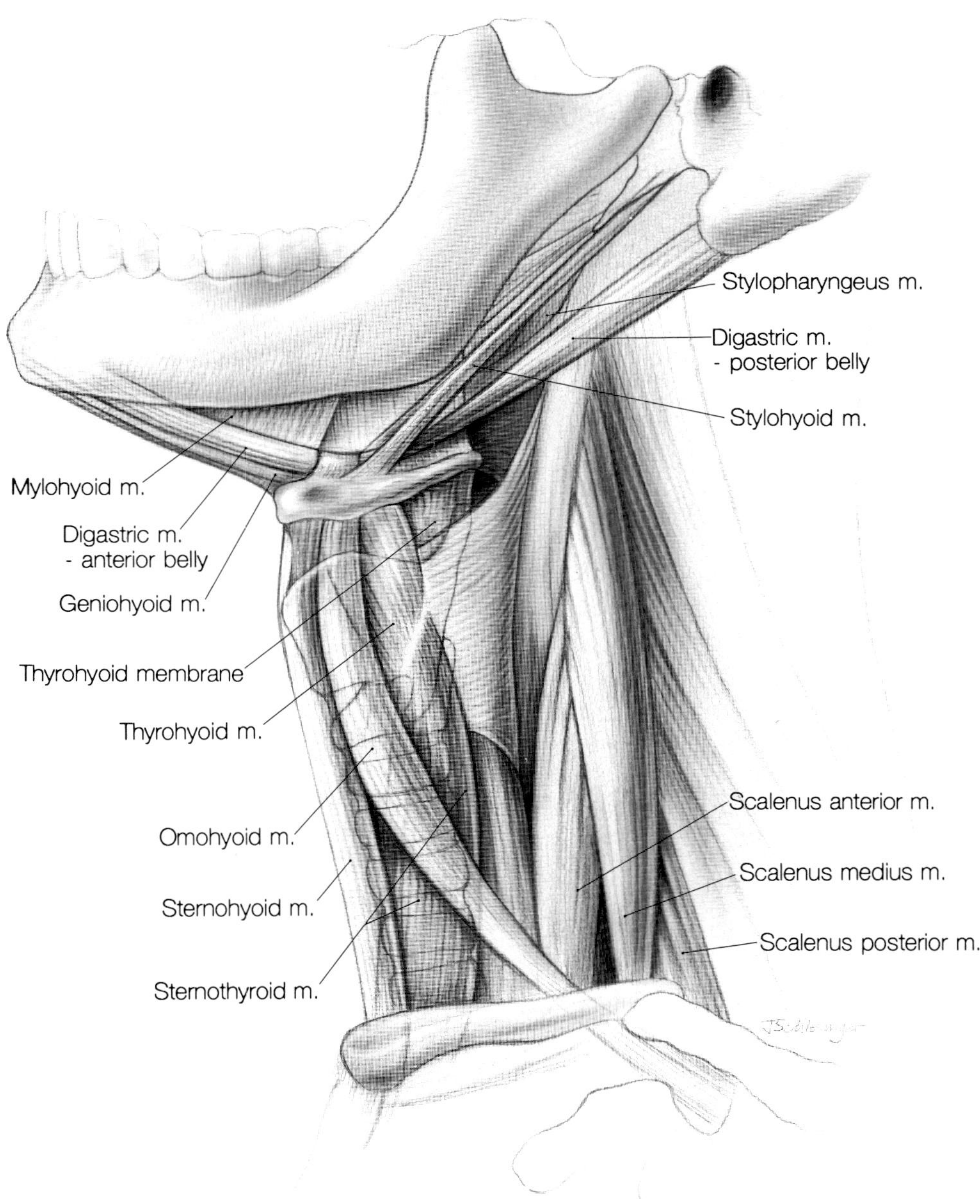

FIG A–3.
Lateral view of laryngeal suspension.

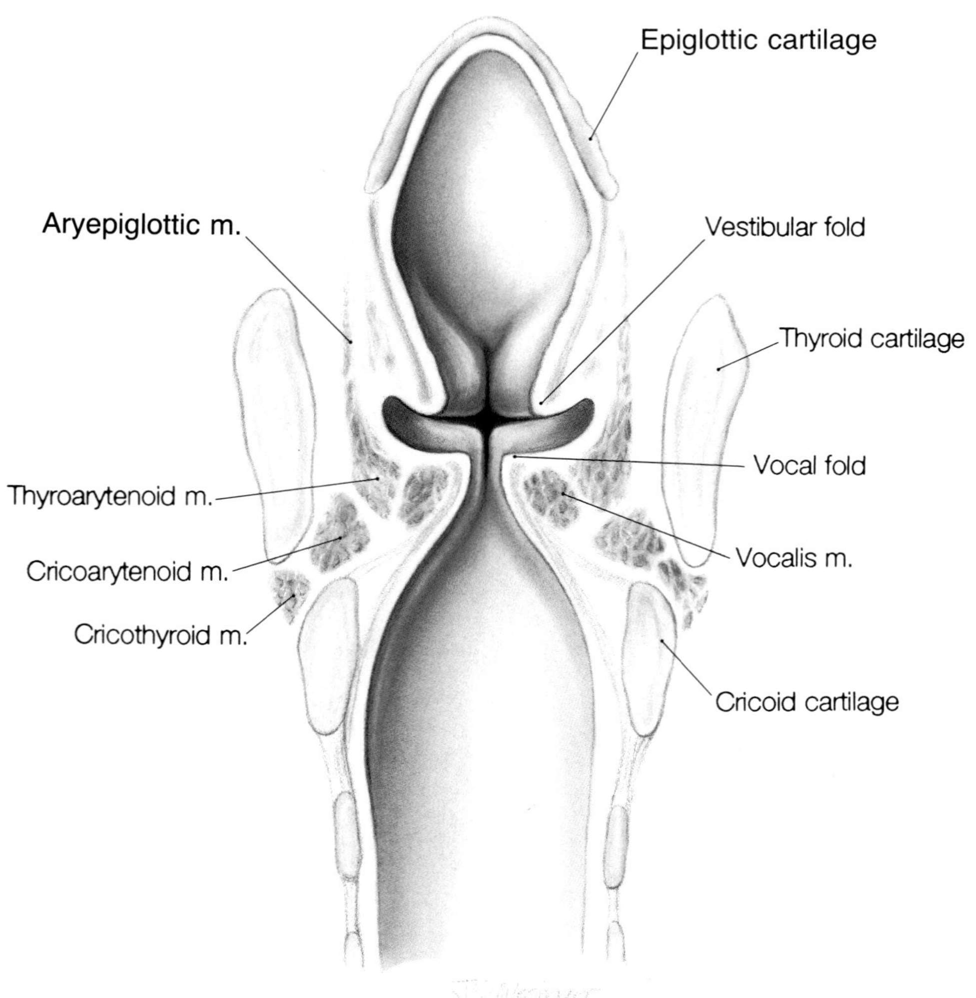

FIG A–4.
Transection of larynx.

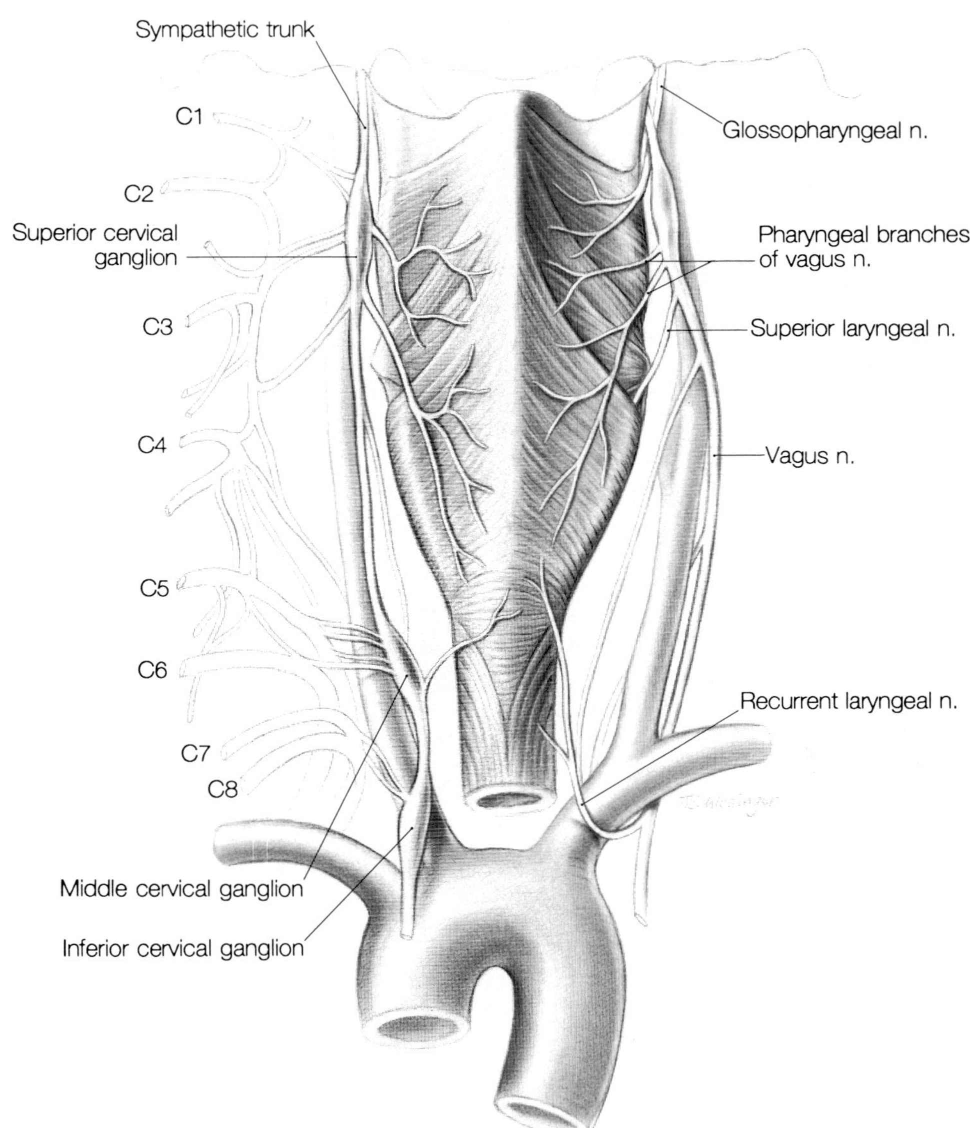

FIG A–5.
Innervation of larynx.

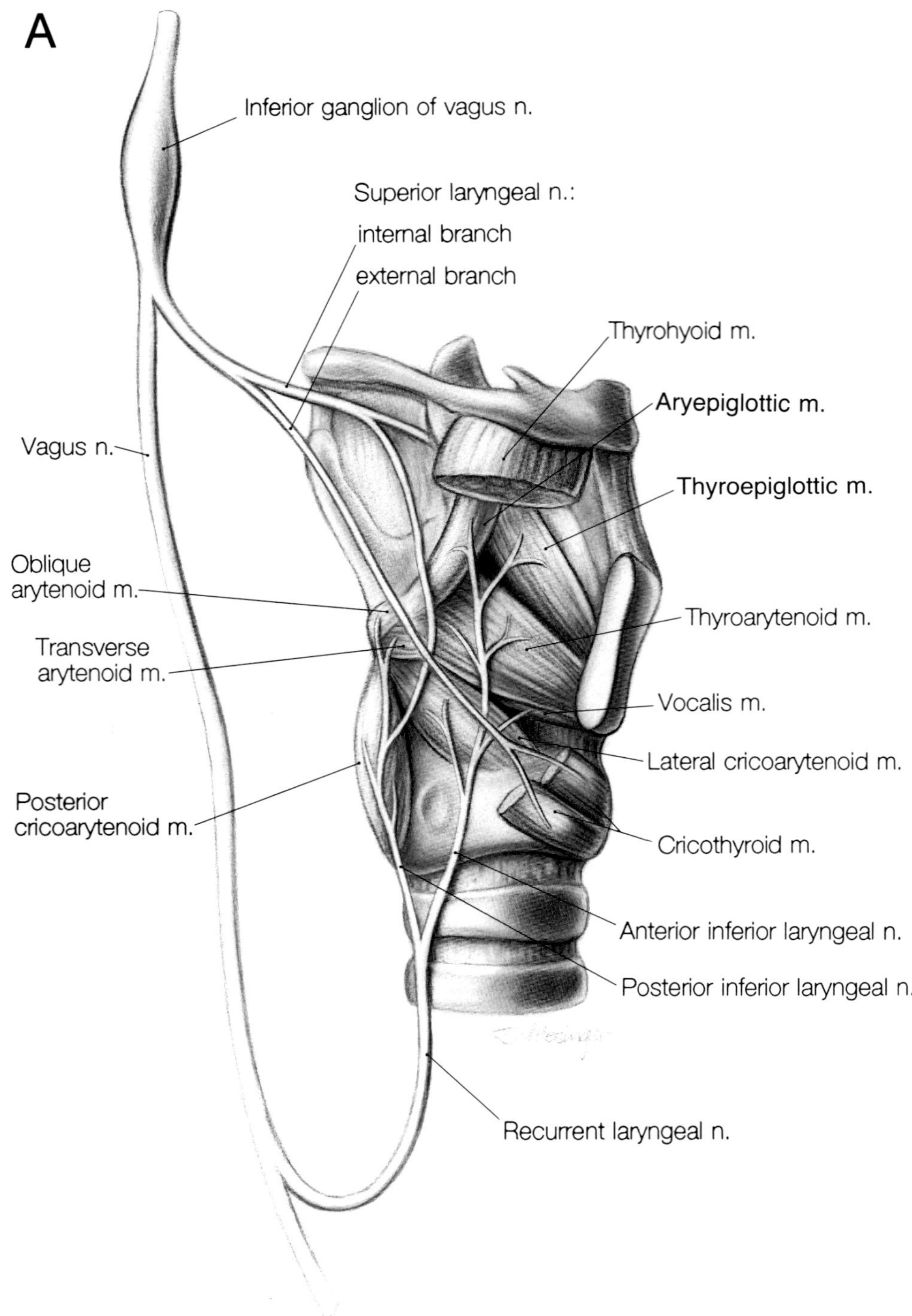

FIG A–6.
A, innervation related to laryngeal musculature. **B,** note cricothyroid puncture site.

B
Superior laryngeal n.:
external branch
internal branch
Omohyoid m.
Sternohyoid m.
Thyrohyoid m.
Sternothyroid m.
Cricothyroid m.
Thyrohyoid membrane
Needle site
JSchlesinger

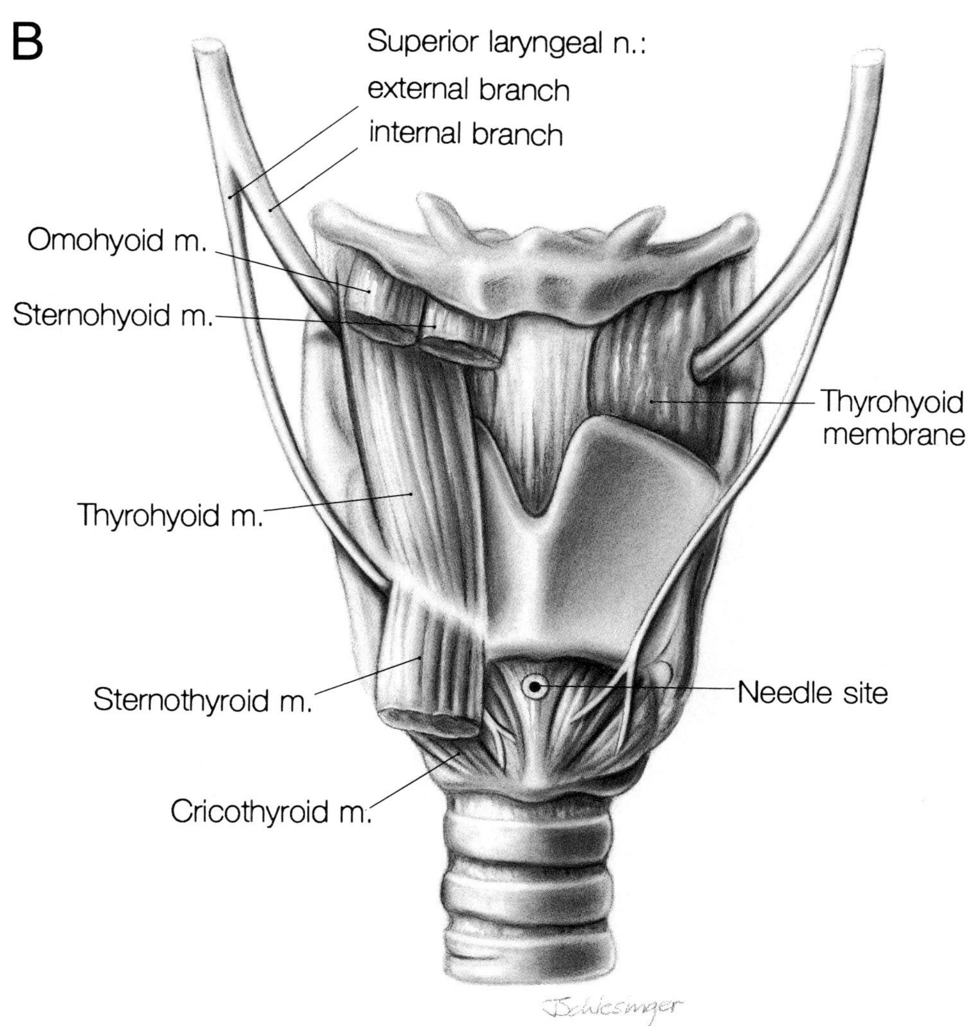

FIG A–6 (cont.).

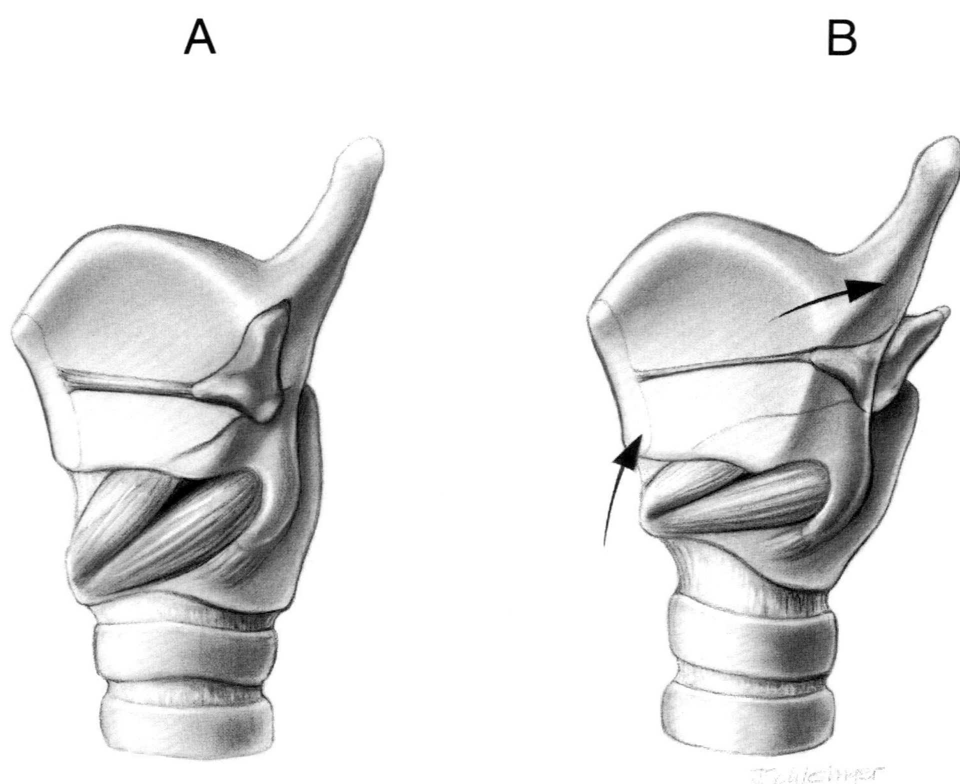

FIG A–7.
A, resting and, **B,** phonation positions of vocal folds.

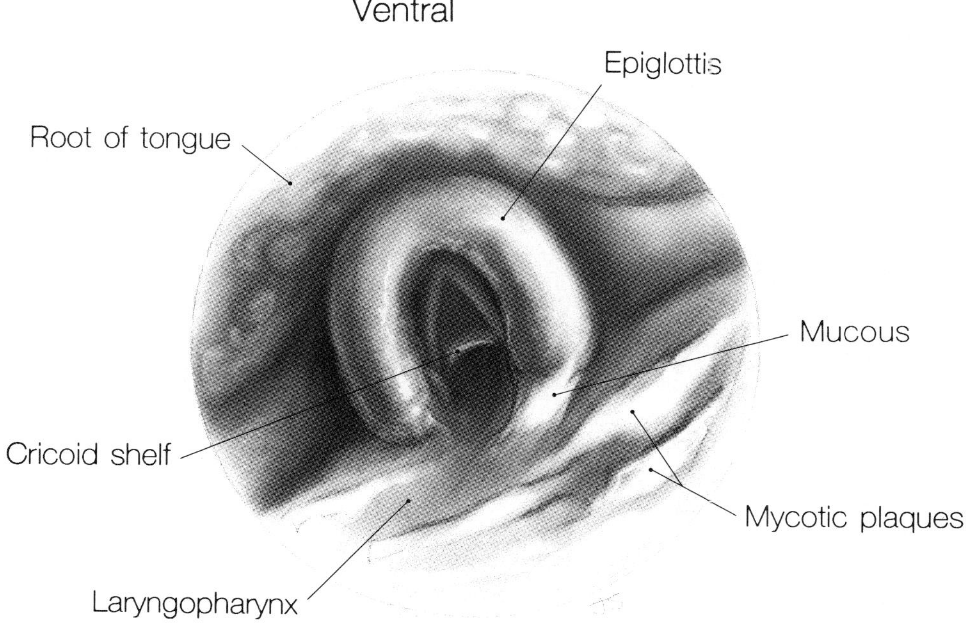

FIG A–8.
Fiberoptic view of additus laryngis.

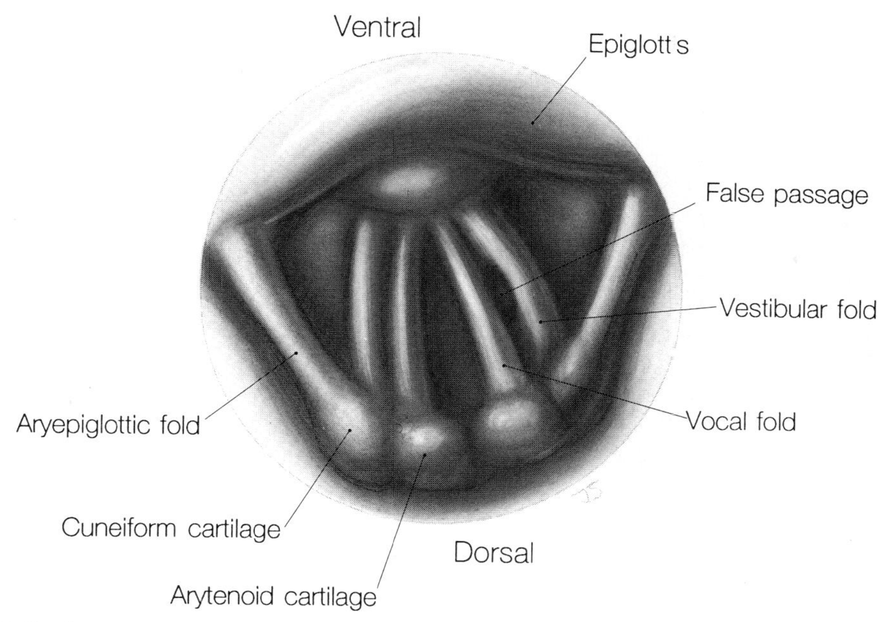

FIG A–9.
Normal anatomy of larynx with postintubation false passage.

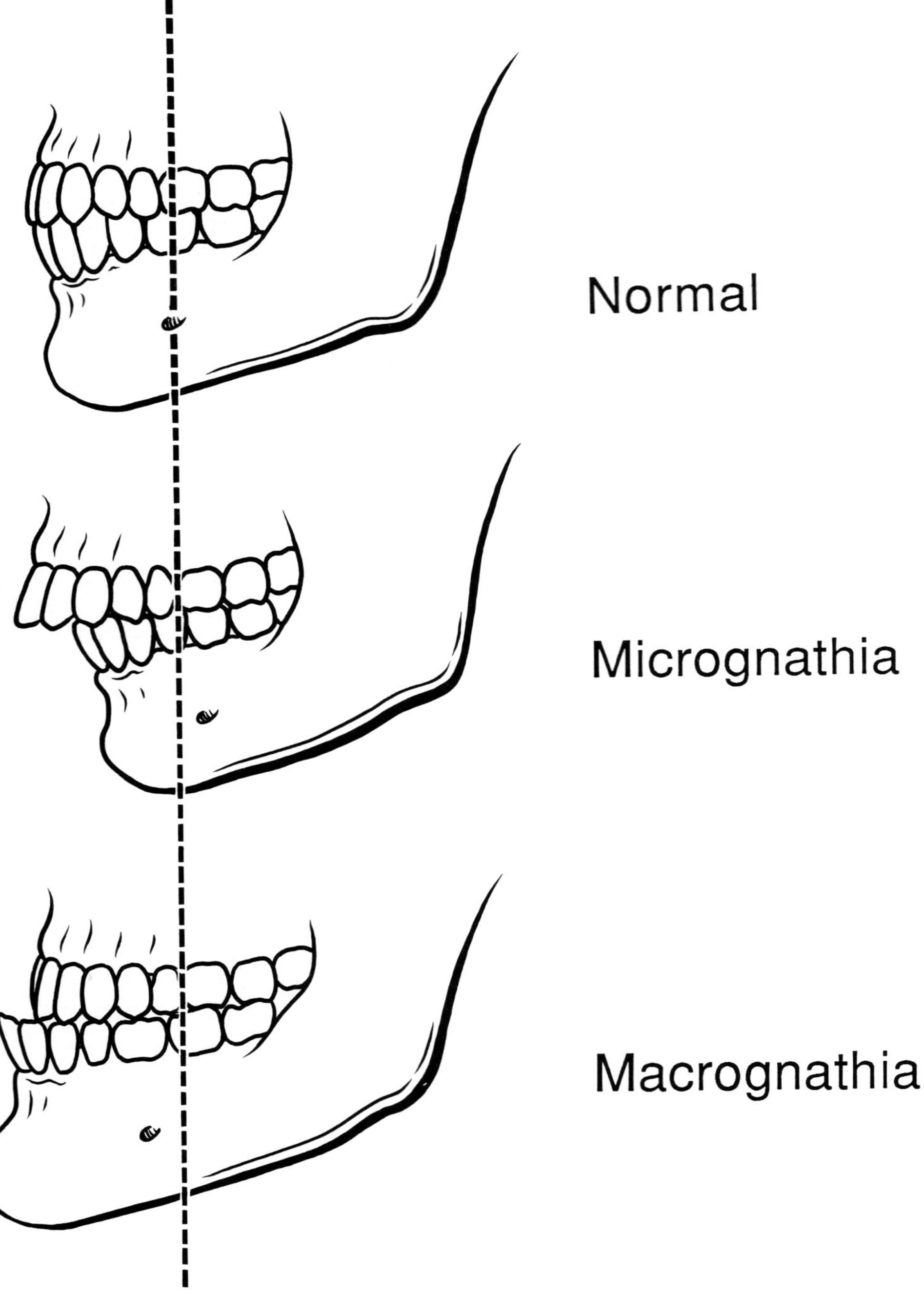

FIG A–10.
Mandibular positions.

Appendix B.

Named Syndromes Related to Potential Airway Problems

Anderson Midfacial hypoplasia, relative mandibular prognathism triangle facies, and kyphoscoliosis

Apert Acrocephalosyndactyly, craniostenosis, symmetric syndactyly of hands and feet, high forehead, flat bridge of nose, maxillary hypoplasia, relative mandibular prognathism, synostosis of cervical spine, visceral malformations, and congenital heart defects

Beckwith Wiedemann Macroglossia and gigantism with neonatal hypoglycemia

Binder Maxillonasal dysplasia

Carpenter Craniostenosis, polysyndactyly of feet, short hands with soft tissue syndactyly, acrocephalopolysyndactyly type II dwarfing syndrome and hypoplastic mandible

Chotzen Craniostenosis and renal anomalies

Christ-Siemens-Touraine Hypoplastic mandible and anhydrotic ectodermal dysplasia

Cornelia de Lange Limb abnormalities, microbrachycephaly, micrognathia, and occasionally choanal atresia

Cowden Multiple hamartomas, hypoplastic mandible, microstomia, and birdlike facies

Crouzon Craniofacial dysostosis, craniostenosis, maxillary hypoplasia, shallow orbits with exophthalmos, relative mandibular prognathism, prominent nose (parrot beak), occasionally increased intracranial pressure, and narrow nasopharynx and oropharynx

Cushing Clinical expression of the inappropriate hypersecretion of cortisol and at times of adrenocortical androgens; disease refers to cases clearly of pituitary origin that usually exhibit a pituitary tumor; obesity is a major concomitant in all types, although pathologic obesity is rare

DiGeorge Hypoplastic mandible and mediastinal and cardiac anomalies

Down Microstomia, protruding tongue, mongolism, hypotonia, mental and motor retardation, and often congenital heart disease

Ellis–van Creveld Abnormal maxilla, cleft palate, cleft lip, hepatosplenomegaly, and a chondroectodermal or mesoectodermal dysplasia

Engelmann Osteopathia hyperostotica scleroticans multiplex infantilis, immobile neck, and limited opening of the mouth

Epstein-Barr A viral infection, a lymphotropic herpes virus with clinical manifestations of infectious mononucleosis developing in approximately 50% of infections, fever, pharyngitis, nasopharyngeal and generalized lymphoid hyperplasia, and splenomegaly; upper airway obstructive symptoms may be severe

Franceschetti-Zwahlen-Klein (see Treacher Collins, Freeman-Sheldon) Craniocarpotarsal dystrophy, whistling face, hypoplastic mandible, a dwarfing syndrome, microstomia, and short broad neck

Freeman-Sheldon Craniocarpotarsal dystrophy, "whistling face," hypoplastic mandible, dwarfing syndrome, short broad neck

Goldenhar Oculoauriculovertebral dysplasia, eye and ear abnormalities, micrognathia, maxillary hypoplasia, cleft or high arched palate, synostosis of cervical spine, and congenital heart defects

Goltz Airway papillomatosis; a focal dermal hypoplasia

Gorlin-Chaudry-Moss Asymmetry of head, a craniofacial dysostosis, and dental anomalies

Gorlin-Goltz Limited cervical motion, hydrocephalus, incomplete segmentation of cervical and thoracic vertebrae, hypertelorism, mandibular prognathism, mandibular prognathism, kyphoscoliosis, multiple jaw cysts, and fibrosarcomas

Greig Macroglossia, webbed neck, ocular hypertelorism, and mental retardation

Gruher (see Hallermann-Streiff) Oculomandibulodyscephaly, a dwarfing syndrome, hypoplastic mandible, microstomia, micrognathia, small pinched nose, and proportional dwarfism

Hallermann-Streiff Oculomandibular dyscephaly, dwarfing syndrome (proportional dwarfism), hypoplastic mandible, microstomia, micrognathia, small pinched nose; also known as Mickel-Hallermann-Streiff

Hallervorden-Spatz Torticollis, scoliosis, dystonia, and trismus

Hanhart Micrognathia and various limb abnormalities

Hunter Gargoylism with mucopolysaccharidosis II; similar to but less severe than Hurler's syndrome

Hurler Gargoylism with lipochondrodystrophy, mucopolysaccharidosis I, dwarfism, frontal bossing, hypertelorism, thick lips, macroglossia, hepatosplenomegaly, exceedingly short neck, deformed thorax, nasal congestion, noisy mouth breathing caused by malformation of the facial and nasal bones, associated with malformation of tracheobronchial cartilages, associated with cardiovascular anomalies, and mental deterioration

Kasabach-Merritt syndrome (thrombopenia-hemangioma syndrome) Capillary hemangioma associated with thrombocytopenic purpura

Kleeblattschädel anomaly Craniostenosis with trilobular skull

Klippel-Feil Short neck resulting from reduction in the number of cervical vertebrae or the fusion of multiple hemivertebrae, low hairline, limited neck motion (torticollis), and often associated with Sprengel's deformity

Kocher-Debré-Sémélaigne Cretinism with muscular hypertrophy, macroglossia, mental retardation, and cardiomegaly

Larsen Dislocations of limb joints, micrognathia, epiglottis, arytenoid and tracheal cartilages, hydrocephalus, and cleft palate

Madelung Multiple symmetric lipomatosis of the neck, shoulders, and back; often associated with congenital dislocation of the wrists; the cervical lipomatoses tend toward an encirclage of the larynx, trachea, and, by extension, into the mediastinum

Male Turner Micrognathia, short neck, short stature, mild mental retardation, and congenital heart disease

Marfan Congenital anomalies of heart in association with multiple somatic deformities, arachnodactyly, recurrent joint dislocations combined with kyphosis, pectus excavatum, and congenital disorder of connective tissues

Marie-Strümpell Rheumatoid arthritis (bamboo spine) and limited spinal motion, especially the neck

Meckel Microcephaly, cleft palate and lip, cleft tongue and epiglottis, micrognathia, congenital heart defects and renal abnormalities, and dysencephalia splanchnocystica

Melnick-Needles Osteodysplasty, exophthalmos, full cheeks, micrognathia, malalignment of teeth, and tall upper cervical vertebrae

Möbius (Moebius) Genetic abnormality characterized by bilateral facial paralysis, abductors of the eye, palsy, occasional oculomotor, trigeminal and hypoglossal dysfunction, and microstomia; because of lack of stimulation of the related muscle groups, mandibular and other facial bony structures may develop in abnormal patterns; often associated with submucous cleft palate, usually not involving the hard palate; other names include oculofacial paralysis, congenital abducens-facial paralysis, and congenital facial diplegia

Morquio-Ullrich Eccentro-osteochondrodysplasia, severe dwarfing, atlanto-occipital subluxation and acute kyphoscoliosis, and mucopolysaccharidosis IV

Noack Obesity, craniostenosis, and digital anomaly

Noonan See male Turner and Ullrich-Noonan

Paget Osteitis deformans

Patau Microcephaly, trisomy 13, micrognathia, and cleft palate or lip (or both)

Pfeiffer Craniostenosis, broad thumbs and great toes, and cutaneous syndactyly

Pierre Robin anomalad Mandibular hypoplasia and micrognathia in association with cleft palate and glossoptosis

Pompe Glycogen storage disease type III, macroglossia, hypotonicity, and mental retardation

Pyle Enlarged mandible, craniofacial anomalies, cranial nerve paralysis, and metaphyseal dysplasia

Riedel's struma Nontoxic thyroiditis with fixation of the trachea and massive space-occupying characteristics

Rieger Associated with amyotonia congenita group, maxillary hypoplasia, and hypodontia

Saethre-Chotzen Craniostenosis, facial asymmetry, low-set frontal hairline, ptosis of eyelids, deviated nasal septum, brachydactyly, and cutaneous syndactylism

Seckel Bird-headed dwarfism, narrow nasal passages, and microstomia

Silver-Russell Dwarfism, micrognathia, and skeletal asymmetry

Smith-Lemli-Opitz Micrognathia, short neck, microcephaly with mental retardation, progressive spasticity, and cleft palate

Soto Acromegalic features and cerebral gigantism

Sprengel's deformity Upward displacement of one or both scapulae with fixation to cervical vertebrae

Stein-Leventhal Obesity associated with anovulatory oligomenorrhea or amenorrhea and mild hirsutism

Stickler Autosomal dominant disorder; a connective tissue dysplasia with midfacial flattening and the anomalad of Robin; associated with submucous cleft palate and abnormal palatal mobility; often associated with sensorineural deafness; joints often enlarged, epiphyseal ossification disturbances, flattening of vertebral bodies, congenital myopia with zones of retinal detachment; very variable

Still Fusion of cervical spine; an arthritis associated with pneumonitis and pericarditis

Treacher Collins Antimongoloid obliquity of palpebral fissures, coloboma, microophthalmia, choanal atresia, hypoplasia of the zygoma, maxillary and mandibular bones, deafness, congenital heart defects, and occasional dwarfism

Turner Small mandible, short neck often webbed, short stature, hearing defect, shield chest, congenital heart disease, and gonadal dysgenesis

Ulrich-Feichtiger Micrognathia, depressed nose, external ear abnormalities associated with deafness, and limb and eye anomalies

Urbach-Wiethe Hyaline deposits in larynx and pharynx, and cutaneous mucosal hyalinosis

von Recklinghausen Neurofibromatosis, nodules arise from nerve sheaths of skeleton, soft tissues, and skin; often invade the head, airway, lungs, brain, and spine; scoliosis is common

Werdnig-Hoffmann Flaccid infant, lesions of the anterior horn cells, and difficulty with swallowing and aspiration.

Wolf Micrognathia and craniofacial anomalies often associated with cleft lip or palate (or both)

Bibliography

Benumof JL: *Anesthesia for Thoracic Surgery*. Philadelphia, WB Saunders, 1987.

Bishop MJ (ed): *Problems in Anesthesia: Physiology and Consequences of Tracheal Intubation*, vol 2. New York, JB Lippincott, April-June 1988.

Converse JM, McCarthy JG, Wood-Smith D: *Symposium on Diagnosis and Treatment of Craniofacial Anomalies*, vol 20. St. Louis, CV Mosby, 1979.

Delbaso AM: *Maxillofacial Imaging*. Philadelphia, WB Saunders, 1990.

Fink BR: *The Human Larynx*. New York, Raven Press, 1975.

Fink BR, Demarest RJ: *Laryngeal Biomechanics*. Cambridge, Mass, Harvard University Press, 1978.

Finucane BT, Santora AH: *Principles of Airway Management*. New York, FA Davis, 1988.

Fried MP (ed): *The Larynx: A Multidisciplinary Approach*. Boston, Little, Brown, 1988.

Healy GB, McGill TJI: *Laryngo-tracheal Problems in the Pediatric Patient*. Springfield, Ill, Charles C Thomas, 1979.

Latto IP, Rosen M (eds): *Difficulties in Tracheal Intubation*. Paris, Bailliere Tindall and Casel, 1985.

McCarthy JG: *Plastic Surgery*, vol 4. Philadelphia, WB Saunders, 1990.

Morgan DH, House LR, Hall WP, et al: *Diseases of the Temporomandibular Joint*. St Louis, CV Mosby, 1982.

Oho K, Amemiya R: *Practical Fiberoptic Bronchoscopy*. New York, Igaku-Shoin, 1984.

Ovassapian A: *Fiberoptic Airway Endoscopy in Anesthesia and Critical Care*. New York, Raven Press, 1990.

Patil V, Stehling L, Zauder H: *Fiberoptic Endoscopy*. Chicago, Year Book Medical Publishers, 1983.

Roberts JT: *Fundamentals of Tracheal Intubation*. New York, Grune & Stratton, 1983.

Shaw JD, Lancer JM: *Fiberoptic Endoscopy of the Upper Respiratory Tract: A Colour Atlas*. London, Wolfe, 1987.

Koopman CF, Moran WB Jr: Sleep apnea. *Otolaryngol Clin North Am* Aug 1990.

Issa FG, Suratt PM, Remmers JE: Sleep and respiration. *Prog Clin Biol Res* 1990; 345, Wiley-Liss Pubs.

Stradling P: *Diagnostic Bronchoscopy*. New York, Churchill Livingstone, 1986.

Index